Galen

This volume offers a comprehensive biography of the Roman physician Galen, and explores his activities and ideas as a doctor and intellectual, as well as his reception in later centuries.

Nutton's wide-ranging study surveys Galen's early life and medical education, as well as his later career in Rome and his role as court physician for over forty years. It examines Galen's philosophical approach to medicine and the body, his practices of prognosis and dissection, and his ideas about preventative medicine and drugs. A final chapter explores the continuing impact of Galen's work in the centuries after his death, from his pre-eminence in Islamic medicine to his resurgence in Western medicine in the Renaissance, and his continuing impact through to the nineteenth century even after the discoveries of Vesalius and Harvey.

Galen is the definitive biography this fascinating figure, written by the preeminent Galen scholar, and offers an invaluable resource for anyone interested in Galen and his work, and the history of medicine more broadly.

Vivian Nutton, FBA, is Professor emeritus of the History of Medicine at University College London, as well as Professor of the History of Medicine at the First Moscow State Medical University. He has published extensively on all aspects on medicine before the seventeenth century, and is the author of *Ancient Medicine*, 2nd edition (Routledge, 2012). He has edited and translated several treatises from the Galenic Corpus including *On Prognosis* (1979), *On My Own Opinions* (1999), and *On Problematical Movements* (2011). His edition and translation of selections from the neglected *On the Voice* is forthcoming in the journal *Galenos*. His recent studies of Renaissance Galenism include translations of *Principles of Anatomy according to Galen* by Johann Guinter and Andreas Vesalius (Routledge, 2017) and *An Autobibliography* by John Caius (Routledge, 2018). A general survey of European medicine from 1490 to 1628 is in progress.

Routledge Ancient Biographies

Herod, 2nd edition
King of the Jews and Friend of the Romans
Peter Richardson and Amy Marie Fisher

L. Munatius Plancus, 2nd edition
Serving and Surviving in the Roman Revolution
Thomas H. Watkins

Agrippa II
The Last of the Herods
David M. Jacobson

Galen
A Thinking Doctor in Imperial Rome
Vivian Nutton

To find out more about this series, visit: https://www.routledge.com/classicalstudies/series/ANCIENTBIOS.

Galen

A Thinking Doctor in Imperial Rome

Vivian Nutton

Routledge
Taylor & Francis Group
LONDON AND NEW YORK

First published 2020
by Routledge
2 Park Square, Milton Park, Abingdon, Oxon OX14 4RN

and by Routledge
52 Vanderbilt Avenue, New York, NY 10017

Routledge is an imprint of the Taylor & Francis Group, an informa business

British Library Cataloguing-in-Publication Data
A catalogue record for this book is available from the British Library

Library of Congress Cataloging-in-Publication Data
A catalog record has been requested for this book

ISBN: 978-0-367-35722-1 (hbk)
ISBN: 978-0-367-35723-8 (pbk)
ISBN: 978-0-429-34138-0 (ebk)

Typeset in Times New Roman
by Taylor & Francis Books

To Christine

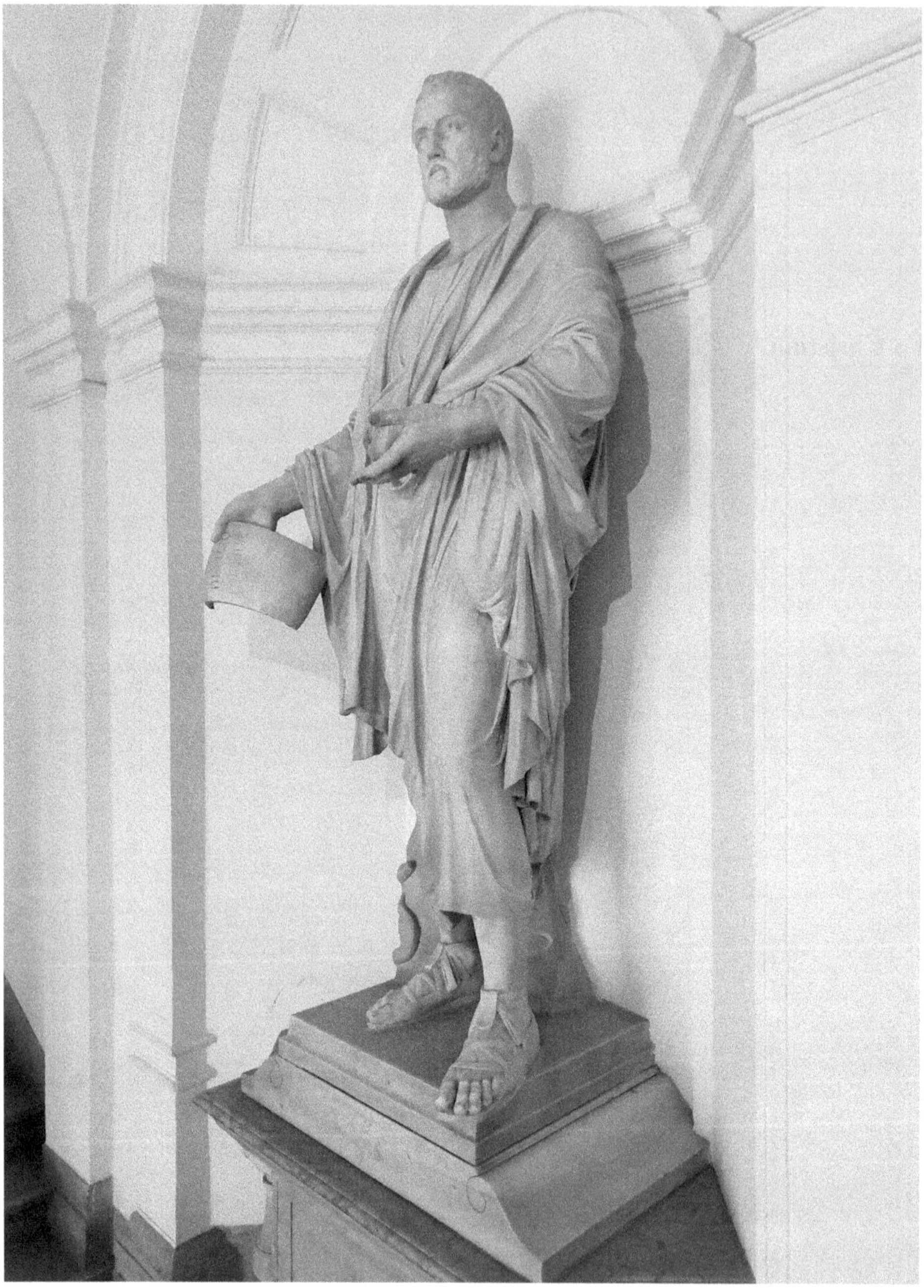

Figure 0.1 Galen holding a copy of *The Use of Parts.* Statue, 1888, by Hugo Haerdtl (1846–1918) at the head of the grand staircase of the new Anatomical Institute of the Vienna Medical School. Photo: Herwig Swoboda.

Contents

Illustrations

Figures

Acknowledgments

A proper record of my acknowledgments to those who have taught me much about Galen, whether by personal friendship or by their books and articles, would be almost as long as a typical Galenic treatise. In my initial forays into the Greek world of the Roman Empire, I was encouraged by my teacher, Joyce Reynolds, and at a suitable Oxonian distance by Glen Bowersock, both of whom have continued to influence me over the succeeding decades. Longevity has been a feature of Galenic scholars. Geoffrey Lloyd was my first Director of Studies in Cambridge, although I did not then know of his interests in ancient science, and he wisely left my faltering steps in ancient philosophy to be guided by others. Owsei Temkin, by his writings and by his humanity, inspired me to think widely about Galen and Galenism. Other *seniores* who were of great help over the years include Philip De Lacy, Nancy Siraisi and Reggie Harris, whose substantial manuscript notebooks of English summaries of Galen I regrettably failed to condense into any publishable form. This book owes much to my work on these notebooks but is a very different survey from what he had planned. Several of the group who assembled in Cambridge in 1979 are no longer with us, including Luis García Ballester, Richard Durling, Zaki Iskandar, Fridolf Kudlien, Paul Moraux and Mario Vegetti, but others continue to publish and investigate Galen and Galenism. My links with the Corpus Medicorum, and particularly with Jutta Kollesch and Gotthard Strohmaier, go back fifty years, and I have enjoyed meeting and working with them and their successors in Berlin. It has been particularly heartening to note that the *odium philologicum* has been absent from Galenic studies, and that personal friendships with fellow Galenists around the world remain strong after decades of collaboration. Among those of longest standing from whom I have benefited for forty years and more I must thank Armelle Debru, Klaus-Dietrich Fischer, my guide and mentor in matters Latin, Ivan Garofalo, Danielle Jacquart, Daniela Manetti, Amneris Roselli and Heinrich Von Staden. Thanks also go to Jacques Jouanna, Véronique Boudon-Millot, Alessia Guardasole, Philip van der Eijk, and the late Antonio Garzya for their organisation of the *colloques* on Galen and Greek medical texts where I have been able to discuss many aspects of Galen with a new generation (and indeed generations) of scholars in France, Germany and Italy, too numerous to mention or to thank individually for providing me with offprints and references. In the final stages of this book several friends volunteered to read my drafts and to make comments and correct them or provided me with information on recent publications. I am particularly grateful to Aileen Das, Stefania Fortuna, Maud Gleason, Ian Johnston, Orla Lewis, Matteo Martelli, Brigitte Mondrain, Lorenzo Perilli, Caroline Petit, Effie Photos-Jones, Antoine Pietrobelli, Julius Rocca, Ralph

Rosen, Herwig Swoboda, Laurence Totelin, Teun Tieleman, Katherine Van Schaik, John Wilkins, and Barbara Zipser. The errors and idiosyncrasies that remain are purely my own.

Hunting for Galen over the world has only strengthened my admiration for the work of archivists and librarians who have allowed me to inspect manuscripts and almost forgotten collections of notes and offprints. I recall with pleasure spending time in the collections in Baltimore, Fermo and Wolfenbüttel in addition to those in the United Kingdom. My main resources since 1977 have been the British Library and those of the libraries of the Institute of Classical Studies, the Warburg Institute, and what used to be called the Wellcome Institute for the History of Medicine. Now, as the Wellcome Library, it has changed its name as well as its priorities, and the bibliographical skills and erudition of several generations of librarians, among whom, *amicitiae causa*, I name Nigel Allan, Eric Freeman, Robin Price, Nikolai Serikoff, Brenda Sutton and John Symons, have almost entirely departed, victims of a touching and misplaced faith in computers and a passion for the ephemeral. I owe a special debt to the librarians of the Cambridge University Library who continue to make a visit to its open shelves a constant delight. I must also acknowledge all those unknown cataloguers and photographers who have made so much material available on the web, at least to those who know where or how to find it. When I first began my Galenic studies, to check up ideas in Galen involved a visit to at least two different libraries, the 1490 *editio princeps* could only be consulted in a visit from Cambridge to London, and at least one volume of the *Corpus Medicorum* was not available in the U.K. Now much comes to our computers at the press of a button, a mixed blessing, since it takes away the opportunity for friendship with librarians and fellow readers.

Above all, this book comes with an immense apology to my wife. When we first met, I told her that I was contemplating writing a book on Galen. It has been long delayed, despite all her gentle enquiries and my equally gentle procrastinations over the years. Now as we approach our golden wedding, I have finally fulfilled my promise to her. Her part in this goes far beyond the customary wifely obligations. Even in the years that she was ill and effectively housebound with three young children, she never complained at my absences in distant libraries, and indeed encouraged them because of the, at that stage, merely epistolary friendships they engendered for her. She has also been my severest critic, not only drawing on her expertise in French and the Renaissance but also going through my drafts line my line, improving my English and pointing out what seemed to her as an intelligent outsider passages that were overly cryptic or inconsequential. For all that she has contributed to my enterprises, to the wider community of Galenists, and to our family life, this book is dedicated to her in love and admiration. I trust that she (and my readers) will find that the long wait has been worth it.

St Albans, 2019

Note on citations and abbreviations of Galen's Writings

A list of titles of Galen's surviving writings is provided in the Appendix, along with brief indications of the editions and translations used or consulted for this book: fuller details are given in the Bibliography. All titles of works by Galen are given in English in the text. In the notes, they are cited by an abbreviated Latin title, following the lead set by Hankinson 2008a and by Peter Singer and others in the new Cambridge series of Galenic translations. Individual books are numbered in Roman numerals, followed by the chapter number; then follow the volume and page numbers in Kühn's standard edition, whose page numbers are almost always given in the much superior modern editions. Where their reading, or indeed the work itself, is not to be found in Kühn, I give instead the reference to the modern edition I have used, as well as, wherever possible, one also to an English translation: relevant editions and translations are listed in the Appendix.

The discovery of the Vlatadon codex of Galen fifteen years ago has had important consequences for some older English versions. Peter Singer has twice published translations of *Affections and Errors of the Soul* and *The Soul's Behaviour Depends on Bodily Mixtures*; only the pagination of the later (2013) publication is here cited. His 1997 English translation of *My Own Books* and *The Order of my Own Books* was made before the discovery of the complete text in the Vlatadon codex, and hence omits several pages first edited by Véronique Boudon-Millot in 2007. My 1999 English version of *My Own Opinions, CMG* V 3,2, was made from a composite text made up from Greek fragments and a medieval Latin translation made from the Arabic; the discovery of the entire Greek text has outdated that translation in many details and, reluctantly, I have decided not always to add references to it. Those without French or Italian who wish for an English translation may still consult it but should be warned that it differs from one based fully on the original Greek in many places and in its overall style.

Abbreviations

ANRW	Temporini, H. and Haase, W. (eds) (1974-) *Aufstieg und Niedergang der römischen Welt: Geschichte und Kultur Roms im Spiegel neueren Forschung.* Berlin: W. De Gruyter.
BJP	Boudon-Millot, V., Jouanna, J. and Pietrobelli, A. (eds) (2010) *Galien. Tome IV. Ne pas se chagriner.* Paris: Les Belles Lettres.
BM	Boudon-Millot, V. (ed.) (2007) *Galien. Tome I, Introduction générale. Sur l'ordre de ses propres livres. Sur ses propres livres. Que l'excellent médecin est aussi philosophe.* Paris: Les Belles Lettres.
BMP	Boudon-Millot, V. and Pietrobelli, A. (eds) (2005) Galien ressuscité: édition *princeps* du texte grec du *De propriis placitis. Revue des Études grecques* 118: 168–213.
CMG	*Corpus Medicorum Graecorum* (1908–44) Berlin and Leipzig: Teubner; (1946–2009) Berlin: Akademie Verlag; (2014–) Berlin: De Gruyter Akademie Forschung.
DR	Daremberg, C. and Ruelle, E. (eds) (1879) *Oeuvres de Rufus d'Éphèse.* Paris: Baillière.
IGRR	Cagnat, R. (1906–27) *Inscriptiones graecae ad res romanas pertinentes.* Paris: E. Leroux.
K	Kühn, K.G. (ed.) (1821–33) *Claudii Galeni Opera Omnia.* Leipzig: C. Knobloch,
L	Littré, E. (ed.) (1839–61) *Oeuvres complètes d'Hippocrate.* Paris: Baillière.

Introduction

To write a study of Galen, his medicine and his influence is almost to write the history of medicine in miniature. Not only did his conception of Hippocrates and Hippocratic medicine determine until recently the approaches of both doctors and historians to their pre-modern past, but his authority also ensured that alternatives to Galenic medicine were quickly forgotten or disappeared entirely for centuries. When choices had to be made in Antiquity and the Byzantine Greek world as to which handwritten and fragile texts deserved re-copying, it was his preferences that were followed almost exclusively. Consequently, apart from writings accidentally associated with his name or with that of his hero, Hippocrates, the only non-Galenic Greek texts from Classical Antiquity surviving in full deal with topics on which he had touched only briefly – gynaecology (Soranus), medical botany (Dioscorides), nosology (Aretaeus), and orthopaedics (Apollonius). Even his great Hippocratic predecessor, Rufus of Ephesus (fl. 100 CE), remains a shadowy figure, whose books have largely disappeared except for those that fill in Galenic gaps, for example his *Medical Questioning* or his book on jaundice.[1]

Galen's later influence was arguably even greater than his immediate achievements.[2] Not only did his ideas constitute the basis of learned medicine in Western Europe from the eleventh until the mid-seventeenth century but his therapeutics remained in use for a further 200 years. The standard collected edition of his works in 21 volumes plus an index volume was produced between 1821 and 1833 by Karl Gottlob Kühn, professor of medicine at Leipzig, as a contribution to contemporary therapy at a time when no medical system commanded universal assent and when remedies and ideas from the remote past had at least the merit of apparently well-documented efficacy.[3] Sixty years later, a leading physician in modern Athens could still read and comment in detail on many Galenic therapeutic tracts, introducing more up-to-date material into the margins of his working copy of the 1538 Basle Greek edition, now in Toronto.[4] In the form of Yunani (literally Ionian, i.e. Greek) medicine as consolidated and developed by Ibn Sī nā (Avicenna) Galenism remains a major medical tradition in the Muslim world of the twenty-first century. At the modern Medical College at Aligarh in India, one may study Galen's treatise on *Elements* alongside biochemistry within an up-to-date and government-funded hospital. Galen's holistic approach also appeals to contemporary Western practitioners of complementary medicine as well as forming one branch of traditional Tibetan medicine. More subtly, Galen continues to influence modern perceptions of medicine and how it should be practised, even if his demands for constant training in philosophy and in dissection can now be fulfilled only with difficulty in a crowded medical curriculum.

This short introduction to Galen sets out to do two things. The first is to repay a personal debt to Galen by explaining why I have found him so fascinating – and continue to do so. Not only had he an extraordinary life, for not many practitioners ever became a doctor to the Roman emperors or remained in that position for so long, but his keen eye noticed things others did not. In addition, when placed in his proper context, he deserves to be regarded as a major independent thinker in many areas of philosophy. But he is, first and foremost, a doctor trying to understand how mind and body work and how one might proceed to a successful therapy on that basis. His conclusions are often misdirected or outdated, something that applies equally to those of his opponents and later critics, but they are rarely foolish. Rather, they are attempts to investigate problems that are still with us at a time when aids to experimentation were almost non-existent and when the doctor had to proceed solely on the evidence of his own unaided senses. This book is avowedly on Galen's side, but not, I hope, so uncritically as to neglect his limitations.

The second aim, and the more difficult, is to show how all the varied aspects of his life and work fit together. Almost everything that is known about Galen comes directly or indirectly from his own writings, in which his information on his own life is heavily skewed towards the period before 176. The lively stories he tells of life in Rome in *Prognosis, for Epigenes*, written around then, together with the much later biographical sections in *My Own Books* focusing on his early career, provide a framework that is largely missing for the events of his later years. Save for the loss of his books in the Fire of Rome in 192, described at length in the recently discovered *Avoiding Distress*, these have to be reconstructed from scattered and often vaguely dated comments, which, like the indications he gives of his date of birth, may involve two apparently conflicting statements. Other details that might be expected in a biography are entirely missing. We read nothing of any siblings or of any partner, or of what happened to his family estates after the death of his father. Faced with these lacunae and uncertainties, the sober analysis of the historian must yield to the imagination of the novelist.[5]

A straightforwardly developmental approach to Galen's intellectual biography, as Peter Singer has argued, is also hard to establish for two reasons.[6] Galen is continually updating his writings, and although one can establish a rough chronology, and at times identify later cross-references and small additions, the full extent of his alterations cannot be known for certain. Besides, Galen claims an almost total self-consistency ever since he began to study medicine, with one exception, his opinion on the order of the development of organs in the foetus.[7] Although, as Renaissance scholars knew well, this is somewhat misleading, for there are many, at least apparent, contradictions throughout his writings, there is no doubt that he retained the same major interests throughout his life and could return to the same theme after a quarter of a century with little more than stylistic differences, as in the two parts of the *Method of Healing*.[8] Treating each aspect of his intellectual life separately, as in the excellent *Cambridge Companion to Galen* or its forthcoming Oxford equivalent, risks obscuring a striking feature of Galen's work, the way in which he can integrate diverse information and apply a consistent methodology to areas of activity that may seem remote from one another. The solution adopted here is to interweave certain topics within the two generally chronological chapters, divided at his first visit to Rome in 162, to show, for example, how his exposure to the classics of ancient literature helped to define his method of commentary on Hippocrates 30 or more years later, or the significance of his being a Greek observer of life in the city of Rome.

The central section of this book is formed by three thematic chapters in part structured according to Galen's own prescriptions for a good doctor. They correspond to the three things that have contributed to Galen's influence and are still relevant to any practitioner of the healing arts today. The first is his remarkable ability to observe, visible not just in his work on anatomy and in his examination of his patients, but also in his recollections of what he had seen during his lengthy travels around the Eastern Mediterranean or in Italy. The fourth chapter begins by unpacking his claim that the best doctor is also a philosopher in order to look at Galen's strategies in presenting his arguments. He has often been criticised for his mistakes in logic and for the insouciant, some might say deceitful, way in which he could slide from plausibility to certainty. He is a master at having his cake and eating it. Many of his complaints about his competitors could equally be levelled at himself, and the viciousness with which he attacks what he alleges are his opponents' view has been turned against him by modern scholars. Yet his overall aim is a laudable one, to find ways of understanding the patient and of devising a successful therapy by applying thought and by utilising some of the standard theories of the time about the workings and make-up of the natural world. Experience was for him useless unless accompanied by thought. Set against the background of the ideas and practices of other doctors in the ancient world, his limitations appear much less culpable. The last of these three chapters deals with his work as a healer, looking at his therapies in the light of what he claimed to be the capacities of an accomplished practitioner. Together, they help to explain why he gained and long maintained his influence over many centuries, the theme of the final chapter. The way in which, time after time, different groups, different generations and different societies have chosen to focus on this or that individual aspect of Galen reveals much about how his authority became accepted, as well as pointing to areas of his work that today's historians have either neglected or condemned in the light of the subsequent development of medicine.

But this record of his achievements masks one important but often forgotten fact. Galen is one of the few individuals from Antiquity of whom it can be said that we can get close to knowing him as a personality. His only rivals are Cicero and St Augustine, either in the volume of material left to us and in their self-revelations and clearly defined views. But no other writer known to us from Antiquity wrote so much about himself in an attempt to make clear to contemporaries and to posterity what he had done and how he wished them to interpret it. His lost work *Slander* contained at least a partial account of his life, while *My Own Books* and *My Own Opinions* were avowedly composed to resolve disputes over what he had written and what he believed. The last section of *The Art of Medicine* includes a catalogue of his relevant works, while in *The Order of My Own Books* he told his readers how best to approach his oeuvre.[9] To penetrate behind his thousands of words to find alternative interpretations to what he would have us believe is no easy task, particularly when the other side of the argument is almost entirely absent, and contextualisation is not always possible.

No one who has studied Galen at all deeply can fail to react to what they find when confronted by his larger than life character, whether they find themselves in sympathy with him or, more often, not. This book attempts to give a sense of what it must have been like to meet and talk with Galen, whether as a friend or a patient. How did those who knew him well respond to the torrent of words sweeping along, if not swamping, the abundant fruits of his learning in a variety of disciplines, or to his constant harping on his own superiority over competitors in a world of charlatans and sophists? Some, we know, acknowledged his authority even if not always accepting it gladly or fully understanding all that he was trying to say, and one must always keep in mind that the social norms of the Roman world cannot be equated with our own – modesty is not a Roman virtue, as my schoolmaster used to say. But in a book that aims to produce a rounded portrait of Galen one must attempt to sketch at least the outlines of his personality, and to restore the life blood to his ghost. Hieronymus Surianus, as we shall see, had a very clear image of the Galen he claimed to have met and introduced to his readers, albeit one that, to modern eyes, is utterly implausible. My own picture may, in the end, be equally fanciful, but there can be no doubt that in the twenty-first century we know far more about Galen, his writings and the society in which he lived than a doctor and editor did 500 years ago. To bring Galen to life for those who have never read him or have heard of him only through his detractors, and to explain why he attained the influence he once had is a challenge that this book attempts to address. Its conclusions would not, I am sure, have satisfied Galen himself, always alert to what he saw as misunderstanding and misrepresentation, and he would have expected a much longer exposition. But he might well have appreciated at least some of the sentiments of its author and be gratified that his ideas are still thought worthy of discussion 800 years later.

Two features mark Galen out from almost all other practitioners of medicine: the sheer volume of his surviving writings and the variety of his interests. To assess fully his achievements in fields as diverse as lexicography, logic, pharmacology, ethics and anatomy requires a range of skills beyond the capabilities of any one individual, to say nothing of the fact that any detailed investigation involves a facility in ancient Greek and Latin, to which the truly committed might add Arabic, Hebrew, Syriac and Armenian, for not everything that survives from what he wrote has yet been translated into any modern language. Besides, in contrast to almost all other ancient authors, our knowledge of Galen continues to increase substantially even today. Over the last 40 years there has been a steady accession of long-vanished treatises, albeit principally recovered in the form of medieval translations rather than in his original Greek, as well as more detailed critical studies, editions and translations than at any time since the sixteenth century. Consequently, today's scholars are more familiar with Galen's works, to say nothing of their historical and cultural setting, than were their predecessors in Early Byzantium or all but a handful of experts in the medieval Islamic world between 850 and 1200.

But this very abundance has proved a stumbling block to any large-scale and coherent account of Galen. There have been several good short introductions to Galen and Galenic medicine, from Lynn Thorndike in 1923, via Luis García Ballester's brief (and never translated) 1972 account in Spanish and Owsei Temkin's magisterial 1973 survey of Galenism (an important change of emphasis signalled by the title) to chapters in Introductions or in wider histories of medicine.[10] Individual themes have been well treated, not least in James Hankinson's *Cambridge Companion to Galen* and in Petros Bouras-Vallianatos and Barbara Zipser's very recent and very substantial *Brill's Handbook to Galenism*.[11] There have also been major studies of aspects of Galen's philosophy by Paul Moraux and Mario Vegetti and shorter essays by Richard Walzer and Michael Frede, to name only authors no longer with us.[12] Galen's biography has been written, from different perspectives, by Heinrich Schlange-Schöningen and Véronique Boudon-Millot, neither, alas, as yet available in English, as well as by Susan Mattern in her exhaustive study of Galen's patients.[13] But, leaving aside prefaces in recent editions and translations, which tend simply to repeat the standard biographical information before passing on to an exposition of the treatise under review, Galen has defied his biographers. The two volumes by Rudolf Siegel bravely try to interpret Galen with the aid of modern medicine, but leave out much, while the eighteen volumes of notebooks compiled by C.R.S. Harris, who went meticulously through the text of Kühn in preparation for a major and never completed survey, remain in manuscript because of their author's Galen-like determination to leave nothing out.[14] Susan Mattern's later attempt to provide an overall survey of Galen and his writings in English becomes thinner the further it moves away from the straightforwardly biographical.[15] Besides, whereas it was possible a generation ago to have read large portions of the secondary literature on Galen, the sheer number of excellent articles in journals, collected volumes and conference proceedings published around the world in a variety of languages, including Armenian and Flemish, and in unexpected places makes this a hopeless aspiration even in the age of computers. If one adds the constant arrival of improved editions and commentaries, to say nothing of new texts or of older ones now recognised as Galenic, any attempt at a synthesis must inevitably be partial and omit many of Galen's fascinating aperçus. Proceeding otherwise will doom it to the fate of the telephone directory, a work in many volumes consulted for individual items but never read as a whole.

This book takes a slightly different approach from its predecessors. It is a distillation of a lifetime's acquaintance with Galen. It began in 1965 when, as a Cambridge research student of A.H.M. Jones, the historian of the Greek cities of the Roman Empire, I tried to put Galen into context as a medical practitioner in the Roman Empire, a task which still continues to exercise me. Not only was he the major source for much of our information on medical life in imperial Rome (and a good deal else), but it quickly became apparent how much basic work still needed to be done before one could be sure that what one was reading was actually Galen's own Greek. Some of his texts had never been edited properly since the Aldine edition of 1525 or its Basle successor of 1538, while others were accessible only in German dissertations from before the First World War. Secondary literature was very variable as well as being hard to find. The frequently cited biography of Galen by George Sarton turned out to be full of error, and not every library within reach housed copies of the *Corpus Medicorum Graecorum* series, let alone of the pre-1914 dissertations and *Schulprogramme* in which the most recent editions of individual works were published. Studies of Galen's medicine and philosophy were long outdated or based on questionable assumptions. Trying to repair some of these deficiencies has occupied me and many colleagues ever since then.

Even more difficult has been the attempt to understand Galen for himself, both because of the complex interrelationship of his ideas (and the consequent need to master a variety of topics for which school and university had in no way prepared me) and because of the general denigration of all that he stood for. Like many other Greek authors of his 'post-classical' period, Galen was more despised than read, condemned for his style as well as for his ideas, and dismissed as a distant shadow of his master, Hippocrates. Today, when so many different colleagues from around the world have made their individual contributions to the study of Galen, it is almost impossible to believe that this was once largely *terra incognita* into which young doctoral students were warned at their peril against setting foot.[16] Finding a fair balance between his undoubted achievements and his equally undoubted faults has been an intellectual challenge, as has the job of reading, re-reading and synthesising such a huge and diverse collection of writings. If this short survey of a most voluminous writer succeeds in persuading others to dip into some of Galen's writings, many now becoming accessible in modern translations made from more accurate Greek, Latin or Arabic texts, its author will be satisfied that he has paid an appropriate tribute to a scholar with whom he has lived for so long.

Notes

1 Pormann 2008.
2 Bouras-Vallianatos and Zipser 2019.
3 Nutton 2002b; Tassinari 2019. Broman 1996 gives the medical context.
4 Gemusaeus H (ed.) (1538) *Galeni Opera Omnia*, Basle: Andreas Cratander, Toronto, Thomas Fisher Rare Book Library, classmark: jah f 00954.
5 Prantera 1991; Magri 2004.
6 Singer PN 2013: 34–7.
7 Debru 1995b.
8 For a substantial investigation into Galen's inconsistencies, Alessandrino 1548. For the dating of the *Method of Healing*, Nutton 1991.
9 Raiola 2015; Petit 2018.
10 Thorndike 1923; García Ballester 1972; Temkin 1973.
11 Hankinson 2008a: Bouras-Vallianatos and Zipser 2019.
12 Moraux 1984: 687–808; Vegetti 2007; Walzer 1962; Frede 1987.
13 Schlange-Schöningen 2003; Boudon-Millot 2012; Mattern 2008. The catalogue of the 2018 exhibition at the Musée de Mariémont (Verbank Piérard *et al.* 2018) contains much valuable information, while Boudon-Millot's 2007 excellent introduction to the Budé series includes a remarkable survey of the manuscript tradition of Galen.
14 Siegel 1968, 1970.
15 Mattern 2013.
16 The 1979 Cambridge conference (Nutton 1981) attempted to bring together as many scholars as possible who were known to be working on Galen. Several contemporaries report receiving the same warning as I did.

1 Galen the Greek

Pergamum and Greek culture

Pergamum, modern Bergama in North Western Turkey, was one of the greatest and most splendid cities of the Roman world. At the end of the third century BCE, a local dynast, Philetaerus, had managed to establish his rule over the region of Mysia, its neighbour to the North, and began a lavish palace complex on the summit of the acropolis that dominates the broad valley of the Caicus. Under his successors, Pergamum became ever more prosperous, thanks to their judicious support for the Romans. Temples, gymnasia, elegant houses on the hillside and, at the top, the celebrated Altar of Pergamum as well as a library of 200,000 volumes that rivalled that of Alexandria, established the city as one of the leading centres of Greek culture.[1] But its independence was hard to maintain in the face of other larger kingdoms like Syria and especially when Rome increasingly interfered in the Aegean world. In the end, the childless Attalus III (ruled 138–133 BCE), who was more interested in carrying out experiments on plants and poisons than in complex political diplomacy, decided to bequeath his kingdom to the Romans, who turned it into their province of Asia.[2]

There followed almost two centuries of decline in both prosperity and status, and it was not until the middle of the first century CE that Pergamum, like many other Greek cities, began to experience a strong revival. The population expanded – Galen gives the number of adult inhabitants, including slaves, as 120,000 – and buildings grew up beyond the walls on the steamy plain by the river and on the neighbouring hillsides.[3] There was a new theatre, a forum, a massive amphitheatre and an equally large stadium, baths, gymnasia, and temples, including the enormous shrine to the Egyptian gods, visible evidence today of Pergamum's continuing connections with Alexandria and Egypt. White stone aqueducts, surpassed, Galen thought, only by those of Rome, stretched for miles through the countryside to bring fresh water to the expanding city as well as to places en route and, in a remarkable feat of engineering, even to the summit of the acropolis.[4] Skilled engineers carefully arranged for its distribution so that the public baths and sacred groves received more than street fountains and private houses.[5] The acropolis was dominated by the new temple of Trajan and a second temple for the imperial cult, along with a gymnasium and baths. Impressive enough in ruins today, these marble buildings would have been visible for miles, announcing the city's renewed wealth and importance perhaps even to distant sailors. In 129 CE, the probable year of Galen's birth, the city must have resembled a building site.[6] New buildings were going up everywhere – large houses on the slopes of the great hill, porticos, temples, fountains, and a variety of monuments, almost all paid for by its wealthier citizens, who provided an important link between Pergamum and Rome, as well as between the city and the neighbouring region where their estates were to be found.[7] Other nearby towns also enjoyed a renewal of prosperity. At Allianoi, some 18 kilometres away, the shrine of Asclepius, familiar to Galen because of its hot spring, was similarly extended and refurbished, and doctors carried out operations in a large and many-roomed building adjacent and possibly even built on to it.[8]

Most spectacular of all was the rebuilding of the shrine of Asclepius some 3 kilometres South West of Pergamum. Although a small temple seems to have been in existence on the site by 400 BCE, the first secure mention of the healing god Asclepius is not for another century and a half, when a major expansion took place led by an otherwise unknown Archias, but undoubtedly with help from the ruler of Pergamum. This temple seems to have been seriously damaged in 201 BCE by the troops of King Philip of Macedon, but it was quickly rebuilt or, rather, restored since it followed largely the same lines as its predecessor. It included three temples, probably dedicated to Apollo, Asclepius and Hygeia, a new altar, and a long colonnaded portico.[9] There were also incubation rooms on the model of Epidaurus where suppliants slept in order to receive healing from the god in a dream. At the centre of the main temple was a beautiful statue of Asclepius made by the famous sculptor Phyromachus. According to a later Pergamene commentator on the Hippocratic *Oath*, the attributes of the cult image corresponded to the ideal properties of the doctor: the staff signified stability, the snake constant alertness and adaptability, while the egg held out by the god represented the doctor's power to protect a fragile world.[10] The whole complex was connected to the city by a long colonnaded street with shops and monumental *exedrae*, semi-circular spaces, often with statues, where people could stop, sit, and talk.

The shrine as it appears today is the result of a further massive rebuilding beginning in the 120s supported by the emperor Hadrian and paid for in part by Cuspius Rufinus, a citizen of Pergamum who had become a Roman consul.[11] As well as new majestic temples looking out over the plain towards the sea, there was a monumental entrance, a library, and a small theatre as well as elegant porticos and a huge circular building whose purpose remains unclear. Asclepius had by this date become *the* healing god throughout the Roman Empire and was widely acknowledged by doctors themselves as the patron of their art.[12] Pilgrims flocked from around the Roman Empire, some like the orator Aelius Aristides, spending a considerable time there, waiting to be healed by the god.[13] It is not surprising that Pergamenes like Galen took a particular pride in their "ancestral god", striking many coins in his honour depicting his image, his temple, and the sacred snake.[14] Galen himself, a "worshipper" of the god, was convinced that Asclepius had guided his life at crucial moments, even recommending treatments for himself and, on occasion, his patients.[15] The god's intervention in 157 to cure him of a dangerous abscess through advocating in a dream the risky procedure of cutting an artery in the finger was so significant in his life that he mentioned it at least three times (each time with slight variations).[16] He excused including a complicated discussion of vision in *The Use of Parts* by invoking a dream in which he was censored for his impiety towards the Creator for leaving unexplained such a great work of his providence.[17]Although many official records of shrines of Asclepius and literary accounts like Aristides' *Sacred Tales* emphasise miraculous or unusual dream healings, Galen was convinced that others were perfectly compatible with standard therapies.[18] In one instance, a man from central Thrace was told in a dream to drink a daily potion containing viper flesh, and as a result his, up to that point incurable, condition was changed into one of curable leprosy. This, so Galen explains, was because viper flesh has an enormous power to dry the body, thus here causing scales of leprosy to form, and so it can be thoroughly recommended in such conditions.[19] He even used the examples of suppliants who preferred to obey the god and fast for a fortnight to following a doctor's advice as proof of the importance of faith in the healer, whether human or divine.[20]

Galen's parents

Although the names of the architects involved in the expansion of the Asclepieion are unknown, this incessant building activity in Pergamum and around will have directly benefited Galen and his family. His father, Nicon, was one of two, or possibly three, architects of that name involved in designing many of these new buildings.[21] One of them, Julius Nicodemus, "also known as Nicon", along with a surveyor, Aelius Isidotus, presented a porticoed building to house the city's *astynomoi*, officials in charge of public order.[22] Another, Aelius Nicon, composed complicated verse inscriptions in which the numerical value of the letters in each line added up to the same total. He was also interested in astronomy, writing a hymn to the sun as well as another in praise of geometry that were engraved on the base of a public monument.[23] Father Nicon shared these interests, which were highly appropriate for the descendant of a land-

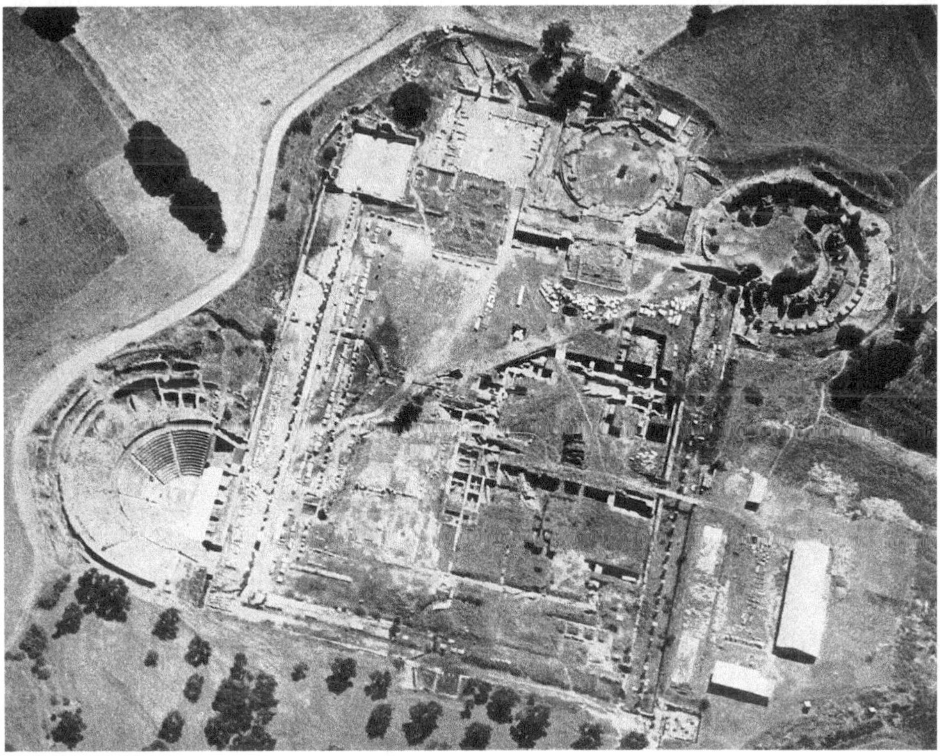

Figure 1.1 The shrine of Asclepius at Pergamum as rebuilt in Galen's lifetime. As well as porticos and, in the centre, cult buildings, it included a theatre (bottom left), a library, and a monumental gateway (top) opening from a colonnaded street that led to the city.

surveyor and an architect.[24] Granted full Roman citizenship by Hadrian or an earlier emperor, he was a member of the civic elite, the well-to-do owner of at least one estate, where he experimented with wine-making and plant-breeding.[25] He held some political office in the city, not entirely to his liking, since Galen claims that he was pushed into local politics because of his sound views and incorruptibility.[26] Given both Nicon's and, still more, Galen's wealth, it may be only chance that has robbed us of secure evidence for an inscription detailing a benefaction to their native city that would allow us to pinpoint further the role of Galen's family within Pergamum.[27]

By contrast with his mother, whom he compared to Socrates' termagant wife Xanthippe for her emotional outbursts, biting the servants, and perpetually fighting with Nicon, Galen always held his father up as a model parent, and not only for his equanimity and high moral values.[28] Indeed, the fact that so much of our information about his father is found in books written at the end of his long life attests his importance as an influence on his son and as an image that may have become even more idealised over time. It was his father who supervised his education right from the cradle, choosing a tutor who spoke 'proper' Greek and, later, accompanying him to school and interviewing prospective teachers.[29] An anecdote preserved in Arabic tells how he chastised a teacher, irritated by Galen's constant corrections, for failing to recognise the boy's genius. Such paternal attention was not unusual – the poet Horace also praised his father for coming to school with him – and would have strengthened the bond between father and son.[30] Nicon played a crucial role in Galen's education, insisting on precision of thought and language, akin to that of geometry, as a way of avoiding fruitless argument.[31] Similarly, Galen acquired the rudiments of his considerable grasp of mathematics and astronomy from Nicon, while the manual dexterity he learned in making little wooden toys would stand him in good stead when he came to practise surgery later and to design his own instruments.[32] When his father was away at his estates, Galen continued to follow his example, studying day and night, far more than his fellow pupils.[33] Even on his way home from school, according to an Arabic biographer, he would revise what he had been taught, preferring to keep on learning rather than join in any children's games.[34] It was this education, a combination of nature and nurture, that enabled Galen, he believed, to overcome any of the unfortunate character flaws that could be detected even in the youngest of children, and to retain his equanimity in the face of what others considered disasters.[35]

Galen's education: language and the cryptic Hippocrates

Pergamum, like its nearby rivals Smyrna and Ephesus, was in the second century a vibrant cultural and intellectual centre. It could boast the presence of a distinguished historian, Claudius Charax, and the reputation of one of its teachers, Aristocles, attracted even the great orator Herodes Atticus to his lectures.[36] This was an age when culture, and particularly Greek culture, mattered. The ability to speak and write elegantly was an indication of social status, as well as literary taste, and might lead to fame and fortune – or to a post in the entourage of the Roman Emperor. It could elevate a man of humble status and, conversely, its absence would mark even more clearly the social decline of a member of the elite.[37] Its leading exponents, often called 'sophists', came from all over the Roman world, from Syria and Egypt to distant Gaul.[38] Galen directed at least three of his tracts against one of them, Favorinus of Arles, who had made a great name for himself in Rome in the 140s, and whose opinion of Socrates Galen regarded as flawed.[39] Greek became the language of high culture throughout the Empire. It was a Greek schoolmaster, Demetrius, who recorded the Northern lights off the Northern coast of Scotland.[40] The surviving Greek authors from this period include some of the most famous names in world literature, such as the biographer and essayist Plutarch and the satirist Lucian, both mentioned by Galen, as well as others less familiar like the miscellaneous writer Sextus Julius Africanus or the medical poet Marcellus of Side, whose poems the emperor Hadrian demanded should be placed in all public libraries.[41] Doctors joined eagerly in this intellectual extravaganza. The fellow-citizens of doctor Heraclitus of Rhodiapolis, a small town in South West Turkey, did not spare the superlatives in their praise of their local celebrity. Heraclitus was "the first doctor of his age", famous around the Eastern Mediterranean as a poet and the author of works on local history and philosophy as well as medicine. This so-called "Homer of medical poetry" was not averse to self-publicity, presenting copies of his treatises and poems to various cities, including his own, to which he also donated a library.[42] Another medical author, the Pergamene commentator on the Hippocratic *Oath*, displays a similarly wide range of learning, in both history and literature, describing the origin of medicine in a variety of regions and quoting unusual traditions about Asclepius and his family as well as a paean in praise of the god by Ariphron and another by an even more obscure poet.[43]

Like theirs, Galen's early education was focussed on the classics of earlier literature – Homer, 'the poet' par excellence, Hesiod, the lyric poets, including Sappho 'the poetess', the great Athenian tragedians, Euripides favourite among them, and writers of comedy down to Menander.[44] They might contain medical as well as literary insights. Two lines from the erudite Hellenistic poet Euphorion are quoted to exemplify the popular belief that pregnancy should last for 300 days.[45] According to a late scholiast, Galen even wrote a book specifically on medicine in Homer, in which he attempted to identify a plant mentioned at *Odyssey* 11, 289.[46] He cites prose writers less often, although his books are permeated with allusions and references to Plato and Aristotle, and Thucydides is his favourite historian.[47] His description of the great plague of Athens Galen regarded as a valuable survey, but one inevitably flawed because he lacked the medical knowledge and judgment of a Hippocrates.[48] Nonetheless, Galen is happy to compare his own experiences with plague in Rome with those of Thucydides when they both appear to agree.[49] He has less time for other historians. Herodotus is to be read for pleasure, and he cites Xenophon's historical writing only for a mention of snow-blindness in his *Anabasis*.[50] The scarcity of reference to Demosthenes and the other Attic orators is easily explained by the genres in which Galen is writing. But a comparison with Plutarch and the consul-historian Arrian, whom he may have met in Athens, shows a similar range of reading that would have been shared with anyone with intellectual pretensions.[51] It looked back to an earlier golden age of Greece, and reinforced Galen's self-identity as a member of the wider Greek world beyond Pergamum.[52]

Galen deployed this literary learning throughout his life in a variety of ways and expected his readers to appreciate his allusions and choice phrases.[53] Literary reminiscences enliven even the most technical of treatises.[54] His moralising writings show clearly the fruits of his education, for they are often illustrated with quotations and stories that can also be found in the writings of other contemporaries, even if he gives them a characteristically independent twist. So, for example, a writer of fables, Babrius, has a slightly different version of Galen's story of the seller of statues debating with himself whether to sell a statue of Hermes to adorn a temple or to decorate a tomb. According to Galen, it was Hermes himself in a dream who said that it was up to the merchant to choose between honouring someone immortal or someone that had already begun to decay, a choice Galen compared to an individual's decision to make his own soul resemble the gods or the beasts.[55] The best demonstration of his rhetorical skills is found in his *Exhortation to Medicine*, a display piece in honour of medicine, and possibly other arts, that combines allusions and quotations in a way that would have delighted his audience.[56] This doctor was indeed an educated man, even if at times he appeared to disdain the arts of rhetoric and etymological fantasy.[57]

Galen also made practical use of the linguistic training he had received as a boy.[58] He could write and, since many of his books were dictated, speak well. He tells a good story, particularly when describing his own cases, and his denunciations of his opponents are at times brilliant in their choice of language. He can turn a phrase and adapt the tone of his composition to the circumstance. His failings as a writer lie more in his prolixity and repetitiveness, something essential in an oral didactic presentation, than in his actual style. He writes on the whole a clear 'common' or *koine* Greek, avoiding, for example, hiatus between words, but not slavishly, as some purists advocated.[59] In the style wars among contemporary sophists he took a middle position. "I myself use the term that people use nowadays, since I think that it is better to teach things clearly than to Atticise in an old-fashioned way".[60] Whereas some, the so-called 'Atticists', refused to use any words not found in the works of Athenian prose-writers of the fifth and fourth centuries BCE, and others championed a more florid, so-called Asianic, style, Galen preached the virtues of *sapheneia*, clarity, and ease of communication, something he derived from his father Nicon.[61] Not only did this help to avoid ambiguity (a topic on which we have a surviving treatise by him) and hence fruitless argument, but it allowed a doctor to communicate better with his patients.[62] While accepting the need for technical terms to give precision, he rejected what he saw as neologisms; these novel coinages could not easily be understood by others, as well as being both unnecessary and confusing to those used to the traditional terminology.[63] A doctor who failed thereby to communicate with his patients was not a good doctor, for effective communication with patients was an essential part of the healing process.[64] Although his education had introduced him to the language of the classical Greek dialects, Ionian, Doric, and Aeolian, he avoided them just as he did local words from modern Cilicia, Syria, Galatia, and Athens or those of traders and tax-collectors. His brand of Asianism, if it can be called that, was no literary affectation, but a reliance on the so-called "common" language of all Greeks that would be intelligible beyond any local boundaries.[65] He wrote for Greeks as a whole, not for "Germans, savages and barbarians any more than for lions or wild boars", although he accepted that even barbarians could become hellenised if they so wished.[66]

This commitment to intelligibility lies at the base of one of his passions – lexicography. In *Avoiding Distress*, Galen devoted a long section to describing his work on Attic Greek and on everyday language.[67] This was not antiquarianism or a frivolous search for rare etymologies, something he condemns in *Examining the Physician*, but had a practical purpose.[68] His writings on foods show his awareness of the difficulties in identifying them across a variety of languages, dialects and social divisions, where the names given them by peasants are as significant as those in sophisticated authors.[69]

But an understanding of words and their meaning had an even greater role to play in Galen's whole medical practice. Given the importance in Galen's eyes of Hippocrates and the medical writings that passed under his name, it was essential to discover exactly what he had intended to say five hundred or more years earlier. Many of his most important works, and especially the *Epidemics* and *Aphorisms*, were frequently obscure, partly because of the summary way in which they were composed, and partly because of the choice and often cryptic language in which they were expressed. Galen was heir to a long tradition of Hippocratic exegesis and commentary that went back to the third century BC and that continued to be vigorously debated in Asia Minor, Alexandria and Rome across the different medical groupings for several centuries.[70] But he seems to have been unusual, if not unique, among doctors in summoning the aid of literary writers as well as of lexicographers to help in understanding earlier medical writings.

The best way, he argued, to discover what Hippocrates meant by a word was to find how his contemporaries used it, in other words to compile a dictionary.[71] Galen's own Hippocratic lexicon survives today, a list of short explanations for Hippocrates' technical terms.[72] It was not the first such guide: Erotian's lexicon survives from the previous century, and modern scholars have unearthed fragments of much earlier Hellenistic dictionaries, but Galen's ambition was on a much larger scale. He planned an enormous dictionary of all Attic writers, not just on medicine. That part devoted to prose writers was in 48 books, each a book-roll up to 30 metres in length, that to the comic writers Aristophanes, Eupolis and Cratinus a mere eleven. The former luckily survived the fire of 192, but the latter was the greatest of all his losses, the fruit of many years' research. In it Galen drew on the 50 books of a Hellenistic grammarian, Dionysius, and his much shorter summary in a single book a mere 6,000 lines long, as well as on his own wide reading.[73] As he explained at length in his *Medical Terminology*, and probably also in his lost works, *The Language of Hippocrates* and *The Value of Old Comedy for Students*, it was important to discover the everyday meaning of the words Hippocrates used. Galen rightly observed that the growth of a technical terminology was a slow process, and that many words were taken over metaphorically from local and daily usage. Comedy was the key to comprehension. The language of philosophers was too technical and too refined, but that of comedy had to be comprehensible to everyone, for a writer whose jokes could not be understood by his audience was bound to fail.[74] Hence, Galen drew on such unfamiliar plays by Aristophanes as *The Merchant Ships* or the first version of *Women at the Thesmophoria* to explain some of Hippocrates' obscure sayings.[75] Only by understanding what the Hippocratic words meant could one fully grasp the therapeutic value of the advice given and decide what came directly from the great healer and what had been wrongly attributed or misrepresented in some way. Galen could then place the Hippocratic treatises along a spectrum of authenticity that ranged from works undoubtedly composed by the master through those written by his family and students to those that merely breathed the spirit of Hippocrates. Part of *Human Nature*, for instance, the most important text for the later doctrine of the four humours, he concluded was not genuinely Hippocratic as it promoted ideas on anatomy that he had found to be incorrect.[76]

The second element in his education was philosophy, a broad term that in Antiquity encompassed metaphysics, cosmology, ethics, and much else. Galen began his studies when he was about fourteen under teachers hand-picked by Nicon to represent all the major groupings, the Stoics, the Platonists, the Epicureans and the Peripatetics or Aristotelians.[77] It was not a success. Although they were all distinguished pupils of famous scholars, their vigorous disagreement on major questions greatly confused the adolescent, who was rescued from his despair only by discovering the virtues of Platonic mathematics and geometry as a way of attaining some certainty.[78] His father's example further encouraged him to trust in his own logical abilities and to refuse to adhere slavishly to any one sect.[79] The experience did little to dispel his sense of his own superiority to his teachers, as well as convincing him that many of the standard themes of philosophical debate such as the eternity of the world or the nature of the human soul and its immortality were incapable of resolution one way or the other.[80] Henceforth he sought to base his conclusions upon solid evidence and cogent argument.

First steps in medicine

What career Nicon had planned for Galen at this stage of his life is unclear. He may have been expected to follow in his father's footsteps as an architect, pursue the life of a wealthy gentleman running his estates, or become a famous sophist.[81] He certainly had the ability, the erudition, and the self-confidence to become a celebrated speaker, to say nothing of the contacts and, some complained enviously, the wealth.[82] He was also determined to succeed. While others wasted their time in trivial pursuits, he was hard at work on his studies "like one inspired".[83] But all this was changed when he was sixteen. His father received several "crystal-clear dreams" as a result of which Galen was directed to the study of medicine and philosophy.[84] At an age when, elsewhere, some young men who died prematurely could already be described on their tombs as physicians, Galen was just setting out on a long educational odyssey that took him around the Eastern Mediterranean.[85]

Galen gained his first instruction in medicine in Pergamum from a variety of teachers, individual doctors rather than professors at a specific institution. The most famous of them was Satyrus, who had been the doctor to the consul Cuspius Rufinus and who was among those who treated the sophist Aelius Aristides, a remarkable example, according to Galen, of a strong soul imprisoned in a weak body.[86] Although Aristides always ascribed his periods of remission to Asclepius, he respected Satyrus, whom he described as a sophist of no humble birth, i.e. a wealthy intellectual like his pupil Galen.[87] Galen's teachers at Pergamum fell into two groups. One, constituted by an old local man, Aeschrion, and a mysterious doctor called Epicurus, followed the so-called Empiricist line.[88] Its proponents eschewed any investigation into the causes of disease, and *a fortiori* into treatments aimed at eliminating these causes, in favour of a careful cataloguing and observation of cases and therapies in order to ascertain an appropriate remedy for the case in hand. Galen was sympathetic to the Empiricists, praising their learning and their powers of observation, although criticising them for their inability to devise a cure when faced with a condition unlike anything seen or recorded before.[89] He was also critical of what he described as their inconsistencies in actual practice, arguing as a student with Aeschrion as to whether or not all the symptoms of plethora needed to be present before one could let blood.[90] On the other hand, he particularly commended Aeschrion for his knowledge of pharmacology, although not everyone will share Galen's enthusiasm for his recipe for rabies, largely made up of ashes of the crayfish.[91] He would also have taken Galen around with him to examine patients like the two young sufferers from epilepsy whom he mentions as seeing with his teachers "in Asia", the man with a severe brain injury he examined with Pelops at Smyrna, or the man with an ulcerated leg treated by another of his Pergamum teachers, Stratonicus.[92]

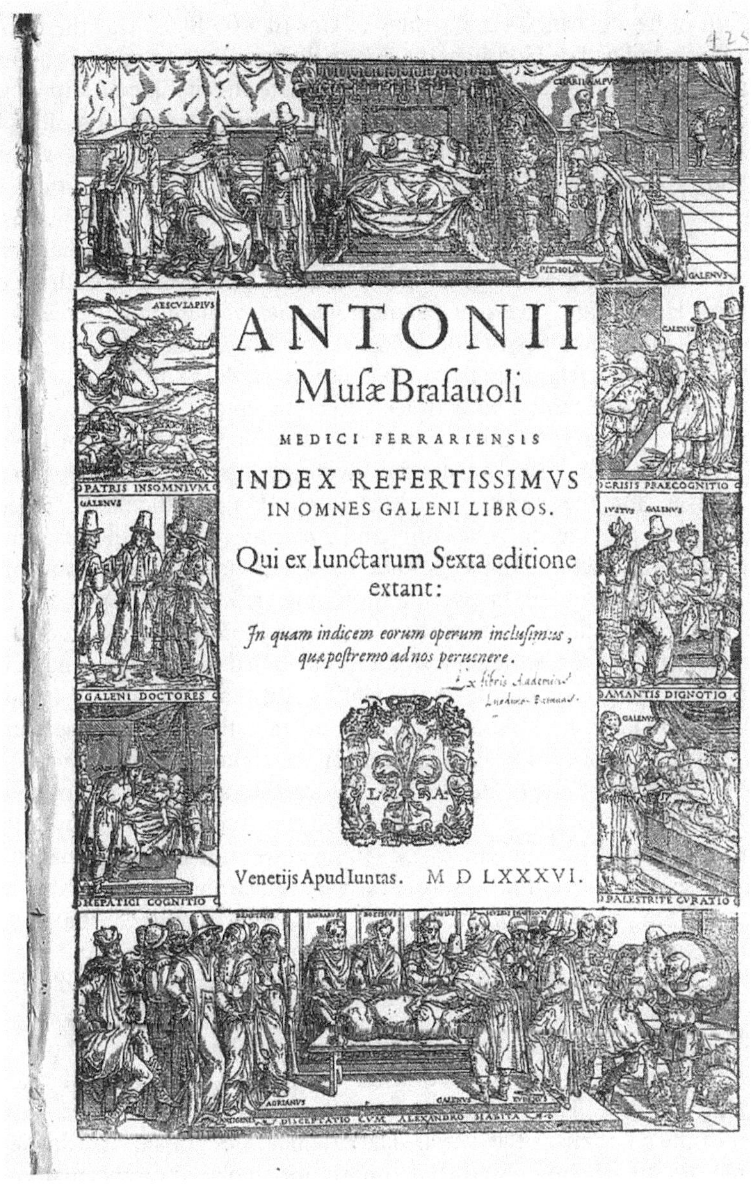

Figure 1.2 Scenes from the life of Galen. Frontispiece to the index to the sixth Juntine edition of the Latin Galen, Venice, 1586. Anticlockwise from top: the cure of Marcus Aurelius; his father's dream of Asclepius; Galen's teachers; diagnosing liver disease; dissecting in Rome; curing an injured wrestler; diagnosing love; prognosing a crisis.

Stratonicus was one of the second group of Galen's masters, physicians who were united in their respect for Hippocrates, even if they differed substantially in their interpretation of his doctrines. Hippocrates of Cos (fl. 400 BCE) was the most famous doctor in Greece in his day. However, the books that circulated under his name and the ideas within them are so diverse that, even if datable to the lifetime of Hippocrates, few, and perhaps none, can be confidently ascribed to the great man himself.[93] Even the most celebrated of Hippocratic notions, the theory of the four humours, with its belief that the body's health depended on an always precarious and constantly changing balance between four humours or fluids, phlegm, blood, bile, and black bile, is ascribed by Aristotle to his son-in-law, Polybus.[94] It was a theory that stressed the individuality of illness, as well as the need for the doctor to know the patient in both sickness and health. These 'Hippocratic' ideas of balance, whether of humours, elements or, more often, simply the four qualities of hot, cold, wet, and dry, formed the theoretical basis of Galen's medical understanding from his youth onwards.[95]

By Galen's day, a substantial body of learned commentary had grown up around the 'Hippocratic' writings, even if not every doctor was prepared to accept them as normative. There were in any case substantial divergences among the Hippocratic physicians themselves, for the variety of ideas within Hippocratic texts, allied to the obscurity of many passages in *Aphorisms* and *Epidemics*, two of the texts most often studied, allowed for a considerable latitude of interpretation. Aeficianus, another of Galen's teachers at Pergamum, favoured a Stoicising view of the Hippocratic body, and he may be the Pneumatist teacher whose views were contested by his combative student. (Pneumatists, like the Stoic philosophers, attributed great importance to an ethereal substance, *pneuma* or spirit, in regulating the balance of the humours and elements.) The Empiricists, although rejecting all investigation into the causes of ill health, shared the Hippocratics' high regard for their master as a practical physician, and the commentaries of one of their earlier leaders, Heraclides of Tarentum, fl. 85–65 BCE, were much appreciated by Galen. His medical education was thus within a tradition that emphasised the supremacy of Hippocrates and his individualist medicine and that had developed over four centuries a body of learning that appealed to Galen's scholarly erudition. Some of his teachers were skilled in observation and in their knowledge of therapeutics, while others stressed the need to understand the potential causes of illness in an individual, something that posed a considerable intellectual challenge to the physician.

It was while studying at Pergamum that Galen wrote his first three books, all different in character, but showing the wide range of interests that he was develop further over his long career.[96] The first, written at the behest of a midwife, was a short description of the anatomy of the womb. The original does not survive, unlike its much later revision. Its title already reveals the importance he placed on the anatomical basis of medicine, although even his later description is based far more on animal than on human anatomy. The second, *The Diagnosis of the Diseases of the Eye*, lost in Greek but with traces surviving in Arabic, was written for a young oculist, and reveals Galen's confidence in his mastery of therapeutics and, one might note, the respect that others already gave him. A later reminiscence of his time as a student stresses his constant efforts both day and night to improve his academic knowledge and, at the same time, to apply it to the treatment of the sick.[97] The third tract, surviving in a later recension in a complete Arabic version, was his private account of a two-day debate at Pergamum between an Empiricist called Philippus and a distinguished Hippocratic, Pelops, over the question of whether one could practise medicine effectively on the basis of one's own and others' experiences alone.[98] This was a question that exercised Galen throughout his life, as can be seen from other works he wrote on the same theme.[99] Although he came eventually to favour Pelops' view that one could not, he always maintained a great respect for those with substantial experience and knowledge, whether physicians, surgeons or midwives.

Academic peregrinations

The death of his father around 137–8 freed him from family obligations (and perhaps also from the tirades of his mother) as well as giving him the money to continue his education elsewhere.[100] He began by moving down the coast to the equally prosperous city of Smyrna (modern Izmir) to study with Albinus, a Platonist philosopher, and with Pelops, evidence for his determination to gain a deeper insight into both medicine and philosophy, and particularly Platonic philosophy. Both men were among the leading specialists of the day. Only traces remain of the writings of Albinus, a pupil of another famous Platonist, Gaius, but they included commentaries on Plato's dialogues, notably the *Timaeus*, of which a later summary survives. Recent scholars, however, have denied him the authorship of a contemporary *Handbook* to Platonic philosophy, preferring instead to stay with the otherwise unknown author named in the manuscripts as Alcinous.[101] How much Galen gained from his instruction is unclear: he refused to involve himself in Albinus' metaphysical questions, but he must have gained greater insights into Plato's thought from so expert a teacher and he placed great importance on his exposition of medically related topics in the *Timaeus*. Plato's assumption, further developed by Aristotle, that the whole universe was created by a divine and purposeful Creator inspired, or confirmed, Galen's later approach to anatomy, and much else.[102]

Pelops, whom he had met earlier in Pergamum, was famous for his exposition of Hippocrates. His commentary on *Nature of the Child* survived in Greek for centuries, and a copy was preserved among the works of Galen down to the ninth century.[103] He had studied, perhaps in Rome, with a certain Quintus, whose enormous reputation among his fellow Hippocratics was qualified by his reluctance to 'publish' his lectures, which were preserved after his death only in the notes and memories of his students.[104] In Smyrna Galen also continued his dissection activities, following Pelops' example.[105] One of the treatises he composed there, and later revised, was devoted to investigating the movement of the lungs and the chest. Its three books summarised Pelops' teaching with, at the end of Book III, a section on Galen's own discoveries, presumably made on living animals. It was written at the request of a fellow student, who died soon after on his way home after a period of study.

Such peregrinations by well-off students around the Greek world were not uncommon. Some might cover only a relatively few miles. A young man from the island of Cythera, off the tip of the Peloponnese, travelled for his medical education first to Boiae, little more than a harbour on the mainland, before moving to the large town in the region, Sparta, neither a place widely famous for its doctors. Alas, he died suddenly, before he could fulfil the hopes of his parents. A similar fate befell another student who died at Smyrna, a considerable way from his home at Tieon on the Black Sea.[106]

It was probably as a result of what he had heard from Pelops that Galen set out from Smyrna for Corinth in order to discover more about the lost teachings of Quintus from another of his hearers, Numisianus.[107] Unfortunately Numisianus may already have left or, indeed, died, so Galen followed his tracks to Alexandria in Egypt, only to find that his son, Heraclianus, was unwilling to release any of his papers to him.[108] This was a check to Galen's hopes, but there were other pupils of Quintus there who could talk about him, and, besides, it was always likely that, given the reputation of Alexandria, someone of Galen's wealth, talent and ambition would make his way to Egypt and to the city that could fittingly be called "the foundation of health for all men".[109]

Alexandria "by Egypt" had been founded by Alexander the Great on an island at one of the mouths of the Nile in 331 BCE to be a Greek bastion in the newly conquered land of Egypt. The new city quickly became also an intellectual and cultural show-piece to rival, if not surpass, Athens as the capital of the new Greek, 'Hellenistic' world. Among its magnificent buildings, including the famous lighthouse, one of the wonders of the Ancient world, two stood out for their ambitious promotion of Greek culture, institutionalising, under royal protection, what had been previously the personal predilections of local rulers: the Museum and the Library.[110]

The great Library (there were also smaller ones elsewhere in the city) was intended to hold copies of all Greek literature, including philosophy, medicine and science. Galen tells the story of ships arriving at Alexandria being searched for books, and any originals taken for the Library and replaced by copies.[111] It is probable, although far from certain, that our Hippocratic Corpus was first assembled there, with some books even coming from Cos itself, which had at one point formed part of the empire of the Ptolemies. Its librarians included some of the great scholars of the period, drawn from all over the Greek world, who investigated and interpreted the texts of Homer and the tragedians. Many volumes were said to have been lost in fires when Julius Caesar captured the city in 48 BCE, but there is ample evidence for the survival of many others into Galen's time and possibly until the Arab conquest in 641, if not beyond.[112] The Museum, or Hall of the Muses, was a complex of buildings around a temple of the Muses headed by its own priest. What took place there, and how many members were entitled to what, in Galen's day, were termed "free meals at the Museum", are difficult questions to answer. In the Hellenistic age, they certainly included distinguished literary scholars as well as mathematicians, but no doctor is named among them, although it is likely, to judge from Museums in Asia Minor three or four centuries later, that some were included. But by the time that Galen arrived, according to inscriptions, administrators and even a champion athlete could be admitted to membership, and one should be wary of assuming that this mix of scholars and non-scholars was present from the beginning. Evidence that the Museum was ever a place for actual teaching, a type of *didaskaleion*, is singularly lacking, although the notion that human anatomies took place within its walls as a sort of sacrifice to the gods is a nice, if unprovable, conceit.[113]

It was teachers and ideas, rather than these two institutions *per se*, that drew aspiring doctors and surgeons to the city – Galen never mentions in any surviving text that he ever entered the doors of the Museum or consulted a manuscript in the Library. During his time there, in the late 150s, Alexandria was a vibrant city, perhaps the largest in the world, with a population drawn from all around the Eastern Mediterranean. Greek influence had stretched well up the Nile, especially in towns like

Oxyrhynchus where there were doctors who read learned volumes of Greek medicine, but Egyptian medicine continued to be practised.[114] There was a constant interchange of remedies of all kinds, some native, others imported from all parts of the known world including Africa, India, and further East. Alexandria was the great entrepôt, and long remained so, with a reputation for medicine that remained high centuries after Galen.

It was famous in particular for two different aspects of medicine, Hippocratic commentary and anatomy. Discussions of some treatises by Hippocrates were certainly taking place there in the early third century BCE in the circle, or 'house', of Herophilus of Chalcedon. This developed quickly into a whole tradition of learned commentary, including lectures, glossaries, and expositions of particular themes that transcended some of the sectarian divisions. Galen reports early explanations of the alphabetic characters that were used as a mnemonic for some of the medical points in the *Epidemics* as well as divergent interpretations and manuscript readings that went back to the third century BCE.[115] The more recent editions of Hippocrates by Dioscorides 'the glossographer' in the first part of the second century and by his contemporary Artemidorus Capito excited considerable debate among learned physicians in Alexandria and beyond. Galen had begun writing his own exegeses of some Hippocratic writings as a private exercise before 162, which were only later made available for others to read. His huge later commentaries are filled with detail about these academic debates, with the result that we know far more about the tradition of the Hippocratic writings in the period before 200 CE than that of almost any other ancient Greek author save Homer.[116]

But it is not easy to determine precisely what Galen derived from his teachers or his reading in this tradition. His comments on teachers such as Heraclianus, the son of Numisianus, or Julian the Methodist, who wrote a commentary on the *Aphorisms* in 48 books, are generally hostile, and he goes into far more detail about points where he disagrees with commentators whom he respects such as Rufus of Ephesus or the much earlier Heraclides of Tarentum than he does when repeating and endorsing their conclusions.[117] A few fragments of commentaries by others survive independently of Galen, but the only complete one, written by Apollonius of Citium in the early first century BCE, is more a meditation on certain aspects of the Hippocratic *Joints* than a systematic point-by-point analysis.[118] Nonetheless, a comparison between some long sections on towns from the commentary on *Airs, Waters, and Places* by Sabinus, the teacher of Galen's teacher Satyrus, and what Galen says in his own commentary reveals the intelligence and clarity of thought of both men, as well as Galen's undoubted dependence on his predecessor.[119] Nor is the pseudonymous Pergamene author of the *Commentary on the Hippocratic Oath* inferior to Galen in learning.[120] But at the same time, as Wesley Smith argued, it would be wrong to assume that Galen's interest in determining which works or even sections were by the hand of the master himself was shared by every commentator or went back much before 120 CE. Galen's passion for Hippocratic authenticity is as much as a defence of his own Galenic medicine as an academic archaeology of Hippocrates. In his search for what the great man himself had said, his linguistic learning takes second place to his conviction that the great doctor of Cos was infallible and its corollary: passages that diverged from what Galen himself had found to be true could not have been entirely original, and could thus be dismissed as only partly valuable to a modern doctor.[121]

Alexandrian anatomy

Although Galen came to Alexandria to learn more about Hippocratic medicine, the medical reputation of the city depended far more on its long tradition of surgery and anatomy. Human anatomy, the deliberate cutting into a human body for the purposes of investigation, had begun there in the early third century BCE. A generation or more earlier the great natural philosopher Aristotle and the doctor Diocles of Carystus had cut up animals to investigate their internal structures, but neither had challenged the religious taboo on touching a human corpse. Similarly, surgeons were familiar with treating fractures and wounds, but their understanding of the interior of the human body is best described as rudimentary, a mixture of metaphor, animal dissection, and occasional fortuitous observation. Why human anatomy for investigative purposes should have taken place first in Alexandria is disputed, but certain factors are well known. The Egyptians had performed mummification on the dead, removing the internal organs and storing them in special Canopic jars around the body, a procedure that aroused in Greek travellers horror and fascination in equal measure. The Greek takeover of Egypt gave them the opportunity to carry out dissections there on natives who themselves allowed something similar for their own relatives. Whether there was any communication between the native Egyptian mummifiers and Greek anatomists is far from clear because of the language barrier, and, at all events, the way in which the organs were extracted in mummification was hardly conducive to clear and detailed observation. There may have been a similar problem of communication with native surgeons, who carried out operations that were arguably more complex than those of the Greeks and had formed part of a learned tradition that went back beyond 1500 BCE. Finally, the status of Alexandria as the Greek capital also gave a measure of protection on the part of its rulers, the Ptolemies, to those who carried out the dissections. If a later Roman source, the encyclopaedist Cornelius Celsus, is right in saying that the earliest anatomical experiments were carried out on condemned criminals, some of them even still alive, this was something that could only have been done with the permission of the monarch.[122]

The first anatomist is traditionally identified as Herophilus of Chalcedon, a pupil of Praxagoras of Cos at the end of the third century BCE. Herophilus provided what might be described as the first map of the previously invisible body, describing and giving names to many of its individual parts, from the duodenum to the torcular, i.e. 'wine-press', a depression in the skull where three great venous sinuses meet. He investigated the eye and the brain, but his anatomy of the womb is that of an animal, not a woman.[123] His contemporary Erasistratus, the son of a doctor at the royal court at Antioch in Syria, is also likely to have carried out his dissections at Alexandria. No medical source associates Antioch with any dissections, and his cure of the lovesick Seleucus is the stuff of legend.[124] Whereas Galen almost always speaks of Herophilus with great respect, his attitude to Erasistratus was ambivalent.[125] In a variety of treatises in his Roman period, he denounced much of his therapeutics and especially his notion that the arteries were filled with air or *pneuma*, and that blood appeared in them only in exceptional circumstances, following a cut or having been forced into them from the veins via tiny anastomoses.[126] But for his belief in the significance of anatomy Galen had the highest praise. To show the importance of constant practice at dissection, he quoted Erasistratus' comparison, in a book on paralysis, of the novice anatomist to an untrained athlete, lacking speed and stamina at first, but steadily improving through training. Structures at first unclear or invisible would become obvious through practice and persistent enquiry, a declaration that Galen, who claimed to dissect daily, took as an inspiration for the rest of his life.[127] Erasistratus had a more mechanistic view of the body than Herophilus, downplaying the humoral theory in favour of seeing the body as a working organism. His experiments on the heart and blood flow, many repeated by Galen often with identical results, remain impressive today, while his investigation of tiny structures in the brain shows his skill with the knife and his acute powers of observation.[128]

This golden age of experimental human dissection lasted for only a couple of generations. Objections were raised to it on the grounds of unnecessary cruelty. Opponents argued that knowing about a dead body was of no help in the treatment of the living, and that repeated dissections added nothing to the sum of human knowledge. Nor were circumstances in Alexandria itself always helpful. Doctors were among the many members of the Museum, "endlessly arguing in a bird-cage of the Muses", according to the satirist Timon of Phlius, who were expelled from Alexandria shortly after 145 BCE by Ptolemy Euergetes II, and the political upheavals in the middle years of the next century will not have aided researchers.[129] Elsewhere, even if there are traces of anatomical investigation, these were fleeting at best. By 100 CE, according to Rufus of Ephesus, who had spent some time in Egypt, anatomy had become merely a question of knowing the technical terms for parts of the body that could then be pointed out on a slave.[130] Some of these terms were only recent, such as the coinages of some Egyptian doctors for parts of the skull that had previously been left nameless or, like the skull sutures, had been given Greek names which they did not recognise because of their weak knowledge of Greek.[131]

According to Galen, a great change occurred "in the time of our grandfathers", i.e. around 130, when a teacher called Marinus, almost certainly in Alexandria, began a series of anatomical investigations that Galen thought sufficiently important to summarise thirty or more years later.[132] Marinus' twenty books, abridged by Galen into four, offered a comprehensive survey of the human body that was more extensive than anything else available at the time. Not only did it provide Galen with a solid textbook, paying particular attention to the brain and nerves, but it also renewed the tradition of dissection that was also passed on to Galen by many of his own teachers.[133] Satyrus, for example, who was also a writer on anatomy, once while examining patients whose arms had been stripped of their skin and sometimes much of the underlying flesh in an outbreak of so-called anthrax, took the opportunity to demonstrate to his students just how the various muscles moved the arm in different ways.[134] The teachers at Alexandria specialised also in teaching osteology from an actual skeleton, something rarely, if ever, done elsewhere.[135] That was why everyone should try to study there.

Galen's relationship with Egypt and Alexandria presents a paradox.[136] Although, like many rich young students, such as his friend Philippus and the man from Adada in central Turkey who died young, he might have been expected to aspire to study there, he describes his arrival almost as an accident, and his comments on what he found are rarely complimentary.[137] His teachers are incompetent, witness their readiness to provide a detailed commentary on an allegedly Hippocratic passage that had been composed as a joke by Lucian, later famous as a satirist.[138] Heraclianus, the son of Numisianus, he heard at first with approval, but soon changed his mind.[139] Another teacher, Aelianus, wrote a useful book on the dissection of muscles, but only considered what was obvious, and even then left much out, while Julian's commentary on

Aphorisms was filled with bombast, stupidity and irrelevance, and the various versions of his *Introduction to Medicine* continued to repeat fundamental mistakes.[140] Galen found little to like on his travels in Egypt, except for some ingenious ways of keeping water cool.[141] The thin Egyptian wine was worse than that of a rough Italian taverna, and the food, with a few exceptions, was almost indigestible.[142] Writers who believed that Hippocrates had recommended Egyptian beans might get away with this nonsense in Asia Minor, but not in Alexandria.[143] Both town and country dwellers lived on nigh-disastrous diets; beer, fish, shellfish, pulses, and lentils engendered a near-incurable thick skin, while it was only habituation that saved those who regularly ate the flesh of camels and donkeys from its most damaging effects. A fellow student who subsisted there for four years on a vegetarian diet without any ill effects was truly amazing, but another, who had eaten some unripe dates, suffered a shaking fever with rigours.[144] Besides, away from the coast, the hot, dry climate made one skinny and dry, a state far removed from the Polyclitan ideal of the well-tempered man.[145] As for relaxation, what could one say about their passion for watching fights between a mongoose and a snake in the theatre of Alexandria?[146]

Why then did Galen stay for four or five years? One possible reason beyond the purely intellectual may lie in Alexandria's role as a centre for the import of drugs from around the world.[147] Visits to the harbour will also have introduced him to members of the seafaring community, from whom he will have gained much information about winds and climate that he put to use in his commentary on *Airs, Waters, and Places.*[148] Like sailors, Egyptian astrologers also had a great knowledge of the heavens, and his comment that their expertise was superior to that of all others is praise indeed from someone who had himself learned much about the stars from his father and who displayed his understanding of the technicalities involved to his advantage in his discussion of the significance of critical days.[149] But like bird-diviners and those who recommended for stomach problems a green jasper stone carved in the likeness of Pharaoh Nechepso, their accurate observations did not justify the conclusions they drew from them.[150] The jasper worked equally well uncarved, while the behaviour of birds and the position of the stars were simply indicators of the climatic changes which alone caused illness in the individual body.

Another possibility is that Galen was keen to improve his skill as a surgeon, for, ever since the days of Herophilus, Alexandrian surgeons had continued to develop new techniques and new operations. The last books of Celsus' *Medicine*, summarising three hundred years of Alexandrian surgery, show how the anatomical discoveries of the third century BC had led to more complex and more daring operations than had been feasible in the time of Hippocrates.[151] Fragmentary papyri from towns in the Nile valley also show a range of new techniques in the Roman period for dealing with fistulae, mutilations and eye-conditions, most deriving almost certainly from surgeons in Alexandria.[152] The city had a reputation for surgery that lasted for centuries, and Galen would have benefited from the cachet that study there gave.[153]

Return to Pergamum

Certainly, it was his expertise in surgery that gained him his first significant job when he returned to Pergamum around 157 after what is the longest medical education on record.[154] He was one of the candidates for the post of doctor to the gladiators who performed at the great provincial games organised and paid for by the wealthy individuals who each year took on the office of High Priest of the imperial cult within the province of Asia. Together with its equivalents at Ephesus and Smyrna, Pergamum's rivals for pre-eminence, this was the most prestigious post in the province, and demanded an appropriately high outlay in providing for the annual celebrations.[155] Gladiatorial games had spread from Italy to the Greek world, where huge amphitheatres were constructed, as at Pergamum, to house the crowds and to display the donor's munificence. Doctor to these gladiators was not a run-of-the-mill job. Not only did it bring its holder into contact with some of the wealthiest men in the whole Roman world, but it offered an opportunity to display one's skills in public. We also know from an imperial inscription only a few years later that gladiators were becoming more expensive than ever, and hence there was an incentive to keep them alive and in prime condition.[156] This was a post for an experienced man, and Galen's appointment came as a surprise to some, not least because he was the sole appointee and at a young age.[157]

The reason for his success he put into the mouth of the High Priest himself. He had himself observed that the young man was constantly studying, never indulging in frivolities, and always occupied in practising something useful. He had also seen him spectacularly successful in a public display.[158] Before his competitors Galen seized a young monkey, slit open its belly, and challenged them to replace its guts and re-stitch the wound successfully. When they hesitated, he took charge and closed up the poor animal's wound. He then gave several examples of how to let blood from a vein, and how to repair a wound, even if it appeared large.[159] The High Priest also seems to have heard about Galen's expertise with drugs, and, of course, would have been already acquainted with his fellow-townsman and his family.[160]

How many gladiators were under Galen's care is not clear, but for the most important games, such as the imperial games held each year in September, the number could reach a hundred or more.[161] Galen was proud of his success in the post. Only two of his charges died in his first year, compared with sixteen under his predecessors, and none subsequently under the next four priests.[162] Most of the wounds he mentions were to the thigh or shins, for which he devised new types of plaster for closing and healing them.[163] Some serious wounds he treated by soaking linen cloths in wine, putting them over the wound and placing moist sponges on top for several days, reusing any excess wine that dripped down. Red wine may have had some antimicrobial effect but keeping the wound moist would also avoid sepsis.[164] Another gladiator, who arrived in the arena mounted on horseback, he successfully treated for a slash across the thigh by suturing the damaged muscles.[165] On another occasion, he was forced to remove a large part of the lower abdomen that had escaped from a wound, and there were always cuts, bruises, and sprains in training to deal with.[166] These professional gladiators, unlike the prisoners massacred in the Roman Colosseum, had to be kept fit and well. Galen fed them a vegetarian diet, heavily based on barley and beans, and remarkably similar to that recently revealed by palaeopathological studies to have been eaten by the gladiators in a gladiatorial training-school at Ephesus at almost the same date.[167]

Galen's career up until this point, 161, had been typical of any wealthy bourgeois in the Eastern half of the Empire. His education, his interests, and his travels had been entirely in the Greek world, of which Pergamum was for him the centre. His father had held some public office there, and he might well have been expected to follow him, or at least to continue his profession there as a highly regarded physician to its wealthy and cultured citizens. Even when he had left for Rome in 162, he remained attached to his home city throughout his life.[168] Like many exiles today, he recalled the delights of his native region – Pergamene hunters in autumn enjoying the taste of meat from foxes who had gorged themselves on late-season grapes, the pine-forests around his home, and the taste of the local sour-milk cheese, perhaps better even than the *vatusicum* cheese preferred by the rich in Rome.[169] The memory of the dreadful diet of the peasants with whom he ate while on a trip with friends also stayed long with him.[170] He often indicated his attachment to Pergamum in more subtle ways. Attalus III was 'our king', and Galen's 'we' refers to the Greeks, and very often solely to Pergamum and neighbouring villages such as Allianoi and Lakettoi.[171]

Other Greek doctors visited Rome but were not impressed. The gynaecologist Soranus of Ephesus was appalled at the way in which tiny Roman children damaged their pliable limbs by being forced to walk on its hard marble floors.[172] None of this need indicate any hostility to Rome on the part of Greeks, however much they might have learned as children about the great days before the Roman conquest when Greece was free and had defeated the Persians by itself. Rather, any nostalgia for the past was balanced by an appreciation of the benefits of Roman rule. Even local indifference to far away events in Italy would have been muted by the ways in which the upper classes had been drawn into the imperial orbit, and it was a rare town that did not maintain links with a citizen who had made good somewhere in the West. Life in larger communities like Pergamum, Ephesus or Smyrna was extremely pleasant, rarely disturbed by wars and rumours of wars, or even by a legion passing by on its way to a distant frontier. When an emperor or a governor did visit, it was likely to result in honours and benefits for the town and its leading citizens.[173] Edward Gibbon's judicious praise of the Antonine peace in the opening paragraphs of his famous *Decline and Fall of the Roman Empire* applies *par excellence* to Pergamum and the environment in which Galen grew up and helps to explain why his attachment to his native city and region remained at the core of his identity throughout his long life.

Notes

1 *HNH* I,44: 15,105 K; II, pref.: 15,109 K; Koester 1998; Coqueugniot 2013; Coarelli 2016; Radt 2016. For parchments, traditionally a discovery of Pergamene libraries, *Hipp.Off. Med.*1,pref.: 18B,630 K.

2 Galen mentions his pharmacological studies with approval: *SMT* X,1: 12,251 K; *Comp. Med.Gen.* I,13: 13,416 K; *Ant.* I,1: 14,2 K.

3 *Aff.Dig.* I,9: 5,49 K; p. 278 tr. Singer PN, including 40,000 male citizens. He gives no figures for children, and his figures may be no more than a guess. For the architectural and settlement history of Pergamum at this period see Koester 1998; Pirson 2017: 95–117.

4 *Hipp.Epid. VI*, iv,11: 17B,159 K; Hodge 2002: 42–5; Radt 2016: 147–58. For the abundance of cooling fountains, *Comp.Med.Loc.* II,1: 12,508 K. Radt 2016: 95–112 gives several examples of the sort of house that a wealthy family like Galen's would have occupied.

5 *UP* XVI,1: 4,265–6 K; II, p. 682 tr. May, although without specifying the place.

6 The exact year of Galen's birth requires a choice between two incompatible statements One, written around AD 176, *Praec.* 2 and 9: 14,605, 649 K; *CMG* V 8,1, 74–5, 118–9, would suggest 129 CE, the other written thirty or more years later, *Lib.Prop.* 1,14: 19,15 K; p. 6 tr. Singer PN, 130 CE. The earlier date is to be preferred. Cf. Boudon-Millot 2012: 286–7.

7 Gleason 2005, an excellent and wide-ranging discussion. For peasants coming into the city, *MM* V,7: 10,334 K.

8 *San.Tu.* VI,9: 6,424 K. Baykan 2012; Nutton 2014b: 389–96.

9 Ziegenaus and De Luca 1968–84; Habicht 1969; Riethmüller 2005: I,334–59; Strocka 2012; Renberg 2017: 138–46, 192–202.
10 Rosenthal 1956: 67–76; Strohmaier 1970; Nutton 2012b; Van Nuffelen 2014; Jouanna 2018: cxxx–cxxxi.
11 *AA* I,2: 2,224–5 K, with the emendation of Garofalo 1991; pp. 4–5 tr. Singer C; Feissel 1999; Riethmüller 2005: I,334–6; Strocka 2012; Van der Ploeg 2018: 115–61.
12 Edelstein and Edelstein 1945, supplemented by Riethmüller 2005; vol. II for the non-literary evidence.
13 Jones 1998; Petsalis-Diomidis 2010; Israelowich 2012: 86–131; Boudon-Millot 2016c; Renberg 2017: 192–202; Van der Ploeg 2018. Galen, *Comm.Plat.Tim.* IV: *CMG Suppl.* I: 33, talks of seeing Aristides, presumably at Pergamum.
14 For Galen, *Lib.Prop.* 3,5: 19,18–19 K; p. 8 tr. Singer PN; p. 142 BM. Cf. the Pergamene author of the commentary on the Hippocratic *Oath*, Rosenthal 1956: 60–76; Strohmaier 1970; Jouanna 2018: cxli. For coins, Riethmüller 2005: II,364.
15 *Lib.Prop.* 3,5: 19,18–19 K; p. 142 BM; p. 8 tr. Singer PN; *Prop.Plac.* 2: p. 173 BMP; pp. 62–3 Garofalo-Lami; p. 188 Vegetti; *San.Tu.* 1,8: 6,41 K; I, p. 61 tr. Johnston. Recent epigraphic discoveries (Petridou 2017; Pietrobelli 2017: 223–9) suggest that Galen's use of the word θεραπευτής indicates that he was a member of a specific elite cult group at the shrine. See also below, p. 14, for Nicon's 'clear dreams'; Frede 2003, Pietrobelli 2017 and Petit 2018 give wider assessments of Galen's prudential theology
16 *Bon.Mal.Suc.* 1: 6,757 K; *Cur.Rat.Ven.Sect.* 23: 11,314–5 K; *Lib.Prop.* 3,5: p.142 BM; Cf. Habicht 1969, no. 139, a man bled "by the order of the god"; Boudon-Millot 2012: 81–4.
17 *UP* X,12: 3,902–4 K; II, pp. 490–1 tr. May.
18 Edelstein and Edelstein 1945: II,152–4, 167–73; Oberhelman 2013: 1–30
19 *SMT* I,1: 12,315–6 K; *Subf.Emp.* 10; pp. 39–40 tr. Frede.
20 *Hipp.Epid.VI*, iv,8: *CMG* V 10,2,2, 199.
21 His father's name is, at present, known only through an entry in the Byzantine encyclopaedia, the *Souda, s.v.* Galen.
22 *IGRR* 504.
23 *Ibid.* 502–3, 506. Ohlemutz 1968: 169–70; Schlange-Schöningen 2003: 49–54; Alexandru 2011; Nutton 2015a.
24 *Aff.Dig.* I,8: 5,41 K; p. 272 tr. Singer PN; for the family, *Ind.* 59: p. 19 BJP; p. 95 tr. Nutton.
25 *Alim.Fac.* I,37: 6,552–3 K; p. 69 tr. Powell; *Bon.Mal.Suc.* 1,16; 5,8 and 11; 6,755, 783–4 K; *Ant.* I,3: 14,17–19 K; cf. *UP* IV,3: 3,270 K; I, pp. 205–6 tr. May, for Galen's expertise in wine-making. The traditional family name, Claudius, is found in only a tiny number of later Greek manuscripts. If correct, this would indicate citizenship for the family from the middle years of the first century CE, perhaps a generation later than that implied by the family name Julius; Aelius, on the other hand, would indicate a grant of Roman citizenship in the time of Hadrian in the 120s or 130s.
26 *Aff.Dig.* I,8: 5,41 K; p. 272 tr. Singer PN. Cf. *MM* I,1: 10,10 K; p. 17 Johnston-Horsley, public speaking should be left only to those of good family, education and morals. For *stasis* at Pergamum, see below, p. 36.
27 *Aff.Dig.* I,8:5,43–4 K; pp. 274–5 tr. Singer PN; Samama 2003: nos. 246–8; Nutton 2013a: 260–2. A fragmentary dedication from the Asclepieion was made by a P. Aelius Nicon (Habicht 1969: 124), but this may have no connection with Galen or the other Nicons. Other acquaintances among the elite include the dedicatee of *Aff.Dig.* I,9: 5,49 K; pp. 277–8 tr. Singer PN and the "great" Pardalas, i.e. probably Ti. Claudius Pardalas, a leading magistrate of the city and a cult official at the Asclepieion, cured of ill health by taking theriac salts (Fischer 2009: 163–5).
28 *Aff.Dig.* I,8: 5,41 (mother), 41–3 K; pp. 272–3 tr. Singer PN; *Ind.* 58–64: 18–20 BJP; pp. 93–4 tr. Nutton; *Bon.Mal.Suc.* 1: 6,755 K.
29 Greek: *Diff.Puls.* II, 4–5: 8,582–3, 587 K; *Aff.Dig.* I,8: 5,42 K; p. 273 tr. Singer PN.
30 Horace, *Satires* I,6,81
31 *Aff.Dig.* I,8 and II,5: 5,42, 80–4 K; pp. 272–3, 299–302 tr. Singer PN; *Ord.Lib.Prop.* 4,4: 19,59 K; pp. 27–8 tr. Singer PN. Cf. *Mor.* III,44: pp. 163, 193 tr. Davies; *Diff.Puls.* II,5: 8,587 K.

32 Astronomy, *Hipp.AWP* G.6,50g Wasserstein; *Sept. Part.* pp. 127–30 ed. Schöne; Toomer 1985; Cooper 2011a; Heilen 2018; instruments *Ind.* 4–5: p. 3 BJP; p. 79 tr. Nutton, with Andorlini 2017: 131–6.
33 *Bon.Mal.Suc.* 1: 6,755 K; *San.Tu.* V,1: 6,308–9 K; II, p. 7 tr. Johnston.
34 Rosenthal 1975: 34; cf. *Opt.Med.Cogn.* 9,1–2: *CMG Suppl. Or.* IV, 100–1.
35 *Mor.* I,29; 31; II,38: pp. 142–3, 144, 155 tr. Davies; *Aff.Dig.* 1,8: 5,43–4 K; pp. 274–5 tr. Singer PN; *Ind.* 60–61: p. 19 BJP; p. 94 tr. Nutton.
36 Charax; Andrei 1984; Aristocles: Philostratus, *Lives of the Sophists* II,3: 567–8.
37 A comment attributed to Galen by the fifteenth-century Egyptian litterateur al-Abshīhī, Rat 1899: I,67. Cf. the story in Aulus Gellius, *Attic Nights* XVIII,10,1.
38 Bowersock 1969; Reardon 1971 remain fundamental. See also Petit 2018: 2–12.
39 Philostratus, *Lives* 8: 489–92; Galen, *Lib.Prop.* 14,21; 15,1: pp. 168–9 BM. His *Against Favorinus, on Socrates*; and *For Epictetus, against Favorinus* are lost; but *The Best Teaching*, 1,40–52 K, has been edited with a commentary by A. Barigazzi, *CMG* V 1,1.
40 Plutarch, *Cessation of Oracles* 18: 419E, cf. 1: 410A.
41 Plutarch, *PHP* III,2,18: 5,300 K;*CMG* V 4,1,2, 183 (his *Homeric Studies*); Lucian, *Hipp. Epid.II*, vi,9: *CMG* V 10,1, 402 (a spoof Hippocratic aphorism); Africanus, Viellefond 1970; Marcellus, *Greek Anthology* VII,158.
42 Samama 2003: nos. 289–90; İplikçioğlu 2014; Nutton 2014b: 385–9. Cf. *Ant.* II,7: 14,144–6 K, for Galen's understanding of the value of medical poetry in appealing to a sophisticated audience.
43 Rosenthal 1956: 73; Jouanna 2018: cxxviii–cxxxvi. Although this commentary is ascribed to Galen, his general lack of reference to the *Oath* and his failure elsewhere to mention this commentary constitute a handicap to accepting it as genuine, Nutton 2012b.
44 Schrier 1995; Nutton 2009a; Coker 2019: for the wider context, Swain 1996; Desideri 2000; Wilkins 2011; Mattern 2017; Petit 2018: 59–63. Note Galen's learned discussion of the digamma in Greek and Latin, Martelli 2012.
45 *Sept.Part.*: p. 348 tr. Walzer, with the discussion, p. 334. This quotation of Euphorion, fragment 100 Lightfoot, is unknown to modern editors of the poet.
46 Scholiast on Oribasius, *Medical Collections* XIV,10,44: *CMG* VI 1,2, 192,15f. For the problem of deciding authenticity, see Kudlien 1965: 295–8.
47 Nutton 2009a. For Galen's Thucydidean exposition of epidemic disease, Petit 2018: 69–75, 140–5.
48 Kudlien 1971.
49 *SMT* IX,1,4: 12,191 K.
50 *AA* III,9: 2,393 K; p. 81 tr. Singer C; *UP* X,3: 3,775–7 K; II, p. 573 tr. May. He quotes Xenophon's non-historical works more often.
51 For Plutarch, Xenofontos 2016, 2018; Arrian, *UP* XI,12: 3,895 K; II, p. 528 tr. May.
52 Swain 1996; Gleason 2005; Mattern 2017.
53 Von Staden 1997a; López Férez 2015.
54 E.g. *Diff.Puls.* III,3: 8,653–6 K.
55 *Mor.* II, p. 40 Kraus; p. 158 tr. Davies; Walzer 1962: 167–9.
56 Boudon 2000; Xenofontos 2016, 2018.
57 *Opt.Med.Cogn.* 8,10; 13,2: *CMG Suppl. Or.* IV, 98–101, 128–9.
58 Manetti and Roselli 1994: 1569–80; Nutton 2009a.
59 The placing of a vowel at the end of one word and another at the beginning of the next (hiatus) was the Greek equivalent of the English split infinitive in the opposition it raised in some quarters.
60 Galen, *Alim.Fac.* II,9,12: 6,579 K; p. 82 tr. Powell; at *Praec.* 5,2: 14, 625 K; *CMG* V 8,1, 94–5, he chides the "over-sophisticated Atticists" for refusing to use the standard modern word for 'chamberlain'.
61 *Aff.Dig.* I,8: 5,42 K: pp. 272–3 tr. Singer PN.
62 *Soph.* 14,582–98: Edlow 1977; Ebbesen 1981.
63 *Nom. Med.*, ed. Meyerhof and Schacht 1931, *passim;* a new edition and English translation of this neglected work is a desideratum.
64 *Diff.Puls.* II,5: 8,584–8 K. Nonetheless, he shows a considerable interest in local terminology, see below, p. 54–5.

65 For clarity as extending beyond mere words and into thinking, cf. Petit 2018: 20–3, 44–8, 134–45.

66 *San.Tu.* I,10,17: 6,51 K; I, p. 75 tr. Johnston. He probably included Favorinus of Arles among these hellenised barbarians: would he have so characterised the satirical writer Lucian the Syrian, whom he knew in Alexandria?

67 *Ind.* 20–30: pp. 8–11 BJP; pp. 84–7 tr. Nutton; Coker 2019. For the possibility of links between Galen and the contemporary lexicographer Julius Pollux, see Pietrobelli 2019a: 13–15. For Galen among possible targets of Lucian's satire on lexicography, Baldwin 1973: 41–59.

68 *Opt.Med.Cogn.* 8,10; 13,2: *CMG Suppl. Or.* IV, 98–101, 128–9.

69 *Alim.Fac.* II,41: 6,628 K; p. 102 tr. Powell; *Vict.Att.* 15: p. 52 Marinone; p. 307 tr. Singer PN; Wilkins, in Powell 2003: xvi–xix.

70 Major studies of this Hippocratic tradition include Smith 1979; Manetti and Roselli 1994; Von Staden 2002; Flemming 2008; Manetti 2009.

71 *Ord.Lib.Prop.* 5,4–6: pp. 101–2 BM; pp. 28–9 tr. Singer PN.

72 *Gloss.*: 19,62–157 K; ed. Perilli *CMG* V 13,1; Manetti and Roselli 1994: 1574–6; Perilli 2007 and in his edition discusses earlier glossators.

73 *Ind.* 20–30: pp. 8–11 BJP; pp. 84–7 tr. Nutton. For the length of some of the book rolls, see my note, *ibid.*, p. 86, note 61.

74 *Nom.Med.* 31–2, with Deichgräber 1956; cf. also *Hipp.Epid.III*, 32: 17A,678 K, for Hippocrates' use of ordinary language.

75 *Alim.Fac.* I,27: 6,541 K; p. 64 tr. Powell; *Nom.Med.* 31–2. Cf. his use of Aristophanes, *Birds* 471 and Theocritus *Idyll* 7.23 to exemplify earlier opinions about larks, *SMT* XI,37: 12,360 K.

76 Smith 1979: 166–72, warning against assuming that this search for the 'real' Hippocrates went back centuries; Manetti and Roselli 1994: 1554–7.

77 *Ord.Lib.Prop.* 4:4: 19,59 K; p. 27 tr. Singer PN; *Aff. Dig.* I.8: 5,41–3 K; pp. 272–3 tr. Singer PN. Boudon-Millot 2007: xxi–xl assembles the relevant texts. For possible identifications of the unnamed Peripatetic pupil of Aspasius (Eudemus or Herminos), Moraux 1984: 226, n. 3.

78 Pietrobelli 2009.

79 *Aff.Dig.* I,8: 5,42–3 K; pp. 272–3 tr. Singer PN.

80 *Aff.Dig.* II,3: 5,70 K; p. 292 tr. Singer PN; *Prop.Plac.* 2,1–3,1: pp. 172–4 BMP; pp. 60–64 Garofalo-Lami; pp. 186–9 Vegetti.

81 Cf. his interest in the planning and siting of buildings and towns in *Hipp.AWP*, quoted in Oribasius, *Medical Collections* IX,10,1–2: *CMG* VI 1,2,11,30–12,5.

82 See below, p. 77, for a discussion of the 'sophistic' character of his moral essays. For envy of Galen's family wealth, *MM* VIII,3: 10,560–1 K; III, p. 393 tr. Johnston-Horsley.

83 *Opt.Med.Cogn.* 9: *CMG Suppl. Or.* IV, 100–1; quote from *DNF* III,10: 2,132 K; p. 205 tr. Brock, a necessary adjunct to native wit and good teaching.

84 *Ord.Lib.Prop.* 4,4: 19,59 K; p. 27 tr. Singer; *MM* IX,4: 10,465 K; II, p. 465 tr. Johnston-Horsley; *Praec.* 2,12: 14,608 K; *CMG* V 8,1, 78–9. He does not explicitly say that they were sent by Asclepius, but the adjective is frequently applied to dreams from Asclepius.

85 For other members of wealthy families at this period who travelled some distance for their medical education, see *Hipp.Epid.II*, vi: *CMG* V 10,1, 401–2; Nutton 2013a: 263, a contrast with the Latin West, where medical members of office-holding families are extremely rare, and slaves and ex-slaves very common.

86 Aelius Aristides, *Or.* 49,8–10; Galen, *Comm.Plat.Tim.* IV,33: *CMG Suppl.* I,33: cf. also pp. 83–4. In general, Boudon-Millot 2016c.

87 *Ord.Lib.Prop.* 3,11: p. 99 BM; p. 27 tr. Singer PN; *AA* I,1–2: 2,217, 224 K; pp. 1–2, 4 tr. Singer C; *Hipp.Epid.VI*, vii: *CMG* V 10,2,2, 412–3.

88 *Hipp.Epid.VI*, vii: *CMG* V 10,2,2, 412–3.

89 Frede 1987; Walzer and Frede 1985; Nutton 2013a: 151–2.

90 *Plen.* 9: 7,558–9 K; p. 60 Otte.

91 *SMT* XI,24: 12,356–7 K.

92 *Loc.Aff.* III, 11: 8,194 K; pp. 94–5 tr. Siegel; *Hipp.Aph.*VI,18: 18A,29 K; *At.Bil.* 4: 5,119 K.

93 Jouanna 1999, 2017; Craik 2015.

94 Nutton 2013a: 82–5.
95 *Prop.Plac.* 4,5 and 12: pp. 174–6, 183–5 BMP; pp. 74–80, 108–18 Garofalo-Lami; pp. 190–6, 208–12 Vegetti.
96 *Lib.Prop.* 2,2: p. 140 BM, with the Note p. 192; p. 7 tr. Singer PN. The second edition of *Ut.Diss.* is edited with a commentary by Nickel, *CMG* V 2,1, 1971.
97 *San.Tu.* V,1: 6,308 K; II, p. 7 tr. Johnston
98 Walzer 1944; Walzer and Frede 1985: 49–106. Greek fragments in Schrenk 1989.
99 *Lib.Prop.* 2: 19,16–17 K; pp. 140–1 BM; pp. 7–8 tr. Singer PN.
100 It may be coincidence that his move allowed him to avoid the gymnasium training associated with ephebes, similarly wealthy young men from the community, which began at age 18, König 2005: 47–68.
101 See the Introduction to Dillon 1993.
102 Petit 2018; Rocca 2018.
103 Lamoreaux 2016: 106.
104 *San.Tu.* III,13: 6,228 K; II, p. 333 tr. Johnston; *Praec.*1,9: 14,602 K; *CMG* V 8,1, 70–1; *Hipp.Epid. VI*, 10 and 14: *CMG* V 10,2,2, 207, 287.
105 *Musc.Diss.*: 18B,959 K (Pelops' dissection of the tongue of an ox). Pelops also preceded Galen in devoting a considerable time to anatomical studies of respiration and the voice.
106 Nutton 2013a: 263.
107 *AA* I,1: 2,217 K; p. 2 tr. Singer C; Grmek and Gourevitch 1988.The Arabic version, p. 82 Garofalo, says that he went to Egypt to seek out a famous student of both Quintus and Numisianus. The variant readings are explained by a simple change in the original Greek behind the Arabic.
108 The papers were later destroyed in a fire, like those of Pelops. *AA* XIV,1: pp. 183–4 Dkw; pp. 1039–41 Garofalo. The ubiquity of fire in the ancient world leaves Galen's suggestion that Heraclianus had deliberately destroyed his father's papers unprovable.
109 Anon. *Description of the Whole World* 37; *Comp.Med.Gen.* III,10: 13,631 K; Nutton 1993b; Harris WV and Ruffini 2004.
110 Fraser 1972: esp. pp. 305–36; Nesselrath 2013.
111 *Hipp.Epid.III*: 17A,606–7 K. Hands 2013, suggests the Library formed part of the Museum, and is sceptical about its contents. Cf. Nesselrath 2013; Zadorojnyi 2013.
112 El-Abbadi 1992: MacLeod 2004.
113 Nutton 2013a: 133.
114 Andorlini 2017: 230–39.
115 *Hipp.Epid.III*, ii,5,9: *CMG* V 10,2,1, 81–3, 91–5; *Lib.Prop.* 9, 1–7: 19,33–5 K; pp. 157–9 BM; p. 15 tr. Singer PN.
116 Jouanna 2018: CLIV–VII, emphasising that Galen began writing 'notes' or 'commentaries' on Hippocratic texts from an early date. The later Hippocratic commentaries contain far more detailed information on his predecessors, the result of retrieving his library from Pergamum, *Lib.Prop.* 9, 1–7: 19,33–5 K; pp. 157–9 BM; pp. 15–6: tr. Singer PN.
117 Below, pp. 21–2.
118 Potter 1993.
119 Oribasius, *Medical Collections* IX,15–20: *CMG* VI 1,2, 15–20; Raiola 2018.
120 Rosenthal 1956; Nutton 2012b; Jouanna 2018: cxl–cxli. Although there are strong parallels with Galen, the fact that Galen never mentions such a commentary and says little elsewhere about the *Oath* is a strong argument against authenticity.
121 Smith 1979; Manetti and Roselli 1994; Von Staden 2009; Das 2018.
122 Nutton 2013a: 130–2; Lang 2013.
123 Von Staden 1989, 1992.
124 *Pace* Fraser 1969. His is not the earliest name recorded in the story, Hillgruber 2010; Ogden 2017: 207–46.
125 Garofalo 1988. A major study of Erasistratus by Von Staden is eagerly awaited. For his ideas on the heart, Harris CRS 1973: 195–233.
126 *Art.Sang.*: 4,703–36 K; tr. Furley and Wilkie 1984: 144–83.
127 *Cons.* 1: *CMG Suppl. Or.* III,12–14 = fr. 247 Garofalo. Galen here links him with Hippocrates as "the most illustrious of doctors".
128 Nutton 2013a: 135–7.

129 Fraser 1972: 317–20, 324–5.
130 Rufus, *Parts* 10: p. 134 DR.
131 *Ibid.* 128–35: 150–1 DR.
132 Von Staden 2004: 209, notes the absence of any unequivocal evidence that places Marinus, Quintus or Satyrus in Alexandria, and is hesitant about an Alexandrian school of anatomy.
133 *Lib.Prop.* 4,9–33: pp. 147–53 BM; p. 113 tr. Singer PN.
134 *AA* 1,2: 2,224–6 K; pp. 4–5 tr. Singer C.
135 *AA* 1,2: 2,220 K; p. 3 tr. Singer C; p. 86 Garofalo.
136 Von Staden 2004: 196–206.
137 Philippus, *Hipp.Epid.II*, vi: *CMG* V 10,1, 401–2: Adada: Samama 2003: no. 338.
138 *Hipp.Epid.II*, vi: *CMG* V 10,1, 402. For other examples, Nutton 1993b: 20–1.
139 *AA* XIV,1: pp. 183–4 Dkw; p. 1041 Garofalo: *HNH* II,6: 15,136 K.
140 *Muss.Diss.* 1,1; 5,5; 19,31 K: 18B,926–7, 935, 986 K; *Adv.Jul.* 18A,246–99 K; *MM* I,7: 10,52–4 K; I, p. 85, tr. Johnston-Horsley.
141 *Hipp.Epid.VI*, iv,10: *CMG* V 10,2,2, 227.
142 *HVA* II,3,8: 15,648 K; *Ant.* I,4: 14,25 K.
143 *Hipp.Aph.* II,20: 17B,493 K.
144 *Trem.Palp.*: 7,635 K; p. 208 tr. Sider, McVaugh; Nutton 1993b; Von Staden 2004: 186–91.
145 *Hipp.Aph.* III,14: 17B,597 K; for Polyclitus, *San.Tu.* II,7,10: 6,127 K; II, p. 185 tr. Johnston (the same applies to Celts, Scythians, and Arabs).
146 Stern 1956: 94.
147 Von Staden 2004: 191–4.
148 Knowledge of mechanical planetaria, *UP* XIV,5: 4,156 K; II, p. 627 tr. May; Jones A 2017: 244–5; Dr Strohmaier kindly tells me that the unpublished commentary on *Airs, Waters, and Places* reveals much about Galen's contacts with seafarers.
149 Toomer 1985; Heilen 2018.
150 *SMT* X,19: 12,207 K; Ryholt 2011; Jouanna 2011; Van Nuffelen 2014; for bird-diviners, Deichgräber 1976.
151 Mazzini 1999.
152 Oxyrhynchus Papyri 5232, 5236–41; Marganne 1998.
153 Augustine, *City of God* XXII,8.
154 He seems to have spent some time on his way back to Pergamum visiting Palestine, Syria, Cyprus, Lycia and possibly other places, collecting information about, and specimens of, various minerals and drugs, although the chronology of his journeys is far from clear, Nutton 1973; Boudon-Millot 2012: 106–19.
155 Robert 1940 remains fundamental. Boudon-Millot 2012: 89–97; Mattern 2013: 81–97. Wörrle 2019: 484–5.
156 Dunkle 2013: 59–64.
157 *AA* I,1: 2,217–8 K; pp. 1–2 tr. Singer C.
158 Such sensational displays were often frowned upon by others, e.g. Plutarch, *Mor.* 71A; Dio Chrysostom, *Oration* 33,6, but cf. Gleason 2009.
159 *Opt.Med.Cogn.* 9,6–9: *CMG Suppl. Or.* IV, 102–5.
160 *Comp.Med.Gen.* III,2: 13,599 K.
161 Mattern 2013: 65–7.
162 Slightly different figures are given at *Comp.Med.Gen.* III,2: 13,600 K and *Opt.Med.Cogn.* 9,6: *CMG Suppl. Or.* IV, 104–5. It is not clear whether these numbers refer only to those injured in training or include those who fought at the Provincial Games.
163 *Comp.Med.Gen.* III,2: 13,564, 600 K; *Ven.Sect.Er.Rom.* 6: 11,227 K; p. 57 tr. Brain. Cf. the recently discovered mosaic of a wounded gladiator, *The Times*, October 12, 2019, p. 45.
164 *Hipp.Fract.* III,21: 18B,567–8 K, with Majno 1975: 395–404.
165 *Comp.Med.Gen.* III,2: 13,600–2 K.
166 *UP* IV,9: 4,286–7 K; I, p. 215 tr. May; *AA* III,1: 2,345 K; p. 62 tr. Singer C. His observations on the swift death of gladiators wounded in the heart (like sufferers from a heart attack) may not have been made in Pergamum, *Loc.Aff.* V,2: 8,304 K; p. 139 tr. Siegel.
167 *Alim.Fac.* I.19: 6,529 K; p. 59 tr. Powell; Curry 2008: 28–31. Note also the fragment preserved in Arabic, von Müller 1895: 475.

168 Cf. *Alim.Fac.* I,28: 6,546 K; p. 66 tr. Powell, a reminiscence from a Carian friend living in Rome of the unusual way in which certain legumes, *dolichoi*, were planted in the fields around his native Ceramos.

169 *Alim.Fac.* III,1: 6,665 K; II,17: 6,591 K; III,16: 6,697 K; pp. 116, 85, 130 tr. Powell.

170 *Alim.Fac.* I,25: 6,539 K; p. 63 tr. Powell. Cf. for other comments on their lifestyles, *SMT* X,22: 12,299 K; *Hipp.Epid.I* 1,3: 17A,210 K; *Comp.Med.Gen.* VII,11: 13,1009 K.

171 Jones CP 2012: 406–9; *Subf.Emp.* 10; p. 40 tr. Frede, "a healing spring in Mysia not far from our city", may be a reference to Allianoi.

172 Soranus, *Gynaecology* II,44.

173 Swain 1996; Gleason 2005; for Ephesus, with its flourishing medical life, Georges 2017.

2 Galen the Roman

Medicine in Rome

Why Galen decided to leave Pergamum and make his way to Rome is a matter for speculation, but for a man of such talent and ambition, as well as independent means, it was hardly surprising. Rome was now a bi-lingual city where, in Galen's own words, the population of a single block far outstripped that of any town where Hippocrates had lived.[1] The "epitome of the whole world", a description borrowed by Galen from a famous sophist from Asia Minor, had long attracted immigrants from all over the Greek world, from millionaires and regional dynasts eager to make their mark in the politics of empire to humble tradesmen and those who simply sought a better life than that of an Anatolian peasant.[2] Those who offered healing had been prominent among them for centuries, for it was no wonder that in such a mega-city illness should be common. Pliny the Elder, writing around 70 CE, had begun the section on medicine in his *Natural History* with a celebrated polemic against the "filthy Greeks" who had introduced the practice of medicine into Rome, undermining Roman self-reliance and contributing to the debilitating growth of luxury. He drew on many lurid examples of greedy and lascivious Greek doctors who cheated their patients and even got away with murder, citing Cato the Elder's warning to his son two hundred and fifty years earlier against putting his faith in doctors like this. Pliny's splendid rhetoric replicated in prose many of the jibes directed against doctors by composers of epigrams in both Greek and Latin, several of them written and circulating in Rome.[3]

Neither diatribes nor jokes had much effect, for Greek doctors continued to arrive in Rome in large numbers, particularly from Asia Minor, and found ready patients in a city far larger than their home towns and big enough for specialists of all kinds to make a good living.[4] An inscription records a young man from the region North-East of Pergamum who died in Rome, "the imperial city", just as his reputation had begun to grow.[5] The great Hippocratic Quintus taught in Rome for a long while until he was forced out, according to Galen, by the hostility of others.[6] By Galen's day, their numbers and thus the importance of Rome as a Greek medical centre had grown to such an extent that some students even came from the Greek East to Rome to study. The authors of two separate tracts preserved in the Galenic Corpus tell of the instruction they had received in the city. One of them had learned how to use the antidote called theriac against the plague from his Roman teacher, Maecius Aelianus, while the other, certainly an immigrant, reported back to his brother somewhere in the Greek world on the remarkable healing properties of the centaury as a universal panacea that he had observed while accompanying his master on his rounds in Rome.[7] Like the Syrian quack dentist who claimed to be a pupil of Galen, they came to make money, secure in the knowledge, so Galen alleged, that once in the anonymous metropolis they could get away with murder.[8] How different, he mused, from the towns of his youth, where everyone knew one another, one's family, wealth, and character were familiar to all, and the pressure of what might be termed a face-to-face society prevented medical incompetence.[9]

Thus, the Rome where Galen arrived in 162 was as much a Greek as a Latin city. Population figures are hard to estimate, and one should take with a pinch of salt the assertion of the satirist Juvenal that the dregs of the Orontes had now flowed into the Tiber, but there can be little doubt that a large percentage of the population was of Eastern origin, even if the number of Greek slaves and ex-slaves was much reduced from what it had been a hundred years earlier.[10] It was by now a Greek cultural centre to rival any of the great cities of the East. Even without Philostratus' biographies of leading sophists, one could easily surmise from Galen's writings alone that Greek philosophers and rhetoricians now flocked to Rome to give public displays and to appear, like modern film and television stars, in the salons of the wealthy. In the opening sections of his *Prognosis*, a treatise that stresses Galen's social importance as much as his medical expertise, he lists several among those who attended his cures and his demonstrations in front of intellectuals famous around the Greek world. Adrian of Tyre, the recipient of a biography from Philostratus, was honoured by the city of Ephesus, and was later the holder of an imperial sophistic chair at Athens. Demetrius of Alexandria, a pupil of Favorinus and a member of the Museum at Alexandria, delivered daily extempore orations on themes suggested by his audience, the test of a brilliant orator. Alexander, described by Galen as coming from Damascus and almost certainly the father of the more famous Alexander of Aphrodisias, was another who went on to hold a chair at Athens.[11] Galen mentions elsewhere others only a little less celebrated such as the orator Diomedes, incompetently treated by the palace doctors, although not by Galen, and Pausanias, a Syrian sophist whose treatment for damaged nerves following a chariot accident Galen cited on several occasions to illustrate the importance of anatomical knowledge in diagnosis and therapy.[12]

Many of these intellectuals were closely connected with the 'new' aristocracy in the Roman senate. Flavius Arrian, for example, the Greek historian of Alexander the Great and of Rome's Eastern Wars, was appointed a consul in Rome by the Emperor Hadrian around 130 before retiring to Athens, where Galen may have met him in his deaf old age.[13] The previous century had shown a steady increase in the number of senators coming from the Greek East, and many Westerners who had spent some time there as travellers or officials returned home with some of the entourage they had acquired. The prayers of a doctor in Cilicia for the safe journey home of his employer, a Roman governor, testifies to his own hopes for preferment as well as to his good wishes for his departing chief.[14]

This hellenisation of imperial Rome was not surprising.[15] The upper classes had long been expected to be fluent in Greek. Many of them studied in Athens, like Aulus Gellius, the Latin author of *Attic Nights*, or the epileptic boy for whom Galen prescribed a regime by letter.[16] But it was further encouraged by the example of the emperors themselves. Hadrian was a passionate Hellenophile, as his buildings in Athens, Ephesus, Pergamum and elsewhere attest to this day, and he is commended in passing by Galen for his approval of the edition of Hippocrates by Artemidorus Capito.[17] His successor but one, Marcus Aurelius, wrote his *Meditations* in excellent Greek. It was a milieu ideally suited to Galen's talents.

Rome: the first visit

When he arrived in Rome in 162, he was no lonely pauper, struggling for a living: he was already among friends. He names two in particular, Teuthras, a fellow student from home with an interest in pharmaceuticals, who commissioned copies of several tracts by Galen, and the Aristotelian philosopher Eudemus, who had been living there for the past ten years.[18] Galen calls him his teacher, although whether this means that Eudemus was the otherwise unnamed pupil of Aspasius who had taught him in Pergamum is unclear.[19] Galen certainly was known to him primarily as a philosopher, for when Eudemus fell ill in winter 162, he was surprised to find that Galen was also an experienced physician. This case was crucial to Galen's success in Rome, for it brought him immediately into contact with the circle around the emperors. It included two prefects of the city, Sergius Paulus and Aufidius Victorinus, Vettulenus Barbarus, the uncle of the emperor Lucius Verus, and Claudius Severus, later the husband of Annia Faustina, the daughter of Marcus Aurelius.[20]

Particularly enthusiastic was a senator from Ptolemais in Syria, Flavius Boethus, who after hearing Galen lecturing in public on anatomy, persuaded him to give a demonstration in front of his friends as well as other philosophers and physicians.[21] These displays proved a great success, despite the criticisms of others, such as Martialius, the most influential student of anatomy among the Erasistratean doctors in Rome, and the Aristotelian philosopher, Alexander of Damascus.[22] Indeed, Boethus insisted that Galen should write up his lectures in a form that he could take with him when he became governor of Syria, a posting cut short by his death. They formed the basis for Galen's most extensive survey of anatomy, *Anatomical Procedures*, and for two other large-scale expositions, *The Use of Parts*, explaining the significance of anatomy for Aristotelians, and *The Opinions of Hippocrates and Plato*, which did the same for Platonists.[23]

Anatomy had become fashionable in Rome in the previous decade. Martialius had made his reputation thereby, but the leading anatomist was Lycus of Macedon, another pupil of Quintus, whose career resembled that of Galen perhaps too closely for comfort. Lycus, who died shortly before Galen's first visit, was also a Hippocratic – Galen devotes a whole treatise to discussing Lycus' (in his own view misguided) explanation of a single *Aphorism* – who had continued the work of Marinus.[24] Despite his assertion that Lycus' high reputation in Rome was not shared by experts in the Greek world, Galen was certainly impressed enough by his nineteen-book survey of anatomy to produce his own summary of it in two books.[25] He praised Lycus as an expert dissector who had also included accounts of discoveries made by his contemporaries, even while accusing him of major mistakes.[26] Lycus' investigations went beyond those of Marinus in paying greater attention to the nervous system and, in particular, to embryology. He devoted one book to a description of the uterus and a second to its condition after the death of the foetus, perhaps the report of a post-mortem dissection. Two more dealt with the anatomy of the foetus itself, one in life and one after death. Whether any based on human dissection is not clear, but this section of his work would appear to be have been far more extensive that anything in this area in Galen or, for that matter, in the works of the gynaecologist Soranus of Ephesus, who, according to Galen, regarded a knowledge of anatomy as no more than polite learning.[27]

Galen's initial demonstrations in Rome, like those of Lycus, were public displays, spectacular and shocking at the same time. A Caesarean operation on a goat was

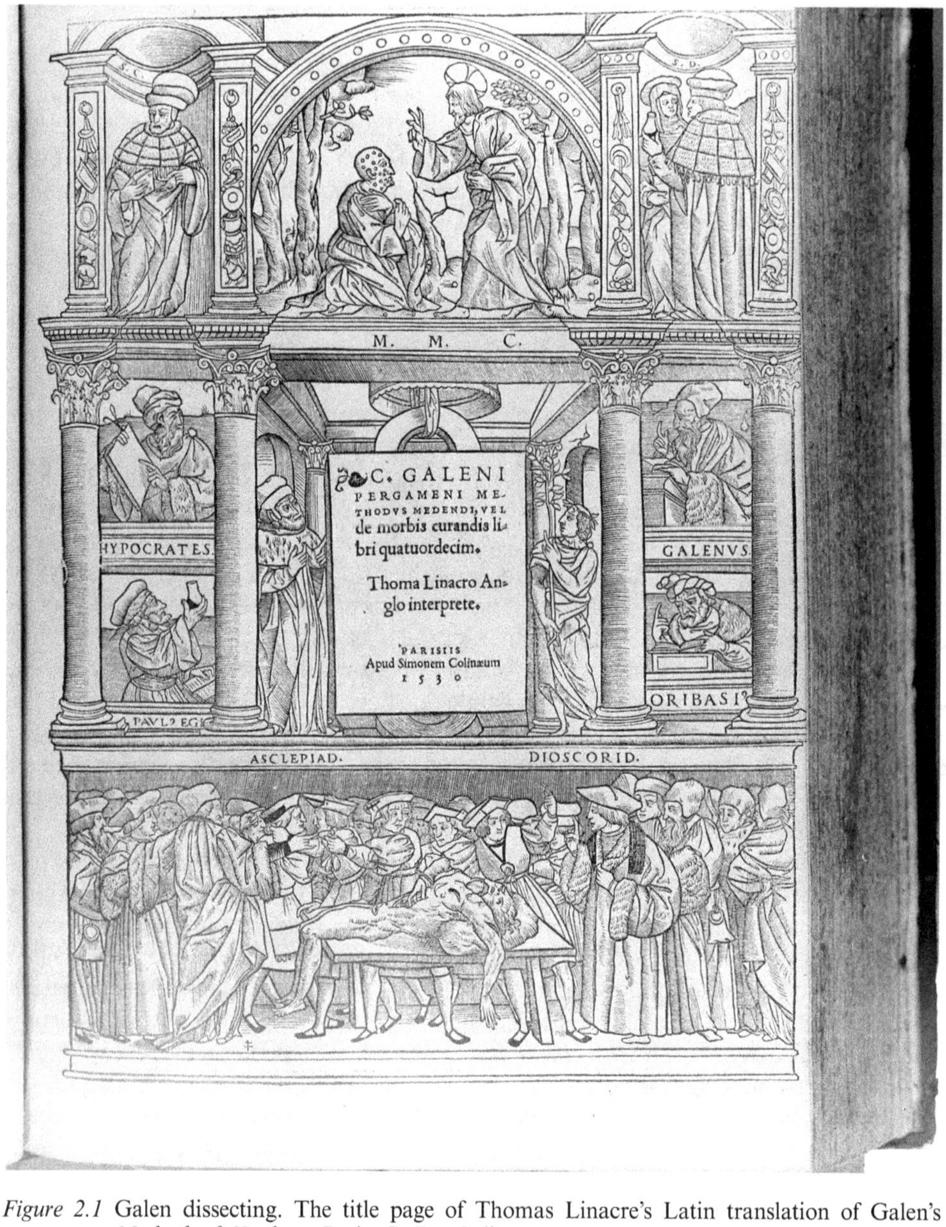

Figure 2.1 Galen dissecting. The title page of Thomas Linacre's Latin translation of Galen's *Method of Healing*, Paris, S. De Colines, 1530. The same plate was reused more appropriately in 1531 as the title page of Johann Guinther's translation of *Anatomical Procedures*, the standard renaissance version of Galen's major anatomical treatise.

cheered when the young kid stood up, fell down, and then stood again to shake off any amniotic fluid.[28] Galen was joined in his examination of the heart of elephant by many other doctors in Rome, eager to see whether Galen was right in claiming that its heart had the same structure as in other animals that take in air.[29] But not everything was so simple. The expression on the face of a monkey as the knife went in was so horrible that Galen recommended that it be turned away from the audience, or a pig used instead.[30] These performances attracted large crowds, eager as much to hear the arguments as to see, if possible, what was being dissected. It was a competition, perhaps somewhat less decorous that those that were taking place at this period within the Museum of Ephesus.[31] One doctor might challenge another to show his skill, bets might even be laid on the result, and it was not only the naive who might be impressed by flashy instruments or fluent patter.[32] Galen's oratorical skills were well suited to this competitive environment.

Medicine in Antiquity was always a public art. Friends might cluster round the bed of the sick in numbers, or a physician arrive in the sick room with an entourage of students and supporters, some even picked up on his way there. In the competition for patients, victory might be gained by a spectacular cure and by discomfiting one's rivals. The significance of Galen's cure of Eudemus lay not only in introducing him into the highest circles of Roman society, but also in his triumph over Antigenes, another pupil of Quintus as well as of Marinus, who was regarded as the best doctor in Rome and who had the most important men in the city as his patients.[33] On another occasion, many years later, Galen laid a trap for his colleague in the palace, Statilius Attalus, who had confidently predicted the recovery of his patient Theagenes the Cynic and had, furthermore, disregarded Galen's advice on appropriate treatment. He allowed Attalus and his friends to arrive almost at the bedroom door still confident of success before they heard the wailing of the mourners around the corpse.[34] The substantial amount of space Galen devotes to this case in the *Method of Healing* says at least as much about his combative nature as about the medical principles involved.

Attalus, a scion of a medical family from Heraclea in Caria and a descendant of a doctor to the emperor Trajan, was a member of the sect of Methodist doctors, one of the three main groupings described by Galen in his own introductory text, *Sects.*[35] Founded in the first century BCE by Themison of Laodicea, it had become by the 150s the most widespread and successful medical grouping.[36] Originally developed in Rome, where its relatively simplistic tenets suited a busy metropolis, it spread around the Roman world, including to Alexandria. Unlike the Empiricists, its adherents believed strongly in first identifying and then removing the cause of any ailment, something which they thought relatively simple. Instead of needing to know the complex humoral balance of the individual patient, the Methodist doctor was taught to proceed on the basis of so-called generalities. Illness depended on an imbalance within the human body between its atoms and its pores, leading to constriction (as in constipation and tumours), fluidity (as in diarrhoea or nose bleeds) or some intermediate state. Simple deduction from the observation of the patient before him would allow the doctor to decide which category applied to the patient, which would in turn easily suggest the treatment necessary to reverse the condition. Careful monitoring of the recovery would permit the treatment to be modified, should it seem necessary. Methodist surgery, about which much less is known, depended similarly on a brief series of surgical generalities. This was a medical system that, in contrast to Galen's prolonged education, some Methodists believed could be learned in a matter of weeks. Such a broad-brush approach to the patient, even if the resulting therapy was very similar to his own, was anathema to Galen, for whom an understanding of the multiplicity of factors that made up the individual condition lay at the very foundation of true medicine. He regarded their rules for treatment, especially the so-called *diatritos*, periods of alternate days given over to fasting, as over-simplistic, and he did not hesitate to feed or bathe a feverish patient at any time, should he think that the patient's individual make-up demanded it.[37]

How far his constant polemic against an apparent multitude of Methodist adversaries reflects the actual situation is not easy to determine. Although he asserts at one point that Hippocratic medicine in Rome was very much a minority preference, it is difficult to reconstruct from his writings what Methodists actually did and thought.[38] He mentions very few Methodist contemporaries by name, although there can be little doubt that some, like Attalus, or the anonymous Methodist who came with Annia Faustina to see the young prince Commodus, were also employed by the emperor and his court, who, perhaps wisely, wished to have a wide range of advice at hand to choose from. There is even a Methodist pharmacological tract, *The Properties of the Centaury*, preserved within the Galenic Corpus. Written by a Greek doctor in Rome, it begins with a quotation from "the famous teacher Themison".[39] But the greatest obstacle to understanding second-century Methodism is that Galen's arguments about Methodist theory are directed largely against Thessalus of Tralles, a flamboyant physician of the age of Nero a century earlier. The opening two books of the *Method of Healing*, written in the 170s, are filled with criticisms of the "Thessalian asses", and of their failure to develop a consistent terminology for ailments and illnesses.[40] Galen may be correct in his analysis of the views of Thessalus himself, but he is also aware that some Methodists, notably Soranus of Ephesus, fifty years later, had modified some of his ideas, although he does not explain how. His attack on all these "unmethodical" Methodists, splendid in its vituperation, is convincing only if one accepts Galen's starting point. To a Methodist his demand for a precise terminology, with its distinction between ailment, condition, illness and the like, was irrelevant to actual treatment, and his complaint about the *diatritos* overlooked the fact that a careful attention to any changes over this short period would also allow a modification of the actual therapy.[41] Galen's insistence on the need to first identify the cause within the individual patient and to concentrate on removing the cause rather than merely the symptoms was in its own way as dogmatic as anything the Methodists proposed.

Galen's first period in Rome, as he described it in the first part of *Prognosis*, was a triumph. He obtained wealthy patients, and enough money to buy a property on the bay of Naples, the summer retreat of leading Romans.[42] However, his abrasive manner and his readiness always to proclaim the merits of Galen did not endear him to his competitors. Their objections to the conclusions he drew from his anatomical discoveries led him to abandon dissecting in public, although he seems to have continued to do so in private for his friends. In late 166 he slipped away, first to Campania and then back home, citing the example of the great Quintus, similarly driven out of Rome by envious opponents, and that of a young man of brilliance who had been poisoned a decade earlier.[43] He had been warned by Eudemus about this inevitable hostility and decided to sell up and go, even though he was on the point of being appointed one of the emperors' doctors.[44] His return home to Pergamum, he claims, was also facilitated by the ending there of what he called a *stasis*, a word used to indicate some civic conflict rather than any external war.[45] There may have been other reasons. At the end of his life, in *My Own Books*, he said that his departure coincided with an outbreak of plague, and, in *Avoiding Distress*, another late work, he recalls the near total loss of his slaves in Rome "during a major attack of the prolonged plague".[46] This may well have played its part in his decision to leave, but the rhetorical trope of the man of genius driven out by vicious and ignorant enemies fits the image that Galen wished to establish in *Prognosis* of an outsider struggling against the hostility of his competitors.

From failure to success

Of the next two years he merely says that he did his "usual things".[47] Apart from a reminiscence of travelling back from Corinth to Athens in the company of an irascible Cretan who nearly murdered his servant for not obeying his orders quickly enough, he is frustratingly imprecise.[48] His trip to Lycia and Cyprus in search of mineral drugs, the latter facilitated by an imperial procurator, may belong to this period but both could equally well have been visited on his return from Alexandria, when he toured Palestine in search of bitumen and swam in the Dead Sea.[49] He implies also that he spent time revising some of his earlier writings, but whether this was on the basis of copies left earlier in Pergamum or brought back from Rome is also unclear. This un-Galenic reticence may, indeed, suggest that he felt that this interlude was a comedown after his Roman triumphs, and contrasts with the detail he then gives for the succeeding eighteen months.[50]

In late 168 he received a summons from the emperors to join them on campaign against the Germanic tribes who had crossed the Danube to invade the Roman Empire. He made his way across the North Aegean, sailing from Alexandria Troas at the mouth of the Hellespont on a boat bound for Thessalonica. He claims to have persuaded the captain to put in at Myrina, a port on the island of Lemnos, to see if he could obtain supplies of the famous Lemnian earth, celebrated as an antidote to plague and poison.[51] Unfortunately, once he disembarked, he found that the harbour that he required, Hephaestias, and the famous tomb of Philoctetes were on the other side of the island, and the captain had no time to wait, so he had to continue his journey.[52] When he arrived in camp at Aquileia in North-East Italy preparations were being made for the spring offensive of 169, but they had to be aborted when one of the emperors, Lucius Verus, died suddenly. A contemporary account, not by Galen, indicates that he suffered a stroke or a heart attack rather than succumbing to plague, whose outbreak there coincided with Galen's arrival.[53] Marcus Aurelius hurried to Rome for the state funeral, leaving Galen and some of the army to follow, and it was not until mid-169 that Galen again reached Rome, which was to become the centre of his professional life for almost half a century. Some twenty-four years later, he remarked that he regarded his time at court with indifference, for he had been forced into it by Fate, and had originally refused the honour several times, a tactful comment that served to distance Galen from any involvement in the murderous activities of the Emperor Commodus.[54]

During the summer he cured one of the emperor's close friends, Sextus Quintilius Condianus, but when Marcus Aurelius asked him to accompany him in his renewed campaign, he demurred, citing the intervention of the god Asclepius who had appeared to him in a dream. His description of the emperor as a good, kind man reveals a certain relief at his acquiescence in the divine command, accepted in part because the campaign was expected to be short.[55] In the event the emperor did not return until late 176, appointing Galen at long distance to be in charge of the preparation of his theriac following the death of Demetrius, the doctor who had previously exercised that role. Marcus had used the drug as a daily tonic and to help him sleep as well as to retain his humoral equilibrium, but there is no evidence that, as some have suggested, he had become addicted to this drug, which contained a small quantity of opium.[56] Elsewhere Galen praised his generally healthy lifestyle, involving regular keep-fit sessions.[57] It was either in the few months preceding Marcus' return North or in the similarly brief period between his return in 176 and the composition of *Prognosis* that Galen treated him for colic with such success that the emperor was moved to declare him the first among doctors and unique among philosophers.[58] (*Fig. 1.2*) This neat appreciation, words put by Galen into the mouth of the emperor, sums up Galen's view of his own achievements.

A crucial role in Galen's relations with the emperor was played by two imperial secretaries, Euphates and Peitholaus. The former conveyed to him the responsibility for the emperor's theriac, the latter kept the emperor informed about Condianus, and arranged for Galen to look after the young prince Commodus while he was in the city and at other palaces in Latium.[59]. Although he gives the impression of an obvious superiority, it is clear that Galen was only one of several court physicians, not all of whom shared his beliefs.[60] Even if, like the author of *Theriac, for Piso*, they too served for decades, this does not mean that they always co-operated harmoniously: Galen complains that Annia Faustina's acid comments on his treatment of Commodus for tonsillitis, "Galen is battling you with deeds, not just words", only added to the hostility felt by other doctors towards him.[61]

Worse was to follow; after the death of Marcus Aurelius in 180, the new emperor Commodus began a reign of terror.[62] Friends of Galen, like Condianus and Victorinus, disappeared or were killed, and those who survived lived in constant fear. The praetorian prefect Perennis was put to death in 185 after his slaves had been tortured to betray him.[63] Many of them refused, setting an example used by Galen in his *Character Traits* to show that virtues like courage did not depend on education or status. Galen planned to leave his home in the centre of Rome for his villa at Stabiae, Castellammare on the Bay of Naples, and to have copies of all his writings specially produced and sent there to form a second library.[64] But before he could send more than a few volumes disaster struck. In early 192 a great fire broke out in Rome which destroyed, among many other buildings, the supposedly fireproof stores near the Palatine in which he, like other wealthy citizens, had kept his notebooks, his instruments, some of which he had designed himself, his gold and silver, and all his financial documents.[65]

For the previous twenty years or more Galen had spent his time when not practising medicine in producing both new texts and revisions of others, like his early anatomical treatises and many texts for students. All were now destroyed, along with his precious dictionary of Attic comedy. Even worse, the imperial libraries had also been burnt, so that it was no longer possible to replace his lost copies of unique texts, like those of Aristotle and the naturalist Theophrastus, that he had been able to consult there.[66] All he could do was to hope that friends of his outside Rome had retained copies that they could in turn recopy for him, and in future make sure that he had duplicates at Stabiae or with friends, whom he encouraged to deposit copies in such local libraries as the library of Celsus at Ephesus or in the small library at Nysa several miles inland.[67] He did not always succeed immediately. He still had not retrieved a copy of *Prognosis* several years later, although one was eventually found.[68] Other books, like his *Properties of Simples*, he expanded from two to eleven books in a revision. The events of 192 were indeed disastrous, but his relatively equanimous reaction resulted in a request

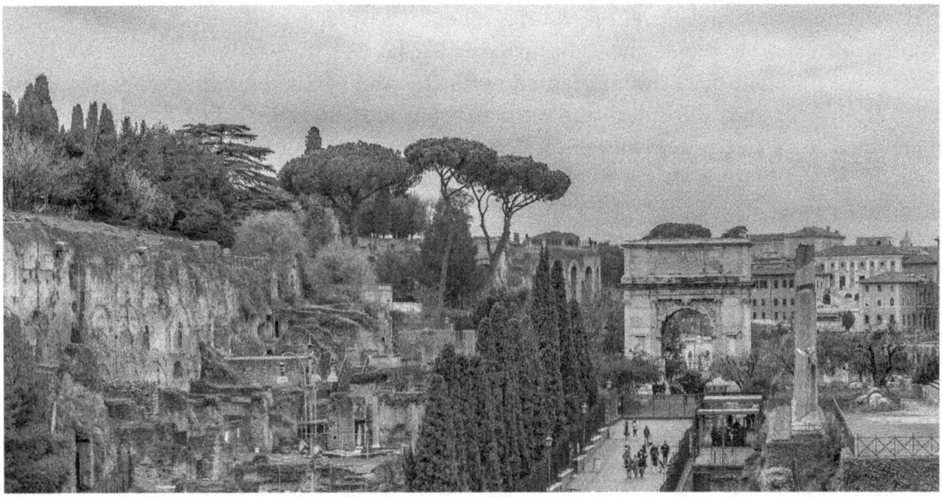

Figure 2.2 The Via Sacra in Rome, looking towards the Forum. The Palatine libraries, on the hill to the left, were destroyed in the great fire of 192, along with Galen's books and valuables stored in one of the repositories further back along the road.

from an old schoolmate for a treatise that would explain how one might follow his example and avoid distress. His somewhat banal response, that one should live each day expecting the worst of calamities, so that one would not be depressed when lesser evils occurred, can be found in other moralists, but also conceals the fact that for a while after the fire, as he tells us elsewhere, he was unable even to open a book.[69]

But the bloodthirsty Commodus did not have much longer to live. Galen, who was in Rome when his successor emperor Pertinax took power in 193, wrote up his reminiscences of "public pronouncements" in his brief reign, which, had it survived, would be a fascinating work for today's historians.[70] He continued in office under the next emperor, Septimius Severus, for whom he once more provided a new supply of theriac, which had fallen out of fashion with the death of Marcus Aurelius. Galen was pleased to be able to rescue for one of its ingredients a cinnamon bush that had languished for decades in one of the royal storehouses on the Capitoline.[71] *Antidotes*, which records this find, was not his last book, for his accounts of his own writings, *My own Books*, and of his major medico-philosophical beliefs, *My own Opinions*, were certainly later, and they cast strong doubt on the tradition, preserved in a Byzantine Greek dictionary, the *Souda*, that he had died aged seventy, i.e. around 199, a date which would also leave little time for him to collect again and sometimes rewrite all the books he had lost in the fire but which are now extant. Byzantine chronographers moreover place his death under Emperor Caracalla, reigned 211–217, which would also fit with the date given in Arabic sources, who have him dying aged 87, i.e. around 216, after seventeen years as a student, and seventy as a physician.[72] This formulation may derive from a comment attributed to Alexander of Aphrodisias that Galen had spent seventy years before coming to the conclusion that he knew nothing, a possible dig at Galen's confession of agnosticism on many philosophical themes that opens *My Own Opinions*, but such polemical statements from late and often fanciful biographers, however intriguing, are to be regarded with scepticism.[73]

Even more unreliable are the stories about the place of Galen's death, which, according to Arabic biographers, occurred while he was on a pilgrimage to the Holy Land. Two different places were pointed out as the site of his tomb, one in Sicily, a few miles from Palermo, the other at Perama, a harbour in Egypt. The latter might be interpreted as a mis-transcription of Pergamum, but none of these locations can be trusted, especially since they are often mentioned in the obviously fictional context of a hunt for drugs in Upper Egypt or a Christian pilgrimage[74] (*Fig*. 3.2).

Galen spent the greater part of his life in and around Rome. He returned at least once more to Pergamum, perhaps in the late 170s or 180s, when he stopped off at Lemnos and at last obtained a large quantity of the Lemnian seals that he had searched for earlier.[75] This may also have been the occasion when he regained much of his personal library, for his later Hippocratic commentaries display a much greater attention to previous scholarship than the earlier ones.[76] Like several of his colleagues at court, he maintained his links with his native city, replying by letter to friends' queries about their health or about his own situation.[77] The advantages of being close to the centre of power, and the wealth and prestige it brought him, easily outweighed any nostalgic pull to return to the life of a provincial doctor.[78]

A Greek view of Rome

What we do have from Galen is a kaleidoscope of impressions of and reactions to life in Rome that are scattered across his writings and together provide a view of how the city appeared to one, admittedly unusual, provincial. However, his coruscating rhetoric often makes it difficult to assess the truth of many of his observations. His treatise on *Examining the Physician*, written around 176–7, begins with a long lament about modern life, dominated by luxury and a disdain for learning. The rich base their choice of their doctors more on fashion than on merit, making them easy prey for charlatans who hunt them down like beasts. Even when they do show an interest in matters intellectual, they prefer studying the useless traditions of the past and dubious chronicles or amusing themselves with etymologising and investigating the most archaic words to the harder tasks of medicine and philosophy.[79] Similar complaints are made in *Prognosis*, written at around the same time and with a more specific focus on the Rome of a decade or more earlier.[80] In it Galen puts many of his criticisms of life in Rome into the mouths of others, notably Eudemus, a neat rhetorical device that ostensibly transfers his views to someone more experienced and more objective.[81] How far this reflects the situation in which he found himself either in 162 or in 176 is impossible to say, although his dislike for the daily *salutatio*, the obligation to pay a morning call on one's patron and social superior, may well reflect the annoyance of a rich citizen from a wealthy and important city at being placed on the same level as humbler tradesmen.[82] But this was a status-conscious society, in which even the act of writing was part of an elite culture of mutual obligation, for Galen insists often that this or that treatise was written in response to a request by a friend, and, in turn, that he expects them to pass it on to others.[83]

Galen's perspective on Rome and Italy comes from within, and is relayed to, a largely Greek community. Most of the persons he mentions are either associated with the Hellenophile court or come from the Greek East, and their words are reported in Greek. His cultural horizon remains resolutely Greek. He cites just one writer familiar today as a Latin author, Scribonius Largus, a doctor with close connections to the court of the emperor Claudius and the author of a drug handbook written in Latin around 48 CE.[84] But, as Alessia Guardasole has shown, Galen is very unlikely to have read it in Latin, for the recipes ascribed to Scribonius seem to be copied at second hand from two earlier drug-books in Greek by two of Scribonius' near contemporaries, Asclepiades the Pharmacist and Andromachus the younger.[85] Whether they translated them themselves or took them from another book written by Scribonius in Greek, for he may well have been bi-lingual, cannot, of course, be known.

Although, like many members of his social class, Galen will have studied Latin, he shows no obvious Latinisms in his Greek style or his vocabulary.[86] A word like λάκκος, 'basin', a phonetic rendering of the Latin *lacus*, had already entered Greek before Galen's time, and as a partly technical term had simply been transliterated.[87] The same may be true of such words as *cestiana, sapo, foliata* and *spicata, decocta* and *candidum*.[88] But it is very unlikely that he communicated only in Greek or through an interpreter with his many patients – he talks of treating four hundred sufferers from fever in a single summer, and he declares that the Galenic lover of truth can disregard the quibbling objections of sophists if he has seen thousands of patients with the same condition, as Galen implies he himself has done.[89] Given the limitations of ancient education, the slaves, women and children whom he treated, and the midwives he helped, would not all have been fluent in Greek, and if the peasants whom he mentions coming to see him from the countryside were Italian, they would hardly describe their symptoms in elegant Greek. Indeed, at one point, he advises his readers, when in Rome, to use 'cerebrum', the Latin word for 'brain', instead of its Greek equivalent, for greater clarity and intelligibility.[90] Not every patient referred to him by local practitioners after suffering dislocations and sprains in the gymnasiums in Rome and at the port city of Ostia would have had Greek, and he is unlikely to have always used only Greek when interviewing boxers and wrestlers about their speed of digestion.[91] It would undoubtedly have been possible, as it is today in a big city, for an immigrant practitioner to have lived his life largely within his own linguistic community, but Galen had larger pretensions and his patients came from a much broader range of backgrounds. Besides, he had a wide-ranging curiosity. A recently discovered passage from his treatise on simples contains a fascinating discussion of the (obsolete) Greek digamma and its relationship to the pronunciation of 'v' in Latin names like Valerius and Severus that implies that he had a more than passing knowledge of Latin.[92]

At times Galen's view of Rome chimes with the complaints of satirists like Juvenal or Lucilius. Sex, gossip, gambling, and booze fill the lives of the wealthy. Cultivated after-dinner discussion and playing the lyre or cithara have been replaced by drinking competitions. Doctors grow rich on flattery, a far cry from the days when they ruled the sick in the same way as generals command armies.[93] He describes with a mixture of glee and revulsion a man who became so drunk at a banquet that he had to be led home staggering all over the road.[94] The unfortunate doctor must accede to the demands of wealthy women unable to bear even the slightest pain, who insist on dressings being made with the softest of Tyrian wool, and refuse a purgative to remove bile.[95] Unlike the peasant women around Pergamum, they flee at the smell of a hair dye including oil and pitch.[96] They demand that Galen should write about beauty treatments, not understanding the difference between the job of a beautician and that of a doctor.[97] Rich men are scarcely better, fobbing off friends in need with the excuse of important business, having their hair done or pampering and prettifying their bodies.[98]

They are frightened off venesection by the words of their servants and prefer their swellings to be treated with warm oil and poultices, which only make things worse, rather than submit to painful bleeding.[99] Some have even died as a result of the large amount of painkillers they took, while others paid hugely for small and useless massages instead of facing up to the knife.[100] But, at the same time, Galen does not shrink from giving advice on how to add expensive, sweet-smelling but entirely useless ingredients to a drug in order to boost its price, for, in his view, the rich would turn their noses up at one that was inexpensive, unable to believe that something so cheap could be effective.[101] They parade the streets with their asses, offering them for mating, and prefer frivolities to sober learning, a prey to the latest fashions in hairstyles.[102] They have eyes only for money-making, falling into despair if they lose even a small fraction of their enormous wealth. When he once asked a billionaire why he didn't share some of it with others or even enjoy it, he was brusquely told that one ought to look after one's money just as carefully as one looked after one's body. Galen was so annoyed at this response that he went off and immediately dictated a treatise on the theme of plutocrats and the love of money. He sent a copy to a friend from Pergamum, but, alas, it has not survived.[103]

The hostility, stubbornness, and ignorance of many of those he meets in Rome is a constant theme. Patients and their carers disregard his instructions, while their doctors take umbrage at any suggestion from Galen.[104] Even when they claim to be following Galen, they misunderstand what he has so carefully said. An egregious example of this incomprehension can be found in a series of treatises on venesection.[105] When he first came to Rome, he was opposed for his views on bloodletting by many of his competitors. The followers of the Hellenistic physician Erasistratus favoured, as an alternative to venesection, starving the patient and using a kind of tourniquet to prevent any influx of blood into the affected part. Galen's first assault on their views was delivered to an audience of philosophers when he argued that the use of bleeding was of long standing and widely practised. It went back to Hippocrates and other great names of the past and was easily justified by comparing the health of women who menstruate with that of sufferers from amenorrhea or the elderly. Besides, in his view, it was far less dangerous than the remedies advocated by the Erasistrateans themselves and could be performed with more precision than the administration of powerful evacuants, another of their alternative therapies.[106] On the right patients, in the right circumstances, and with appropriate safeguards it was foolish not to take advantage of bleeding. The failure of Erasistratean doctors to bleed a twenty-one-year old with a cough and apnoea, even when its benefits were obvious to the non-medics at the bedside, was a clear demonstration of their stupidity.[107]

In the debates that followed in Rome the Erasistrateans at first persisted in citing chapter and verse from the writings of Erasistratus, much to the annoyance of Galen's friend Teuthras, who sent a slave to copy down from Galen's own lips what he had earlier said, so that he could have the information with him when he returned to Asia Minor. But details of this transcript soon leaked out, and once it was widely circulated, readers found its arguments so compelling that, Galen claims, many of the leading Erasistrateans changed their views completely, espousing venesection with the same inordinate zeal they had shown in opposing it.[108] They attempted to justify Erasistratus' silence about it on the grounds that it was such a universally accepted procedure that its employment could be taken for granted, even if it was not specifically mentioned.[109] Galen's response to this volte-face was to show by a careful exposition of the texts of Erasistratus that he had never carried out any venesection, and then to emphasise the limits within which it should be performed.[110] Many years later Galen returned to the subject of when, how and in what circumstances to let blood, this time presenting a rather less combative account, although it still contains a vigorous set-piece contrasting Galen's careful cure of a young steward on a country estate with the failure of his Erasistratean physicians to let blood.[111] The response of the rich owner when greeted by the recovered slave after only two days, was to seek from Galen an explanation for this miracle cure, which he, of course, was only too delighted to provide.

Such public confrontations between doctors were not, of course, unique to Rome, but a regular occurrence in a society that lacked any effective control over medical practice. How best to choose a physician may have been a particularly acute problem in Rome itself simply because of the enormous range of choice available. Galen's solution, propounded in *Examining the Physician*, was to provide the patient with the questions he should put to any potential practitioner before engaging him, a wonderfully optimistic proposal that reflects the wealthy, literate and leisured clientele at which he aimed.[112] But, equally, he never shrank from arguments in public spaces such as the Forum or the Temple of Peace, where Rome's intellectuals often congregated. It may have been here that he encountered the centenarian teacher, Telephus, the slightly younger physician Antiochus, still walking around the city to see his patients at over eighty, and the mime-writer Marullus, the owner of a slave whose cure by excision of a suppurating breastbone Galen regarded as one of his greatest triumphs.[113]

Friends and patients like these were rich and well-connected, and his association with them would have enhanced his reputation. About his finances we know nothing specific, but they must have been considerable. He mentions only one monetary payment he received, 400 gold pieces, as a present from Boethus for curing his wife, but he would also have been paid for his attendance at the imperial court.[114] This might have brought in some 200,000 *sestertii* a year, the sum posited for the salary of the contemporary imperial doctor Gellius Maximus, which was equivalent to that of a minor provincial governor.[115] Imperial service, it is also clear, did not preclude him from seeing other patients. He will, presumably, have also continued to derive some income from his family estates around Pergamum, whether they were managed by another family member or by a bailiff acting for their absent owner. Galen may not have been a billionaire like Herodes Atticus or some of his fellow Pergamenes, but not everyone would have agreed with his self-description as a man of only "moderate wealth". The feeble attempt he makes to refute the charge that he had achieved what he did because of his family wealth suggests a certain embarrassment at least.[116] His boast elsewhere that he provided books, instruments and money to his fellow professionals in need, and, if necessary, waived any fee from his poorer patients is a further indication that he did not lack for funds.[117] Several of his treatises are subtitled 'for beginners', but any suggestion that he took pupils, and still more, that they paid him, founders on the ambiguities of some of the Greek terms he used.[118] The same word *hetairos* can be used to mean a pupil or a friend, while the injunction he gave to his *hetairoi* to watch carefully his dissection could apply equally well to students and to those interested senators and intellectuals who were often in attendance. The doctor Glaucon, who was taken along by Galen to see the case of Theagenes, and to whom Galen dedicated his shorter *Method of Healing* and much else, straddles both categories.[119] Curiously, the only person whom he mentions specifically as claiming to have been taught by him was a Syrian quack dentist, whose pretensions depended on the widespread assumption that a leading physician would take pupils who would accompany him on his rounds.[120]

It is not just the varied inhabitants of Rome who emerge from Galen's writings. The recently discovered *Avoiding Distress* provides remarkable new information about Roman libraries and their contents, including the imperial collections on the Palatine and those at the Temple of Peace and at the House of Tiberius.[121] The destruction of the imperial libraries he regarded as the single biggest disaster occasioned by the great fire of 192. Not only had they contained extremely rare material but also copies of common works that were of special merit for their beauty, accuracy or association with famous scribes, scholars and owners. They included the (allegedly) autograph copy of the editions of Homer by the Alexandrian critic, Aristarchus (c. 216–144 BCE) and a copy of the works of Plato brought to Rome around 145 BCE by the Stoic philosopher Panaetius of Rhodes, as well as autographs by other famous scholars, doctors, and philosophers. In his own researches in the Palatine libraries he had discovered some books not described in the so-called *Catalogues* and others that were clearly not the work of the author whose name they bore. They included writings by Aristotle and rare books on science by Theophrastus, alongside his two big treatises on plants that were "familiar to everyone".[122] The riches of these Roman libraries had delighted Galen, eager to have his own copies made as exactly as possible, down to the last jot and tittle. They also allowed him to exercise his ever-enquiring mind as well as the scholarly discrimination that enabled him, on grounds of style and content, to distinguish between genuine works and those circulating pseudonymously.[123]

But the presence of books and libraries was not only thing that made Rome so attractive to Galen. It lay at the centre of a vast Empire that stretched from Scotland to the Sahara, and from the stormy shores of the Bay of Biscay to the stony desert of Syria. News of Galen's successes brought him letters asking for help from Gaul and Spain in the West (or, less likely, on another translation, from Iberia and Galatia in modern Turkey) and Asia Minor and Thrace in the East.[124] However, he shows little knowledge of or interest in the world beyond the Alps. He mentions Spain for its excellent fish, especially tuna, its prunes, its tarts, and "a little animal that resembles a hare and which they call a rabbit".[125] His description of the Germans bathing their new-born offspring in cold water to toughen them up could come from a literary source, and his comments on their constitution and their hair colour are simply extensions of Hippocratic climatology.[126] Apart from a recipe involving dock collected by Axius, a doctor in the British fleet, the ingredients of his compound remedies come from Italy or, overwhelmingly, from the Eastern Mediterranean and further East.[127]

As a royal doctor, he was at the centre of a whole network of information. He knew where in Rome to find the best thin cord for suturing, that brought from Gaul and sold cheaply in the stores on the Via Sacra between the Temple of Rome and the Forum; and he expected his friend Glaucon to have observed the Marsi, peasants from the Apennine mountains, at work in the city slicing up vipers for use in the treatment of consumption and presumably also making up their own antidotes.[128] He waxed lyrical about the opportunities that living in Rome brought in obtaining substances from all over the world, from Syria, Palestine, Egypt, Cappadocia, Pontus, Macedonia, from Gaul and Spain in the West and from the land of the

Moors in the South.[129] Still more were native to Italy, or were imports processed in Italy such as copper at Pozzuoli on the bay of Naples or litharge (lead monoxide) in Rome itself.[130] Some were available all the year round, others came only in summer from places like Sicily and Libya. Galen himself was also able to rely on travelling friends as well as on officials, and even provincial governors, to ensure that he was provided with the best quality products. He had access to the botanical riches of the island of Crete, a veritable garden of Eden where the emperor kept a staff of plant gatherers. These experts collected the many medicinal plants and packed them in wicker baskets for the voyage to Italy, where they were made available to the general public. Indeed, so prolific was the island in medicinal herbs that there was little need for its inhabitants to resort to adulteration, as was the case with substances from elsewhere.[131] The perfumiers of Rome were taught how to recognise adulterated substances when they made their annual bids for these baskets, as well as to distinguish those plants that were in prime condition from those liable to rot quickly, even if, unlike Galen, they could not recognise useful herbs growing just outside the city walls.[132] Others were less scrupulous, improving the appearance of their merchandise by stuffing the stems with substances that would soon rot and decay. But at least in Rome one had the opportunity to see these cheats at work and take precautions against them. Similar deceits were also practised by sellers of honey purported to be scented with thyme.[133] As an imperial doctor Galen had access to the best quality ingredients, including plants which were kept in a storehouse on the Capitoline. It was there that he came across a cinnamon bush that had been lying neglected for years after theriac, for which it was a main ingredient, fell out of fashion under Commodus. It may also have been through his Roman connections that he was able to visit the imperial mines of Cyprus with the permission of the local procurator and bring back a store of rare minerals.[134]

Profiting directly from his status, Galen took full advantage of what Rome and its empire had to offer. His view of the Roman emperors is positive, save for Commodus and one critical anecdote about Hadrian who damaged the eye of a servant when he struck him with a pencil. Asked by the penitent monarch what he would want in recompense, the man replied, "Only an eye".[135] In a memorable simile, Galen went so far as to compare the achievements of Hippocrates and himself with the road-building programme of the emperor Trajan (ruled 98–117). He had driven paved roads across mountains and marshes, levelled hills and valleys, bridged rivers, cleared forests and thickets, and protected travellers from dangerous beasts by creating a flourishing network of highways. This is praise indeed, but in an unusual context, that of self-praise: Galen had done likewise in his *Method of Healing*, marking out "the entire road to healing …., a project which needed great care to bring to fulfilment". The pathway cut by "the ancients" which had become muddy and strewn with rocks, infested with thorns, laboriously steep, frequented by wild animals, and at times impassable because of collapsed bridges, Galen had now repaired, making things clear, going straight to the point, and sweeping away entirely any errors and misconceptions.[136]

Not surprisingly, his attitude towards Rome evolved in many ways over time, as can be seen in the difference between the two parts of the *Method of Healing*. Part I was being planned during Galen's first absence from Rome, around 167, and must have been completed no later than the first months of 175, while, to judge from cross-references, he did not resume writing and finish Part II until some twenty years later.[137] It is not simply that far more of the cases in Part II come from Rome, whereas in Part I he presents himself as a newcomer, willing to defer to Roman practice and, for example, leave cranial surgery to surgeons.[138] There is also a more subtle change of perspective. Many more of the observations made almost in passing by Galen in Part II relate now to Rome and Italy; the alum springs of the Aquae Albulae in Latium, the tricks of punters wishing to discover a horse's condition before placing a bet, and the quality of Italian nard compared with that of Laodicea.[139] His lists of wines are headed by the Italian, and his sympathies can extend even to peoples further West such as the Celts or Germans. He is still a Greek writer, writing for fellow Greeks, but at the same time he is readier to explain carefully some of the things he saw in Rome and Italy. He is an interpreter of Rome to those who do not know it, while stressing his own successful career in the largest of all cities.

Nonetheless, his attitude differs noticeably from that of the contemporary authors of two treatises surviving under his name, the two texts on theriac, which both contain markedly more fulsome praise of Rome and the emperors. One, written by a man who had learned his medicine in Rome, was dedicated to a Cretan, Pamphilianus, who seems to have held some official post in Egypt.[140] The other was composed by a man who had enjoyed a similar career to that of Galen, and was equally long-lived as an imperial physician.[141] Writing in the first decade of the third century, this author waxes eloquent about the generosity of the benevolent emperors, Severus and Caracalla. They are delighted to share their goods with their subjects, for the common weal is the greatest part of kingship. They are always at hand to help those whom they know are sick, letting them use drugs from the royal stores, and even prescribing and administering remedies themselves.[142] This enthusiasm for the emperors, by contrast with Galen's more sober comments in the genuine *Antidotes*, is but one of the many reasons which have led recent scholars to conclude that, despite the chronological overlap, this treatise cannot have been written by Galen. Another is the Roman focus of the three exempla that this pseudonymous author gives when discussing poisons and antidotes, namely the deaths of Hannibal, Cleopatra and Mithridates, the last pair in some detail.[143] While none of these stories would have been unfamiliar to any Greek who knew their Plutarch, and Galen himself refers briefly to the death of Mithridates in *Antidotes*, the way in which they are here described at length is entirely from a Roman perspective. Three such exempla in a few pages, as well as the lavish encomia of the emperors, indicate a substantial difference of tone from Galen's genuine writings.[144]

Nonetheless, Galen deserves to be called a Roman. He spent the greater part of his life in Rome, fully engaged in its intellectual life and a shrewd observer of everything around him. He served the members of the imperial court for some fifty years, something he saw as a mixed blessing and one that led him, in the reign of Commodus, to live in constant fear of what the next day would bring. But he wrote for Greeks outside as well as inside Rome, and he expected that his books would be made available to readers throughout the Greek world. Particularly in his later writings, one can see how he interprets life in Rome for those who have little or no knowledge of the capital, even if sometimes his comments appear as afterthoughts.[145] But advertising Rome is always secondary to advertising Galen, who, in his own specialty, could portray himself as the equivalent of a Roman emperor.

Notes

1 *Hipp.Art.* I,22: 18A,348 K. Figures are hard to come by but an estimate of 15–20 per cent of Rome's population of a million is plausible. In general, Tacoma 2016.
2 *Hipp.Art.* I,22: 18A,347 K, a celebrated comment by the sophist Polemo of Laodicea.
3 Nutton 1986.
4 *Part.Art.Med.* 2,3: *CMG Suppl. Or.* II, 28–9. For a doctor possibly contemporary with Galen who moved from Pergamum to Falerii, South Etruria, Samama 2003: no. 500.
5 Samama 2003: no. 184.
6 *Praec.* 1,9: 14,602 K; *CMG* V 8,1, 70–71. Cf. the Latin tombstone of a doctor from Cappadocia who died around this time near Rome and was commemorated by his pupil, *L'Année Épigraphique* 1989: no. 307.
7 [*Ther.Pamph.*] 1: 14,299 K; [*Virt.Cent.*] 1: Galen 1490: sig. yy.viii (= f. 159); ed. Nutton 2015: 161.
8 Meyerhof 1929: 83 (from *Diseases Hard to Cure); Opt.Med.Cogn.* 1,12: *CMG Suppl. Or.* IV, 46–7.
9 *Praec.* 4,6–15, 18: 14,620–4 K; *CMG* V 8,1, 90–1. Cf. *AA* IV,10: 2,470 K; p. 117 tr. Singer C, for the implication that one could gain a reputation in Rome that one would not have had among the Greeks.
10 *Hipp.Aph.* VI,31: 18A,47 K. Juvenal, *Sat.* III,62. Tacoma 2016 gives the wider background.
11 *Praec.* 5,9–11: 14,627–8 K; *CMG* V 8,1, 96–9.
12 *Praec.* 3: 14,625 K; *CMG* V 8,1, 94–5; Pausanias, *AA* III,1: 2,343–5 K; IV,10: 2,470 K; pp. 61–2, 117 tr. Singer C; *Loc.Aff.* I,6: 8,56–9 K; pp. 38–9 tr. Siegel; III,14: 8,213–4 K; p. 102 tr. Siegel; *Opt.Med.Cogn.* 9,12–13: *CMG Suppl. Or.* IV, 108–9.
13 *UP* XI,12: 3,895 K; II, p. 528 tr. May.
14 Samama 2003: no. 364.
15 Cf. for a nuanced interpretation, Woolf 1994.
16 Aulus Gellius, *Attic Nights*; Galen, *Puer.Epil.* 1: 11,357–8 K; pp. 180–2 tr. Temkin.
17 *HNH* I,2: 15,21 K; Spawforth and Walker 1985, 1986; Boatwright 2000.
18 Teuthras, *Ind.* 34: p. 12 BJP; p. 88 tr. Nutton; *Ven.Sect.Er.Rom.* 1: 11,193 K; p. 41 tr. Brain; he was the dedicatee of *Pulses for Beginners, Puls.* 1: 8,453 K, and the *Hippocratic Glossary, Gloss.* 1: 19,116 K. Eudemus, *Praec.* 2,1–4,18: 14,604–24 K; *CMG* V 8,1, 72–95; *AA* I,1: 2,218 K; p. 2 tr. Singer C.
19 *Aff.Dig.* 8,4: 5,42 K; p. 273 tr. Singer PN. Galen's reference at *Praec.* 3,2: 14,613 K; *CMG* V 8,1, 80–1, cf. 4,17: 14,624 K; *CMG* V 8,1, 92–3, implies that he had studied under Eudemus, and the identification is not entirely certain, cf. Boudon-Millot 2012: 312, n. 33. Galen's use of the pluperfect at *Praec.* 2,12: 14,608 K; *CMG* V 8,1, 76–7, also suggests that Eudemus had heard of Galen's change of career only after he himself had left Pergamum.
20 *Praec.* 2,24–7: 14,612–3 K; *CMG* V 8,1, 80–4; Victorinus, *HVA* III,55: 15,722–3 K; *Di. Hipp.Morb.Ac.* 1: *CMG Suppl. Or.* II, 77.
21 *Praec.* 2,24–7; 5,9–20: 14,612–3, 627–8 K; *CMG* V 8,1, 80–4, 96–8; *AA* I,1: 2,215 K; p. 1 tr. Singer C; *Lib.Prop.* 1,7: 19,13 K; p. 138 BM; p. 5 tr. Singer PN. For his cure of Boethus' son, *Praec.* 7,1–18: 14,635–41 K; *CMG* V 8,1, 104–11.
22 Martialius/Martianus *Lib.Prop.* 1,7–9: 19,13 K; p. 138 BM, with the note on the name, pp. 185–6; p. 5 tr. Singer PN; *Praec.* 3,6–4,3: 14,614–20 K; *CMG* V 8,1, 84–91; Alexander, *Praec.* 5,9–16: 14,627–9 K; *CMG* V 8,1, 96–9; *AA* I,1: 2,218 K; p. 2 tr. Singer C. If this Alexander was the philosopher father of Alexander of Aphrodisias, which is likely on chronological grounds, this will have provided an additional reason for the latter's hostility to Galen the philosopher, see below, p. 77. Neither Boudon-Millot (2012) nor Mattern (2013) was aware of the relevant recently discovered inscription, Chaniotis 2004.
23 *Lib.Prop.* 1,7 and 17: 19,13 and 16 K; pp. 138–40 BM; pp. 5–6 tr. Singer PN; *AA* I,1: 2,215 K; p. 1 tr. Singer C.
24 *Adv.Lyc.*: 18A,196–245 K.
25 *AA* IV,10: 2,470 K; p. 117 tr. Singer C: *Lib.Prop.* 4,34–7: p. 153 BM.
26 *AA* I,3; IV,6; 7; 10: 2,227, 449, 458, 470 K; pp. 6, 107, 111–2, 117 tr. Singer C.
27 Soranus, *Gynaecology* I,1 and 3.
28 *Hipp.Epid.VI*, V,4: 17B,245 K. For anatomy as spectacle, Gleason 2009.

29 *AA* VII,10: 2,620–1 K; p. 187 tr. Singer C. Cf. *UP* XVII,1: 3,348–9 K; II, p. 725 tr. May, for his dissection of an elephant's trunk. Mattern (2013: 150–4) discusses the types of animals used and Galen's methods of preparation.

30 *AA* VIII,8: 2,690 K; p. 218 tr. Singer C.

31 For the Ephesus contests at the Great Asclepieia, Samama 2003: nos. 210–5.

32 *AA* VII,16: 2,642–5 K; pp. 197–8 tr. Singer C. For a sceptical description of such performances, Dio Chrysostom, *Oration* 33,6; Lucian, *Against an Ignorant Book-buyer* 29. Cf. *Diff.Puls.* I,1: 8,494–5 K for fisticuffs in an argument over grammar.

33 *Praec.* 3,3 and 6: 14,613–4 K; *CMG* V 8,1, 82–3.

34 *MM* XIII,15: 10,909–16 K; III, pp. 371–81 tr. Johnston-Horsley. For speculation that he could be the author of the tract on the centaury, Nutton 2015b. For Methodist doctors at court, *Praec.* 12,7: 14,663 K; *CMG* V 8,1, 132–3.

35 Samama 2003, nos. 2478, cf. for Crito, doctor to the emperor Trajan, nos. 205, 246.

36 Tecusan 2004; Nutton 2013a: 191–206.

37 Leith 2008.

38 *Opt.Med.Cogn.* 2,1: *CMG Suppl. Or.* IV, 46–7.

39 Nutton 2015b.

40 Hankinson 1991a.

41 Leith 2008.

42 *Praec.* 5,2–3: 14,624–5 K; *CMG* V 8,1, 94–5 mentions a servant of Charilampes an imperial chamberlain and Diomedes, an orator, as among his earliest patients.

43 *Praec.* 9,1–4; 9; 4,16: 14,648–9, 602, 623–4 K; *CMG* V 8,1, 116–9, 70–1, 92–3.

44 *Praec.* 9,1: 14,648 K; *CMG* V 8,1, 116–9. The opposite of *stasis* is concord, *homonoia*, a word found frequently on civic coinage of this period but also applied to individuals; which of these meanings was uppermost in Galen's lost treatise *Concord, Lib.Prop.* 16,4: 19,46 K; p. 170 BM; p. 21 tr. Singer PN, cannot be determined.

45 *Praec.* 9,2: 14,648 K; *CMG* V 8,1, 116–7. What this concerned is unclear, although Galen implies that it was well known, at least to Epigenes, his dedicatee. For an earlier example of stasis on Cos, mediated by the emperor Claudius on the advice of his physician, Stertinius Xenophon, Van der Ploeg 2018: 97.

46 *Lib.Prop.* 1,16: 19,15 K; p. 139 BM; p. 61 tr. Singer PN; *Ind.* 1: p. 2 BJP; p. 78 tr. Nutton. Galen's wording suggests that this was the 'Antonine plague' (cf. *Praes.Puls.* III,4: 9,357 K for the same term), in which his friend Teuthras died (*Ind.* 35: p. 12 BJP; p. 89 tr. Nutton). The plague was raging in the East by mid-late 165 and could easily have reached Rome before the return of the army in mid-166, the traditional catalyst for the outbreak in Rome, see Gourevitch 2013; Duncan-Jones 2018; Flemming 2019; for problems of identification Mulhall 2019.

47 *Lib.Prop.* 3,1: 19,17 K; p. 141 BM; p. 7 tr. Singer PN.

48 *Aff.Dig.* I,4: 5,18–20 K; pp. 254–5 tr. Singer PN. He may also have met the historian Arrian in Athens then or in Rome, *UP* XI,12: 3,895 K; II, p. 528 tr. May.

49 Above, p. 29, n. 154. For the Dead Sea, *SMT* IV,20: 11,690–1 K. For the possible dating of his travels, Nutton 1973; Harig 1987–8; Boudon-Millot 2007: LI; 2012: 106–19; Jones CP 2012. Given that he makes no reference to Boethus, its recent governor, a visit to Palestine in 166–8 is unlikely.

50 *Lib.Prop.* 3,1: 19,18 K; p. 141 BM; p. 8 tr. Singer PN. The addition of the adverb 'immediately' when describing how the emperors sent for him, also deliberately truncates this time he spent away from Rome.

51 *SMT* IX,2: 12,171–3 K.

52 This probably excludes this visit as the occasion of his cure of a young man wounded in a sword fight, *Loc. Aff.* I,1: 8,4 K; p. 17 tr. Siegel. This may be when he trekked through deep snow in freezing winter weather, *SMT* IV,2: 11,625 K.

53 *Praec.* 9,6: 14,649–50 K; *CMG* V 8,1, 118–9; Aelian, fr. 206 Hercher, with the possible reference to an earlier similar attack around 166, Fronto, *Letters* II,6. For other accounts, Augustan History, *Life of Marcus* 15,5–6; Cassius Dio, *Histories* 71,3,1.

54 *Ind.* 49; p. 16 BJP; p. 92 tr. Nutton, with note 92 for the translation problem. For Commodus, see above, pp. 38–9.

55 *Praec.* 9,10–19: 14,651–6 K; *CMG* V 8,1, 120–27; *Lib.Prop.* 3,2–6: 19,18–19 K; p. 142 BM; p. 8 tr. Singer PN.

56 *Ant.* I,1: 14, 4 K. Cassius Dio, *Hist.* LXXII (LXXI),6,3. For theriac, Mattern 2013: 215–9; Boudon-Millot 2016a: XXXIV–XLI.

57 *San.Tu.* VI,5: 6,406 K; II, p. 151 tr. Johnston.

58 *Praec.* 11,1–8: 14,658–60 K; *CMG* V 8,1, 126–9.

59 *Ant.* I,1: 14,4 K: *Praec.* 10,2–12,10: 14,652–65 K; *CMG* V 8,1, 120–33.

60 Cf. *Praec.* 2: 14,625 K; *CMG* V 8,1, 94–5, "the most famous of the palace doctors". Galen may well have been one of the court doctors who according to Herodian, *History* I,12,2, advised Commodus during an epidemic in 188 to leave Rome for Laurentum, whose laurel groves would purify the tainted air.

61 *Praec.* 12,10: 14,663 K; *CMG* V 8, 170–1, 132–3, probably from the early 170s.

62 *Ind.* 54: p. 18 BJP; p. 93 tr. Nutton: his crimes are "the worst in recorded history". *Mor.* I; p. 147 tr. Davies, with the fuller version in the fragment, p. 180 tr. Davies; Schlange-Schöningen 2013; Nicholls 2019. Cf. *Caus.Symp.* I,2: 7,157–8 K: someone appearing before a terrifying ruler is likely to tremble and speak in a quavering voice, not noted by Rothschild 2014.

63 See my comments at Singer PN 2013: 50.

64 His house in Rome is some way from the suburbs, *Cur.Rat.Ven.Sect.* 17: 11,299–300 K; p. 91 tr. Brain. For the probability of his villa being in the still unexcavated villa area of Stabiae, see Raiola and Mascolo 2014; Petit 2018: 150–1, noting *MM* V,12: 10,362–5 K; II, pp. 87–91 tr. Johnston-Horsley, a lyrical description of Stabiae and its environs.

65 Tucci 2013: 291–300 discusses at length the descriptions of the libraries and storage places mentioned in *Ind.*; Nicholls 2014 offers a judicious assessment of the possibility that some of these losses occurred in an imperial library at Antium,

66 *Ind.* 6–7; pp. 3–4 BJP; p. 79 tr. Nutton. For Galen's notes on anatomy that were also lost, *AA* XI,12: pp. 107–8 Dkw. For other treasures of the Palatine libraries, *Ind.* 16–19: pp. 5–6 BJP; pp. 81–2 tr. Nutton.

67 For a friend depositing the books of another writer, probably Phlegon of Tralles' *Wondrous Stories*, in a library, see Robert 1938: 45–51. Galen also claims to have used books in friends' libraries, *Hipp.Epid. VI*, iv,22: *CMG* V 10,2,2, 233.

68 *Hipp.Epid. VI*, viii: *CMG* V 10,2,2, 495.

69 *MM* VII,1: 10,456–7 K; pp. 237–9 tr. Johnston-Horsley. Cf. Rothschild and Thompson 2014: 91–158.

70 *Lib.Prop.* 15,5: 19,46 K; p. 170 BM; p. 21 tr. Singer PN, included in his list of writings on ethics. Whether referring to official decrees or, more likely, 'public opinion' in early 193, this would have been highly unusual. In it he would have emphasised the links between Pertinax and Septimius Severus, the ultimate victor in the civil war that followed, as well as playing down his own long service with Commodus. For a modern novelist's recreation of Galen's reminiscences, Prantera 1991.

71 *Ant.* I,13: 14,65–6 K.

72 Nutton 1995b; Boudon-Millot 2012: 241–4.

73 Fazzo 2002; Pietrobelli 2019a: 21.

74 Amari 1897; Strohmaier 2007; Boudon-Millot 2012: 244–5.

75 *SMT* IX,2: 12,171–3 K.

76 *Lib.Prop.* 9,4: 19,35 K; p. 160 BM. The alternative, advocated by Jouanna, 2013: CXL–CXLI, is that he arranged for the transfer of most of his library to Rome when he left to join the Emperor in 168, but this suggestion is also not without its problems.

77 Attalus gave money to the association of young men at Heraclea (Samama 2003: nos 247–8); Gellius Maximus was a notable benefactor at Antioch in Pisidia (*ibid.* nos 331, 332, 337, 337bis; Christol and Drew-Bear 2004). If his Greek cognomen is rightly restored as [Poly] histor, it suggests at least hopes or pretensions to wider cultural learning. Galen, *Aff.Dig.* I,9: 5,51 K; pp. 278–9 tr. Singer PN; *Ind.* 1: p. 2 BJP; pp. 77–8 tr. Nutton. Both men as court doctors would have had a long relationship with Galen.

78 For his wealth, above, p. 43.

79 *Opt.Med.Cogn.* 1,1–13, 8,1–4, 13,2–4; *CMG Suppl. Or.* IV, 42–46, 92–5, 128–30. *MM* I,1: 10,1–5 K; pp. 3–9 tr. Johnston-Horsley opens with a similarly florid description of medical life in Rome. Cf. the denunciation of ivory-footed couches, gold, silver or glass vessels, and lots of beautiful slaves as irrelevant to a healthy lifestyle, *Thras.* 18: 5,837–8 K; p. 68 tr. Singer PN.

80 *Praec.* 1,1–16; 4,5–18: 14,599–605, 620–4 K; *CMG* V 8,1, 69–75, 90–3.
81 Lehoux 2017.
82 *Opt.Med.Cogn.* 9,2: *CMG Suppl. Or.* IV, 102–3: *MM* I,1 and IX,4: 10,2 and 609 K; I, p. 5 and II, p. 465 tr. Johnston-Horsley; *Praec.* 1,1: 14,600 K; *CMG* V 8,1, 68–9 with the parallels listed there and on p. 148 for this common complaint of satirical writers. The Greek adjective in the compliment paid him by Marcus Aurelius, "a man of considerable independence", *Praec.* 11,8: 14,660 K; *CMG* V 8,1, 128–9, carries both social and intellectual connotations.
83 König 2009: 38–44, 50–8.
84 Sconocchia 1993: 856–9, 890–908; Langslow 2000: 51; Nutton 2013a: 174–8; Jouanna-Bouchet 2016: VIII–LXXIV. The reference to the Elder Pliny's *Natural History* XX,24,264 at *Ant.* II,14: 14,183 K is an interpolation by Chartier in his edition, repeated by Kühn.
85 Jouanna-Bouchet 2016: LXXIV–V; Guardasole 2014, 2015.
86 Boudon-Millot 2012: 32.
87 *SMT* IX,34: 12,239–40 K; cf. *Comp.Med.Gen.* I,16: 13,435 K, claiming that since the Roman conquest, Greeks all used the Latin word '*sextarius*', but for different local measures.
88 Respectively, *MM* XIII,15: 10,911 K (interpreted for the Greek reader but not at VII,5: 10,469 K); *MM* VIII,4: 10,569 K; *MM* VIII,5: 10,574 K; *MM* VII,4: 10,467 K; III, pp. 375, 255, 405, 413, 253 tr. Johnston-Horsley; *Ant.* I,3: 14,49 K.
89 *Di.Dec.* II,7 and 6: 9,873, 868 K.
90 *UP* VIII,4: 3,629 K; I, p. 394 tr. May.
91 *Hipp.Art.* I: 18A,348 K; von Müller 1895: 475, a fragment of *Demonstration* preserved in Arabic.
92 Martelli 2012. For a Latin term superseding local terms throughout the Empire, *Alim.Fac.* I,2: 6,483 K; p. 40 tr. Powell.
93 *MM* I,1: 10,2–4 K; I, pp. 5–7 tr. Johnston-Horsley.
94 *MM* VIII,6: 10,581–3 K; II, pp. 423–5 tr. Johnston-Horsley.
95 *MM* VIII,5; XIV,16: 10, 573–4, 1007–8 K; II, 412–3; III, pp. 517–9 tr. Johnston-Horsley.
96 *Comp.Med.Loc.* I,3: 12,440–2 K.
97 *Comp.Med.Loc.* I,2: 12,435 K.
98 *UP* XI,14: 3,902 K; II, p. 531 tr. May.
99 *MM* IX,5; XI,15, 17; XII,7: 10,620, 784–5, 797, 856 K; II, p. 481; III, pp. 185–7, 205, 293 tr. Johnston-Horsley.
100 *MM* XII,1, 15: 10,816–7, 783 K; III, pp. 233–5, 185 tr. Johnston-Horsley; cf. *Praes.Puls.* I,1: 9,218 K.
101 *Comp.Med.Loc.* VI,2: 12,909 K.
102 *Ind.* 62, with the emendation of Raiola 2011; p. 94 tr. Nutton; *Praec.* I,13–4: 14,604 K; *CMG* V 8,1, 72–5. *Hipp.Epid. VI*, iv,9: 17B,150 K.
103 *Ind.* 83: pp. 25–6 BJP; pp. 98–9 tr. Nutton.
104 *MM* II,5: 10,109 K; I, p. 171 tr. Johnston-Horsley.
105 On Galen and venesection, see further below, pp. 111–12.
106 *Ven.Sect.Er* .7: 11,173 K; p. 30 tr. Brain.
107 *Ven.Sect.Er.Rom.* 1: 11,187–90 K; pp. 38–9 tr. Brain.
108 *Ibid.* 2: 11,194–5 K; pp. 41–2 tr. Brain; Teuthras' copy is presumably the basis for *Ven.Sect. Er.* 11,147–86 K; pp. 15–37 tr. Brain.
109 *Ibid.* 3: 11,211 K; 7: 11,57 K; pp. 50, 57 tr. Brain.
110 *Ibid.* 11,187–249 K; pp. 38–66 tr. Brain.
111 *Cur.Rat.Ven.Sect.* 17: 11,299–302 K; pp. 91–2 tr. Brain.
112 Nutton 1990a.
113 *San.Tu.* V,5 and 12: 6,332–3, 379 K; II, pp. 31–2, 111 tr. Johnston; *AA* VII,12–13: 2,631–3 K; pp. 192–3 tr. Singer C; *PHP* I,5,1–13: 5,181–2 K; *CMG* V 4,1,2, 76–8.
114 The equivalent of 40,000 sestertii: *Praec.* 8,20: 14,647 K; *CMG* V 8,1, 116–7. Larger sums were reportedly charged by other elite doctors, and several non-imperial physicians amassed huge fortunes (Nutton 2013a: 260–2, for parallels); Galen lost gold and silver plate and many financial documents in the fire of 192, *Ind.* 4: p. 3 BJP; pp. 77–8 tr. Nutton.
115 Christol and Drew-Bear 2004.
116 *MM* VIII,3: 10,561 K; I, p. 393 tr. Johnston-Horsley.

117 *Aff.Dig.* I,9,15–16: 5,47–9 K; pp. 276–7 tr. Singer PN; *SMT* X,15: 12,286 K, for slaves, peasants, and travellers. He may have made a similar claim in a work now lost, adding there that he had recommended some individuals for service with governors and other wealthy patrons, Meyerhof 1929: 84.

118 Boudon 1994.

119 *Loc.Aff.* V,8: 8,361–6 K; pp. 161–3 tr. Siegel; Galen had planned to give him other books before his death, *MMG* II,13: 11,145–6 K; I, p. 559 tr. Johnston.

120 Meyerhof 1929: 83. Cf. the author of *The Properties of the Centaury* 1: p. 165 Nutton, who had learned about this panacea from accompanying his distinguished master on his rounds.

121 Nicholls 2011.

122 *Ind.* 13–18: pp. 5–9 BJP; pp. 81–4 tr. Nutton. This section remains the most controversial. While the general sense of the passage is clear, the text needs emendation in several places, see the various solutions put forward at Garofalo-Lami 2012: 124–9; Nutton in Singer PN 2013: 100–6; Singer PN 2019a: 22–6.

123 *Lib.Prop.* 1,1–4: 19,8–9 K; pp. 134–5 BM; p. 3 tr. Singer PN; *Prop.Plac.* 1,1: p. 172 BMP; pp. 58–9 Garofalo-Lami; p. 186 Vegetti.

124 *Loc.Aff.* IV,2: 8,224 K; p. 107 tr. Siegel. At *San Tu.* III,6: 6,196 K; I, p. 285 tr. Johnston, Galen says that Iberia is the equivalent of the Latin *Hispania.* He could also secure a ready supply of monkeys and other animals for dissection purposes, and even some exotica.

125 *Alim.Fac.* III,5; II,31; III,1: 6,728–9, 613–4, 666 K; pp. 143, 94–5, 117 tr. Powell.

126 *San.Tu.* I,10: 6,51 K; I, p. 75 tr. Johnston; *Temp.* II,5 and 6: 1,618, 629 K; pp. 134–5, 142 tr. Singer PN. More can be expected from the forthcoming publication of Galen's commentary on *Airs, Waters, Places.*

127 *Comp.Med.Loc.* IV,7: 12,786 K. Cf. *Ant.* II,15: 14,197 K, the juice of a British plant mentioned in a poem on theriac by Damocrates, fl. 50 CE.

128 *MM* XIII,22: 10,942 K; III, p. 421 tr. Johnston-Horsley; *MMG* II,12: 11,143–4 K; p. 557 tr. Johnston. Note also the professional viper hunter, *SMT* XI,1: 12,316 K, and an imperial servant employed to catch vipers, *Loc.Aff.* V,8: 8,355 K; p. 159 tr. Siegel.

129 *Ant.* I,2: 14,8–9, 23, 25 K; *SMT* VI,6,2: 11,880 K (ginger from among the barbarians). Touwaide 2012: 32; cf. 2014: 86. argues that the contemporary pseudo-Galenic *Substitute Drugs* shows a distinct change to a metropolitan from a local or regional environment.

130 *Ant.* I,2: 14,9 K.

131 *Ant.* I,2: 14,8–10 K.

132 *Ant.* I,5: 14,30–31 K.

133 *Ant.* I,2: 14,8–13 K.

134 *Ant.* I,13: 14,64–7 K.

135 *Aff.Dig.* I,4: 5,17 K; p. 253 tr. Singer PN.

136 *MM* IX,8: 10,632–3 K; II, pp. 499–501, tr. Johnston-Horsley; Petit 2018: 146–9.

137 Nutton 1991.

138 *MM* VI,6: 10,455 K; II, p. 235 tr. Johnston-Horsley.

139 Respectively *MM* VIII,2; VII,6; XI,16: 10,536, 478, 791 K; II, pp. 355, 269; III, p. 197 tr. Johnston-Horsley. Cf. also VII,4; 6; 7: 10,467, 483, 501 K; XII,4: 831–4 K; II, pp. 253, 277, 303; III, pp. 257–61 tr. Johnston-Horsley, and the reference to the Aquae Domitianae at Vigarello, below, p. 71, n. 19.

140 [*Ther.Pamph.*]: 14,298–9, 304, 295 K, probably of Severan date.

141 [*Ther.Pis.*]: 14,216–8 K; he was in Rome in the early third century, 14,212–4 K; and had studied at Alexandria 14,237 K, and was, like Galen, an opponent of the Methodists, 14,223–4, 250–5, 281, 285 K. Probably written around 206–7.

142 [*Ther.Pis.*] 2,7–14: 14,216–8 K; pp. 7–9 Boudon-Millot.

143 [*Ther.Pis.*] 5, 8, 16: 14,231, 235–6, 283–4 K; pp. 19,37–8, 83–4 Boudon-Millot.

144 For authenticity, Swain 1996: 430–2; Nutton 1997; against, Leigh 2015; Boudon-Millot 2016a: lxxiv–lxxx; ci–cxx; and forthcoming. Nathalie Rousseau in a paper at a 2016 Warburg Conference, forthcoming, presented a very convincing linguistic case against authenticity.

145 *Alim.Fac.* III,17: 6,697 K; p. 130 tr. Powell. Cf. *HNH* II,6: 15,137 K, where he uses the contrast between the single acropolis of Athens and the seven hills of Rome to illustrate different types of mistake.

3 Galen the observer

In 1862 the German professor Ludwig Friedländer (1824–1909) published the first volume of a multi-volume work, subsequently translated into English as *Roman Life and Manners under the Early Empire*, which went through eight editions before 1910.[1] It was a remarkable survey of everyday life in imperial Rome, based on a broad knowledge of the literary, epigraphic, and archaeological sources. Friedländer, an expert on the Roman epigrammatist Martial, naturally drew upon him and other satirists for much of his information, but he also relied considerably on Galen's evidence. In this he was unusual, for most classicists of his day left Galen to doctors or to a handful of philologists interested in editing Greek texts. Friedländer, by contrast, had seized upon what distinguishes Galen from almost every other ancient author: his insatiable curiosity and his remarkable powers of observation. One might also add his ability to let his impressions stimulate new thoughts, for not every doctor seeing a large crowd impeded by narrow exits as they rushed to leave the theatre after a performance would be moved to consider the possible damage to health if the body's small pores became blocked, invoke wooden puppets moved by strings as an example of art imitating nature in the placement of muscle, or when describing diarrhoea in humans, think of a bird called locally in Pergamum the *seleucis*, which, after gorging itself on grasshoppers or locusts, swiftly evacuated all that it had eaten.[2]

What Galen saw in the world around him is only one facet of his ability to observe. He had a similarly sharp eye for interpreting the results of his dissections both in his careful descriptions of organs like the brain and in applying them to an understanding of the workings of the body. Even when he is wrong, as in his explanation for the pulse, he is not foolish, and he errs in his interpretation of crucial phenomena more often than in any failure to notice them. Above all, his observations are rarely random but are subordinated to a medical purpose, to identify appropriate foods, drinks and therapeutic substances, to diagnose a patient's condition and understand its future development, and to take appropriate measures to restore it to its natural, healthy state, if at all possible.

Galen the traveller

Galen's books are filled with stories and reminiscences. Some of them are second-hand, for instance, that of the Bithynian poisoner who discovered that a common plant could cause unstoppable bleeding, or simply folklore, like the mention of human flesh fed to unsuspecting travellers in place of pork by rascally inn-keepers, or of the huge animal, half bear, half pig, roaming in Lucania, in S. Italy, although at least one such story mutates over the years to suggest that he was in some way involved in it.[3] But most seem to derive directly from his own experiences. He has seen slave dealers tone up the bottoms of skinny or flabby slaves by beating them with rods or even by making small incisions and coating them with pitch, "a good medication for increasing flesh".[4] The account of a house fire in the countryside near Pergamum is so vivid as to suggest that Galen had been present. A pile of pigeon-droppings outside a newly painted window frame caught fire in the hot sunshine. The blaze quickly spread to other doors and windows that had been freshly painted, and the flames, which reached as high as the roof, rapidly consumed the whole house.[5] In his similarly detailed reminiscence of his visit to the mines near Soloi on Cyprus he describes not only the mine buildings and the varied colours of the lodes, but also the dreadful conditions in which the miners worked. Naked and in chains, they hurried down a passage some 200 metres long to fill their jars from an underground pool of thick, warm, pale green water before returning to empty them in settling tanks. It was hot and dangerous work. The air in the tunnel was almost as hot as in a sweating room at the baths, it smelled of copper and Verdigris, and was so thick that it was almost impossible to keep the lamps lit. It was safest to spend as little time underground as possible, for a tunnel might collapse at any moment, killing everyone in it. The precision of Galen's information is matched by his sympathy for the slaves or convicts.[6]

Some of his observations are almost casually tossed into an oral presentation, others are carefully chosen to exemplify the point at issue, as in his work on foodstuffs, and to support his own credibility as a witness. He has examined "carefully" the saffron growing at the famous cave at Corycus (South Turkey). His comment on the habit of peasants (and others) in his native region of Mysia coming into town each spring to be bled emphasises the dangers of letting an inexperienced doctor open a vein (and his own expertise in repairing the damage caused by the inadvertent incision of an artery).[7] The oars in the three banks of a trireme, like the fingers of the hand, are made of different lengths, just like fingers, the middle row being the longest, so that they all reach the water-line together.[8] Sometimes his reminiscences are artful compositions. The validity of his advice in *Affected Parts* or the last sections of the *Method of Healing* is strengthened by the abundance of detail that is added to the stories in order to confirm the truth of what he has just asserted. The theory he has just propounded is thereby shown to work in practice beyond any doubt.

Sometimes the personal details have a largely stylistic purpose: to break up what would otherwise be a dull catalogue of drugs or cases. The account of his second visit to the Aegean island of Lemnos to collect seals of the famous Lemnian earth can stand for several other digressions. Galen begins with a detailed description of his two voyages to Lemnos, carefully noting the distances from Philippi, the main town in the region of Macedonia, to the coast, from there to the island of Thasos, then on to Hephaestias, and finally from there to Alexandria Troas on the mainland, so that future visitors will not make the same mistake as he did and land at the wrong port.[9] The bare hill near Hephaestias, onto which Hephaestus, according to Homer, was said to have fallen, Galen describes as being typical of the island in its tawny colour. He was fortunate to arrive there at a festival, when earth from the hill was consecrated in a special ceremony before the seals were made.[10] A priestess, who alone was permitted to touch this earth, cast wheat and barley on the ground in exchange for what had been dug, performed various rituals, but without making any animal sacrifice, and then escorted a cart-load of earth into town. Next she gradually applied water (presumably in a settling tank), letting the useless stones and heavier sand sink to the bottom. She then removed the clear surface water before taking out the thick, greasy suspension of earth and water, which was allowed to dry until the mud reached the consistency of soft wax. She then took small portions, formed them into little seals and imprinted on them the figure of the goddess Artemis before finally drying them out completely. These round seals, which were now red in colour (possibly as a result of the action of talaromyces fungus in the soil) and, unlike the red ruddle he had glimpsed elsewhere in the island, did not stain the fingers of those who touched them, were then put on sale in this easily transportable form. Galen took away some twenty thousand, with an estimated weight of 50 kg, enough to fill two large amphorae, which he used as an antidote to poisons as well as for treating ulcers and chronic wounds. As a further guarantee of efficacy, he questioned the Lemnians about the constituents of the seals, even obtaining a book from a local healer setting out their many medicinal uses.

This incident is typical of Galen in many ways: his persistence, his inquisitiveness, his learned references, his precision and his assistance to his future readers in giving the distances on the island and the details of preparing the earth.[11] Similarly, in a recently discovered passage, he gives both the Syriac and Armenian terms for a medicinal earth found on mount Agarak on the borders of Eastern Cappadocia and Armenia in the territory of a place called Bagawan.[12] Linguistic exactitude matters to

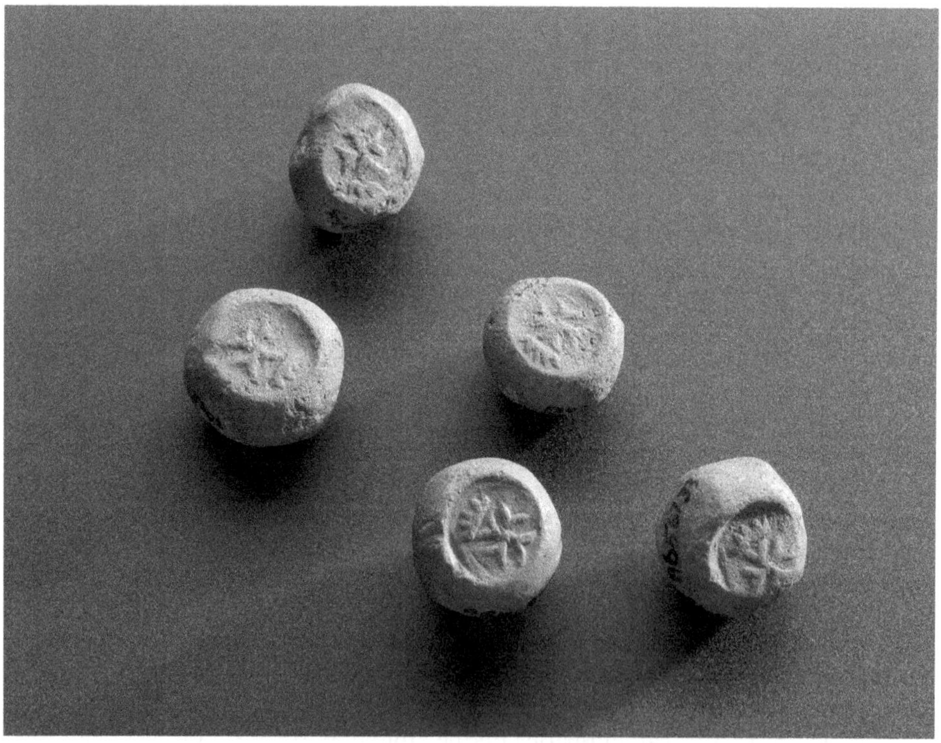

Figure 3.1 Late medieval seals of Lemnian earth/ terra sigillata.
Copyright: Science Museum, London.

Galen. He has no objection to the use of a Phrygian word for bread, *bakos*, provided that it is one everybody knows or is explained. But piling up words from different dialects, three from Cilicia, four from Syria, five from Galatia, six from Classical Athens, is a waste of time. Besides, one should always remember that some languages and local pronunciations often sound dreadful – like pigs, frogs, jackdaws, or someone snoring or whistling. He is interested in languages, but he takes exception to those who have no wish to learn the beautiful and euphonious Greek in which he was reared and brought up and would instead compel him to abandon it.[13]

It is not just words that attract his attention. He notices small differences in the vegetation as he moves from place to place, such as the various types of wheat and barley he observed on his passage through Greece and the Balkans, the marjoram growing in profusion near Cyzicus on the shores of the Black Sea, or the peasant preference for eating radishes with bread, in contrast to townsmen who eat them on their own with garum, a fish sauce, or vinegar as a first course.[14] He records local peculiarities of vocabulary. Some people call pears and peaches Armeniac or Armenian apples, while the names of the months differ from region to region.[15] He is particularly interested in different kinds of water, as befitted a learned commentator on the Hippocratic *Airs, Waters and Places.*[16] Hot springs are rare but there are several within a kilometre or so of the town of Bursa, whereas one must travel much further from Pergamum to find the closest to it, at Allianoi. In the suburbs of Bursa there is also a mineral healing spring, similar to that at Lakettoi, a village in the hinterland of Pergamum.[17] The salt lake at Tragasai in the Troad, North of Pergamum, produces a rare type of salt, while fish that can flourish in the two rivers flowing into the Dead Sea die as soon as they enter it.[18] Drinking from a spring near Rome containing traces of copper and iron helps sufferers from kidney or colon pains, but is harmful if continued for a long time.[19] Rome's water supply, although generally excellent, is not as good for cooking as that of Pergamum, while the Tiber, like the rivers of other huge cities, becomes extraordinarily polluted by all the filth that is discharged into it from sewers, baths, kitchens, and laundries. The proof can be easily seen in the fish that are caught in the estuary and sold cheaply in the market. They are scrawny and lacking in nutritious value, very different from the plump fish that are found in the upper reaches of the Tiber and in its tributary, the Nar.[20] Besides, the frequently damp Roman climate leads to colds and similar phlegmatic diseases.[21] Like Alexandria, Rome is an unhealthy place.

The countryside, however, is not much better. In times of famine, which were not uncommon, the inhabitants were reduced to eating grasses and shrubs, with dreadful consequences.[22] They also slaughtered their pigs so that they themselves could eat the acorns they would normally have fed to them, or resorted to eating oats, which Galen regarded as food for draught animals rather than humans.[23] No wonder that at one point he compares peasants to donkeys in their physical make-up.[24] But he is also aware of the peasants' justified suspicion of the bosses from the town who carry off all the wheat and barley immediately after the harvest, leaving them only various kinds of less nutritious pulses, and sometimes not even these.[25] It is not surprising that they in their turn try to get the better of these unscrupulous landlords. When they bring their grain to market, they often place jars of water in their carts so than the grain can absorb some of the moisture and thus weigh more when the time comes for it to be exchanged for money.[26] When the harvest is poor, they do not trouble to sieve out any darnel that has got into the grain, a situation also accepted by the public bakers and resulting in headaches and ulcers among those who eat the bread.[27] But at the best of times, their food is far from satisfactory, being rough and often almost indigestible to those unused to it.[28] Even the bread they use for their favourite meal of bread and soft cheese becomes quickly uneatable after three or four days.[29]

Galen takes pains to describe how each region has its own type of cereal. There is a particular kind of white barley in Cappadocia (Central Turkey) that is called 'naked' by the locals, while in Thrace and Macedonia a type of rye, *briza*, grows that produces a nasty-smelling black bread.[30] This grain is as inferior to the winter barley from Bithynia and Phrygia (North West Turkey) as that is to wheat.[31] A celebrated type of parsley comes from Astraia in Macedonia, although less is now grown there than formerly, and the name 'Macedonian parsley' is now often applied to that grown elsewhere and merely exported through Thessalonica.[32] He is amazed that although Cypriot peasants cultivate wheat, they still prefer to eat barley, especially when the Roman army had long ceased to use barley meal on the grounds that it does not provide enough nutrition for those in heavy training.[33]

Wine and honey likewise vary from place to place. Some of the best honey is so localised that it is all consumed on the spot, and hence has no wider reputation. He recalls with evident delight the thyme-scented honey, at least the equal of that of Hymettus, that comes from a hillock on the left of the road from Pergamum to its port of Elaea. Even more remarkable was a very sweet honey carefully produced at Brittos, not far from Pergamum, by a farmer on a small rocky hillside covered with thyme and oregano and close to clumps of cytisus, for other honey from the same district was absolutely awful.[34] As might be expected from the son of a father who took great care with his vineyard, Galen was a connoisseur of wines, particularly of those produced near Pergamum at Perperene, Aegae, Titicaza, and on the adjacent Aegean islands, and, later on, of those near Rome.[35] He remembered his first taste of Falernian, a famous Italian vintage but one which seemed to him inferior to the best of his native region, that coming from Mount Tmolus, near Sardis.[36] He is particularly interested in methods of producing and storing wine. He explains how sealing wine jars with a leather cover which is then smeared with pitch or gypsum keeps out the air, and that storing the jars in a warm environment induces early maturity and reduces acidity.[37] His father was an expert at this, improving on the typical peasant custom of having special outbuildings nicely heated by fire or simply by the warmth of the animals in adjacent stables by building a special store with individual rooms upstairs, rather like an inn, with one wall pierced with holes to allow the warm air to circulate.[38] Nicon never stored his wine in new jars, but always in ones that had been emptied of a mature vintage, something Galen had also observed in Naples and its environs where the hills produced the Trifolinum wine. It was also, so he had been informed, common practice elsewhere in Italy.[39]

Some of these observations provide detail to illustrate a wider argument. So, for instance, the common custom of patients taking puppies or small children (or slaves) to bed with them as hot-water bottles illustrates how heat can dry up pus.[40] The three books of his tract on the properties of foodstuffs are filled with records of his own experiences.[41] As well as giving details of how they may bring about or correct resulting imbalances in the four Hippocratic humours he also identifies a variety of situations and qualities that can impede proper digestion, a theme taken up in such treatises as *Good and Bad Juices, Barley Gruel* and *A Thinning Diet.*[42] The last is not a book on slimming, as unwary Italian readers of Marinone's 1973 Italian translation assumed, but on how one can choose a diet that will thin any thick, glutinous mixture of humours that impedes proper nutrition. Galen's recommendations include avoiding liver, kidneys, boiled eggs, mushrooms, shellfish, milky foods like cheese, and heavy red wine in favour of the meat of animals and birds from the mountains and rosé wines, which are less diuretic than whites.[43] But he has seen very many people who follow a bad diet improve through drinking a mixture of vinegar and wine with scilla in it, and the inhabitants of the plain around Aegae in Aeolis and Perperene, both near Pergamum, do not appear to him to suffer from drinking the local heavy reds, presumably because they have become habituated to them.[44]

His observations are often used for comparative purposes or to clarify for the uninitiated things otherwise hard to understand. For example, the fatty grease generally applied to the axles of wagons and chariots to make them run better graphically explains the similar role of fluid around the joints or the larynx.[45] The inability of a lion to see someone in front of it if a flaming torch is held between them helps to explain night-blindness and why those who can see very well in moonlight may do so less well in bright sunlight.[46] It is not surprising that many of his images of animals occur in discussions of rational and irrational behaviour, for Galen had precedents for this in both Plato and Aristotle, and his examples are often standard.[47] But they are not entirely confined to what his predecessors have written. His simile of a hunter and his dog aiming to catch a wild bear is an unusual extension of a famous simile in Plato about how to train the soul.[48] Most striking of all is a long passage preserved in a tenth-century Arabic writer on zoology, al-Marwazī, from the book *Character Traits*, in which Galen uses the example of the enmity between a snake and a mongoose to argue that some traits are innate.[49] Having been offered some poisonous snakes by a friend in Egypt who had been given them as an unwanted present, Galen conducted an experiment, introducing a young mongoose into the presence of one of the snakes to see if the two would fight, even if they had never been trained to do so or even seen the other species before. He describes the fight in graphic detail, noting their moves as each tried to get into position to deliver the killing bite until they ended by each grabbing half of the open jaw of the other. His servant, forewarned of this possible ending, then cut off the snake's head, and saved the mongoose by pouring a draught of the theriac antidote down its throat. Even in Arabic and the subsequent English translation the vigour, precision and relevance of Galen's observations stand out clearly.[50]

Seeing inside the body

The use of comparisons with familiar objects had been a feature of ancient writings on anatomy ever since the days of Herophilus, for they allowed the observer to describe, and the reader to imagine, parts of the body that had not been viewed before or only with difficulty.[51] Galen's own investigations into the normally invisible parts of the body constitute one of his greatest achievements, and formed a significant element in what has been called his theology.[52] No other surviving medical writer from Antiquity discusses dissection to a similar extent or makes such use of anatomical findings in dealing with patients. The contrast with his predecessor Rufus of Ephesus is marked. Although for Rufus knowledge about the body, or at least the names of its parts, was an essential element in the doctor's tool kit, he does not appear to have dissected personally, and he made little or no use of his anatomical knowledge in treating patients.[53] By contrast, in Galen's view, an understanding of how the human body was put together and how it functioned, both included in his use of the word 'anatomy', was essential for the proper practice of medicine. It required more than mere book learning, although that did not stop him from writing a major dissection manual, *Anatomical Procedures*, several shorter texts for students on the anatomy of bones, veins and arteries, muscles, and nerves, and further books, notably *The Use of Parts*, in which he explained the significance of his discoveries for non-medical readers.[54] One would not expect a helmsman to steer simply by a book, so why should one expect a doctor to navigate the body likewise?[55] One required constant practice, both to obtain the necessary manual skill and to become accustomed to observing correctly what was revealed by the knife. Galen provided further guidance on the actual technique of dissection in two small tracts, *Dissection* and *Vivisection*, both later translated into Arabic, of which only the former survives today although it has not yet been fully published.[56]

Anatomy in the time of Galen was controversial. There was a long tradition, going back centuries to Hellenistic times, of antagonism to it. Opponents argued that it was cruel and unnecessary, for repetition of dissection was subject to the law of diminishing returns. Evidence from a dead body was at best a fallible guide to the living, and animals were not identical to humans.[57] Galen's main opponents in Rome, the Methodists, could see no virtue in dissection, believing that its conclusions could indeed be learned from a book, and that careful observation of the external body of the sick patient could by itself swiftly reveal the underlying causes of any illness that needed to be removed. Even so eminent a practitioner as Soranus could assert that anatomical knowledge was valuable only in as much as it provided a doctor with a reputation for learning.[58] But at the same time, as we have seen, public anatomy displays using animals became popular in Rome and elsewhere in the generation before Galen, gory spectacles attracting eager crowds to witness almost gladiatorial contests between rival dissectors.[59] At least two of his own writings on anatomy were overtly polemical; his *What Lycus did not Know about Anatomy*, in four books, and the three books dedicated to *Disputed Points in Anatomy*, both alas now lost.[60]. In addition, his treatises on the anatomical ideas of Hippocrates and on those of Erasistratus both derived from his public arguments with Martialius in Rome.[61] Participation in these controversies required technical and rhetorical skill, both of which Galen possessed in abundance and did not hesitate to deploy.[62]

Whether writing, debating or dissecting in public, among a small circle of friends, or in private by himself, Galen believed that he was participating in a tradition of anatomical investigation that went back to Hippocrates himself, as he explained in the six (lost) books of *Hippocrates' Anatomy*.[63] Modern scholars are not convinced he was right, for although there are a number of short texts found in the Hippocratic Corpus and known to Galen by their anatomical titles, there is no evidence for systematic dissection in the age of Hippocrates or for any regular use of anatomical information in clinical cases.[64] But Galen had been educated by teachers who looked back to Hippocrates, many of whom were themselves interested in anatomy, and his belief in Hippocratic precedent would not have been unique. He also had a great respect for the Alexandrians Herophilus and Erasistratus, writing a book on the latter's understanding (or misunderstanding) of anatomy, and, as we have seen, in his youth he had made his own summaries of the anatomical textbooks of Marinus and Lycus.[65] What precisely he gained from earlier authorities is far from clear, apart from the impetus to repeat several of Erasistratus' experiments on the body in action, but one must be wary of assuming that everything that he describes derives solely from his own dissections.[66]

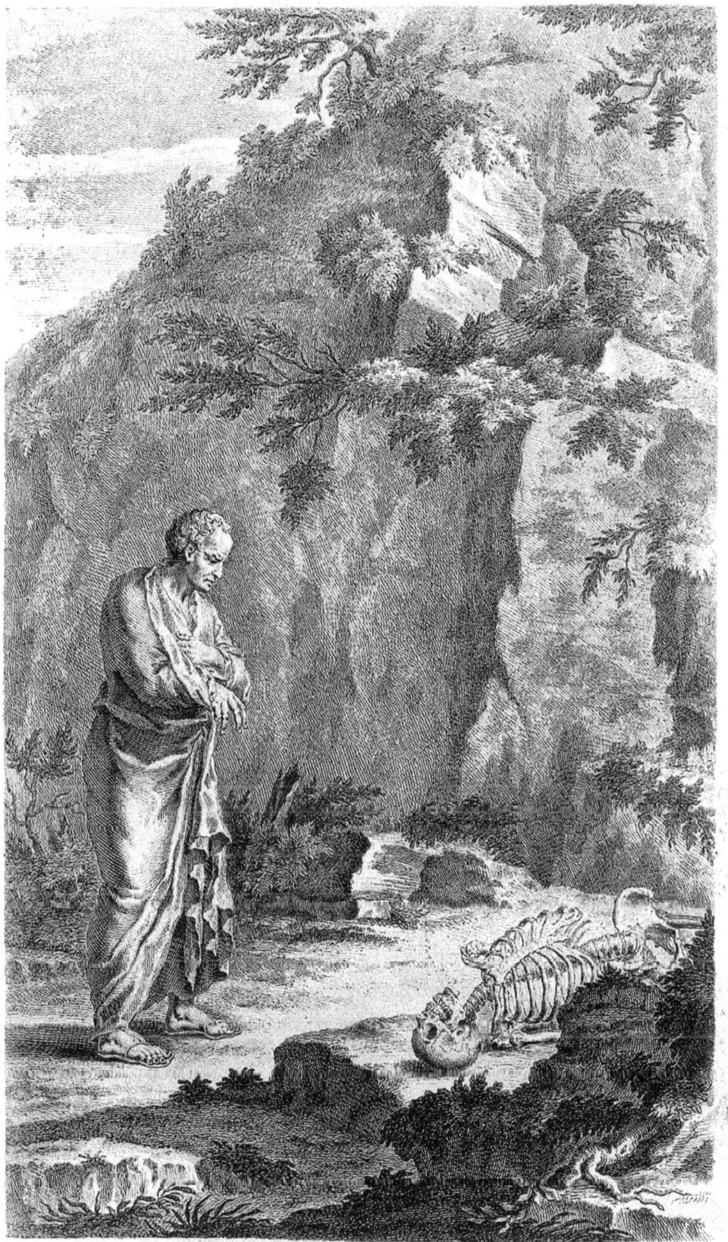

Figure 3.2 "The Conversion of Galen". Originally the frontispiece to William Cheselden, *Osteographia or the Anatomy of Bones*, London, 1733, this image of Galen contemplating a human corpse was frequently recopied and circulated as a print in the eighteenth century. The title alludes to the false tradition that Galen had become a Christian. Private Collection. Compare also *Figs 1.2, 2.1*, and *7.1.*

He did not lack experience of the interior of the human body, as his supporters in the sixteenth century were quick to point out. But dealing with sprains, fractures, wounds and necroses would have taken him only so far, and he was well aware of the limits of what could be done with human subjects alone. The best one could hope for was 'chance' or 'empirical' anatomy, the opportunity to inspect a corpse washed from a tomb damaged in a flood or that of a brigand killed by his intended victim and left by the roadside to be stripped clean by birds.[67] These were rare occurrences, and he criticises severely as knowing no more than chefs those army doctors who failed to take advantage of a massive defeat of the invading Germans in the 170s to look at the insides of dead warriors.[68] But chance by itself was not enough, for one needed continued familiarity to identify and recall the structures one saw, and operating as a surgeon, especially on the battlefield or, more often, when dealing with corpses of condemned criminals or those killed in the arena, did not always allow time for a careful inspection.[69] *Faute de mieux*, one had to dissect animals, choosing where possible those most like humans and extrapolating carefully from them to the human body.[70] Galen relied most often on monkeys, but also used dogs, sheep, pigs, and, particularly when dealing with such small structures as the hyoid bone or the interior of the brain, large animals such as cattle.[71] On one famous occasion, he had the opportunity to examine the heart of a recently killed elephant to see if it contained a bone, but although he and his many colleagues could discover its presence by feel, he was persuaded by them not to proceed with an actual dissection in the face of dissenting opponents. Instead he sent an experienced colleague to beg the emperor's cooks, who had removed the heart, to allow him to take out the bone. Having done so, he presented it to Galen, who kept it as a souvenir.[72] Galen was not to know that in elderly elephants the fibrous triangles separating the atria and the ventricles often ossify and give the impression of a bone.

Bodily systems

His dissections confirmed him in his conviction that Plato and, before him, Hippocrates were correct in their belief in a body that was made alive by the presence of a soul distributed among its three major organs, namely the liver, the heart and the brain, each of which had its own near-separate system of conduits.[73] Although at first he thought that each organ was formed simultaneously in the foetus, he later came to believe that the liver developed first.[74] He thus rejected the view of the primacy of the heart as advocated by Aristotle and the Stoics, reserving much scorn in the opening books of *The Opinions of Hippocrates and Plato* for the cardiocentric views of the Stoic Chrysippus and especially for his ignorance of anatomy.[75]

In Galenic theory the liver was responsible for nutrition. In it, 'digested' or 'concocted' food received from the stomach and intestines, like a city receiving food along roads from the countryside, was turned into nutritious blood, which was then transported via the veins to provide the essential nutriment for the whole body, like water flowing through conduits in a garden.[76] This nutritious venous blood, produced in the flesh of the liver, was taken up into the various parts of the body as each required.[77] Some of the venous blood that reached the right side of the heart then passed through perforations in the interventricular septum to the left side, where it met air coming from the lungs via the pulmonary vein. Galen was aware that the pulmonary artery carried blood from the heart to the lungs and that some of this blood returned in the pulmonary vein, but he seems to have regarded this means of transit as secondary to that via the septum.[78] He may have been strengthened in this belief by his discovery that in the foetus there is a direct connection between the two sides of the heart via the *ductus arteriosus* and the *foramen ovale*, which closes at birth, and by his correct observation of pittings within the actual septum. It would have been simple for Galen to conclude that one connection replaced the other after birth, although he himself never states this explicitly.[79] Similarly, although he accepted Erasistratus' view that the arterial and venous systems were linked by invisible capillaries, he considered that they allowed only for the transfer of a small amount of nutritious venous blood and refined air, *pneuma*, between the two systems, and were fully opened only in unusual or abnormal circumstances.[80] Although Galen provided much of the anatomical data upon which, fifteen centuries later, in 1628, William Harvey was to base his theory of the circulation of the blood, Galen's own discoveries in no way entailed that conclusion and could be easily explained on the basis of his own physiological theories.[81] Given his conviction that the functions of his three Platonic systems were separate, Galen was hardly likely to have searched diligently for a means to unify two of the three into a single circulation of the blood.[82]

According to Galen, the mixture of blood and *pneuma* in the left side of the heart was then further concocted by the heat of the heart to produce a thinner, red blood that then flowed within the arteries to energise or vivify the body by its 'vital spirit'.[83] That the arteries contained blood was the theme of another of his anatomical demonstrations, designed to confute the Erasistrateans, who thought that they contained only *pneuma*.[84] As with venous blood, a small proportion of this arterial blood was passed on for further refining, which took place in a vascular network, the *rete mirabile*, at the base of the brain where a 'psychic *pneuma*' was produced that circulated in the ventricles of the brain and throughout the nervous system.[85] Also nourished by air breathed in through the nostrils (shown by the speed at which people died if their air supply was cut off), this 'psychic *pneuma*' was responsible for consciousness, sensation and voluntary movement.[86]

Galen's belief in a tripartite system of vessels and his consequent failure to discover either a significant pulmonary transit of blood or the Harveian circulation has coloured many accounts of Galenic anatomy. Even the sympathetic Margaret Tallmadge May prefaced her assessment of Galen's positive achievements with an equally long account of his errors, notably his placing of the kidneys with the right higher than the left (which is true of the ape) and his description of the thyroid cartilage as if it were that of a pig. He misunderstood how tendons are formed, and his description of a channel leading from the infundibulum of the brain to the palate seems to have been wishful thinking. But many of his errors were shared with Aristotle, Herophilus and Erasistratus, to say nothing of other anonymous writers.[87]

These mistakes can be balanced by the discoveries to which Galen lays claim. His descriptions of many of the bones of the body would be acceptable today, and his errors in his reports of the heart and vascular system are far more the result of working with animals and of mistaken interpretation than of incompetent dissection. His studies of the nerves and muscles are remarkably accurate, especially given that they were performed without modern aids and involved at times structures that are hard to see with the naked eye. He made important discoveries concerning the ducts of the sublingual glands, the Achilles tendon (although his description more closely resembles the tendon in monkeys) and the muscles of the face. He was also prepared to change his views if presented with new anatomical evidence.[88] The muscles that flex the first joint of each finger and toe, the *musculi interossei*, were for a long while unknown to him, but he describes them at length in books from the mid-160s onwards, including *The Anatomy of Muscles, The Use of Parts* and *Anatomical Procedures.*[89]

Observation and experiment

Particularly impressive both in their methodology and in their results are his dissections involving the brain and the nervous system. In a complex series of experiments, he traced the pathways of the nerves from inside the brain and down the spinal cord, ligating and cutting the spinal cord at each vertebra to discover just what effect would thus be produced. The sudden cessation of a very loud noise from a pig when the nerves and muscles that produced vocalisation were tied or cut, and its equally noisy resumption when a ligature had been removed, provided an immediately understandable proof of the correctness of his ideas.[90] He contrasted the common experience at public sacrifices when one might see the animal on the altar not only breathing and bellowing but even trying to escape before dying from lack of blood with the immediate cessation of movement, breath and vocalisation when the neck of the bull is cut at the first vertebra. (The heart and arteries continue to pulsate a little longer.)[91] His own series of dissections of the neck, alluded to here, firmly established the interrelationship of nerves and structures in articulating the cartilages of the throat, as well as the chronological order of the movements involved in swallowing. In the four books of *The Voice* he extended his investigations to voice production and to explaining the reasons behind different types of vocalisation.[92] He was particularly proud of his discovery of the recurrent laryngeal nerves, whose complicated paths he traced from the point of branching from the vagus nerve to the larynx.[93] These were not random findings, but part of a sustained and coherent research programme, to use a modern term: Galen identified interesting problems, and then devised appropriate means to resolve them.

These results depended on two complementary skills, Galen's experimentalism and his powers of observation and description, best appreciated by those who, like Wynfrid Duckworth and Julius Rocca, themselves repeated some of his dissections. Both scholars found his *Anatomical Procedures* to be a remarkable textbook of dissection, for in it Galen gives clear instructions on how to dissect and observe what has been revealed, as well as what to avoid. One should obtain ox brains from a butcher and use a strong chisel or an axe made of hard iron (soft iron becomes useless after a few blows) to remove any excessive bone from the skull, taking care not to damage the brain by repeated blows, for a fresh bovine brain is a delicate structure.[94] One is told exactly how to cut, and, more importantly for the neophyte, what one should be looking out for. For example, if one holds a dissected portion of the dura mater over the cribriform plate up to sunlight, one can see a pattern of tiny holes in some of it, but not throughout.[95] Clarity, accuracy and concision are here combined. Rocca also draws attention to Galen's description of the plexuses in the (ox) brain and particularly the *rete mirabile*, resembling fishermen's nets heaped one on top of the other, which are not always easy to disentangle and thus are best removed all together. He also gives a precise indication of where to look for it. Although scholars have long wondered why Galen believed so strongly in this non-human structure as an essential element in his understanding of the body's three systems, there is no doubt that he had found it described in earlier literature and had himself carefully observed it in ox brains. Since he does not appear to have dissected human brains but, instead, many other animals in which this structure is found, he may well have regarded its absence from apes, and *a fortiori* from humans, as anomalous, if, indeed, he ever dissected the much tinier and more fragile ape brain.[96]

In his experimentalism Galen had a precedent in the work of Erasistratus centuries earlier, whose views on blood flow he challenged by repeating some of his experiments. On at least one occasion Galen inserted a cannula into an artery to see whether pulsation continued beyond the cannula and what happened if the artery was ligated.[97] His erroneous conclusion that pulsation was a movement within the actual walls of the arteries and not the result of blood being forced out from the heart may be excused by the difficulty of performing the experiment without the aid of modern technology. Investigating the movement of the heart and arteries in warm blooded animals is not easy, and William Harvey was enabled to make his discovery of the circulation and of the sequence of cardiac movements only through his many vivisections of cold-blooded creatures, as well as of animals on the point of death when the actual movements of the heart are slowed down.

In another series of experiments, Galen ligated the carotid arteries to see whether this would have any effect on sensation and motion, as some people believed it did. He gave careful instructions about how to lift the vagus nerves clear of the arteries before tying them, and, somewhat against his initial expectations, he discovered that ligation had little or no effect.[98] His conclusion was that it was the nerves coming from the brain, and the psychic substance they contained, that were responsible for sensation and movement rather than the blood supply in the arterial system, a further confirmation of his belief in a tripartite rather than a unitary Aristotelian cardiocentric system. A similar experiment with the ventricles of the brain, pressing down upon them or incising them, also led him to be more precise about their functions in an interesting foreshadowing of the localisation of brain functions.[99] At other times he used experimentation to disprove the theories of others. His experiments on the kidneys and ureters refuted the ideas of Asclepiades by demonstrating that fluid flows in only one direction, downwards.[100] The last part of *Problematical Movements* also shows how a knowledge of the anatomy of the neck and throat, partly obtained through dissecting subjects that have been specially emaciated, can disprove any theory that relies on the assumption that the larynx is moved upwards by the action of the tongue.[101]

Dissection and experiment were clearly passions of Galen, but they had a very practical purpose. Not only did he believe it impossible to diagnose correctly without an understanding of the anatomy of the body, but the two main sites of Galen's experiments, the brain and the heart, were directly linked to major clinical concerns. The former set of dissections confirmed his belief in the crucial interrelationship between mind and body, in both health and illness, as we shall see, and have been generally praised. The latter are harder to appreciate today for two reasons. The development of technical aids in medicine, particularly since the later nineteenth century, has changed the role of pulse-taking, by providing quantitative explanations for phenomena that Galen preferred to explain in qualitative terms that depended on the diagnostic skill and touch of the individual doctor. Today one can see and measure the workings of the heart in ways that Galen could scarcely have imagined. Secondly, and more significant, his understanding of the role of the heart involved a major misunderstanding: Galen believed that he had demonstrated that a major diagnostic feature of illness, the pulse, was not directly related to the heart, but depended on the nature of a property in the walls of the arteries which allowed them to pulsate. The heart processes and transforms venous blood but does not itself pump it out except for a very short distance in the aorta. But this substantial error in his theory of pulsation does not detract from the accuracy of his observations.[102] He is happy to accept the standard categories for describing pulses – their size, strength, speed or frequency, regularity and any hardness or softness – and he takes over many of the familiar metaphorical names for pulses that went back centuries to Herophilus and Aristoxenus (around 200 BCE), such as the gazelle pulse, the mouse-tail pulse, the ant-like pulse, or the double-hammer pulse.[103] These names, which continued in use at least into the early twentieth century, served a valuable diagnostic function: the double-hammer pulse, for instance, was rightly seen by Galen as indicating a life-threatening condition.[104] Typically, however, he sought a greater precision in these descriptions, wondering whether the ratios between pulse beats would not best be expressed in both musical and verbal terms, something suggested long before him by Aristoxenus but not fully developed.[105]

Prognosis and the creation of authority

Where Galen differs from other surviving writers on pulses is in the amount of attention given to what he calls prognosis, a term which for him also encompasses many aspects of diagnosis. Like them, he notes what he calls the natural changes in pulses between old and young, male and female, before and after exercise, after taking a bath or eating a large meal, in different regions and over the seasons, but he goes beyond them, at least in the length of his exposition, in considering the different kinds of pulse in relationship to the causes of disease.[106] Not only does he describe the sort of pulse to be found in a variety of illnesses, from bronchitis and pleurisy to dropsy and even poisoning with hellebore, but also explains how the indications from the pulse reveal not only possible disease conditions, but can also help to predict their outcome.[107] The pulse is the best indicator of the body's own forces and whether they are likely to overcome whatever morbid conditions are afflicting it either as a whole or in a particular part when only the arteries in that region are affected. Many of his observations will have derived from his clinical practice.[108] One, placed at the end of the first section of Book I of *Prognosis from the Pulse*, has a function that goes beyond the straightforwardly medical.[109] By taking the pulse Galen was able to diagnose that his patient, a wealthy man who knew enough about medicine to attempt to treat his own servants, had been taking a drug contrary to Galen's orders, a diagnosis that he maintained even in the face of the man's initial denial. Galen ostensibly uses this story to show that knowledge of the pulse can reveal changes brought about even by drugs, particularly if one is familiar with the habits of the patient, but the language he chooses to describe his consultation carries other implications. The patient is described as contentious, frequently deriding others for their lack of "secure knowledge" (a phrase commonly used by Galen), and unwilling at first to accept Galen's diagnosis, even to the extent of considering lying under oath. Galen thus triumphs over the steadfast refusal of the man to follow his advice, a rare occurrence in his case-histories, for patients usually co-operated with Galen, and their compliance only enhances the image of supreme competence that he wishes to convey.

This story, and others like it in *Prognosis*, neatly exemplify an aspect of prognosis singled out by Tamsyn Barton when she compared it to other methods of forecasting such as astrology or physiognomics.[110] Like his insistence on the precision of his observations and calculations, prognosis is a weapon in a power struggle for authority, in this instance over a recalcitrant patient of wealth and status.[111] Other descriptions of successful cases cured through his prognostic skills often include words like 'amazing' (sometimes put for added effect into the mouths of others), emphasise the high status of the patient, or highlight the incompetence and ignorance of other doctors, sometimes in spectacular fashion.[112] On one occasion, Galen, who had predicted the death of Theagenes if the treatment recommended by his colleague Attalus was not altered, allowed the unsuspecting doctor and his friends, to reach almost to the door of the sick room before the wailing of the mourners apprised them of the death of the patient.[113]

Prognosis, along with anatomy, was one of the skills that Galen emphasised in his struggle to acquire or retain patients. His opponents, and especially the Methodists, derided it as mantic prophecy, the hallmark of the charlatan or magus, but this only showed their ignorance of a Hippocratic text whose author had firmly declared, "I am no prophet".[114] But it was not only Methodists who had forgotten what the Master had said. Even contemporary Hippocratics had abandoned what for Galen was the simple and rational application of a method set out by "our guide to all that is good" in what should have been to them a familiar text, *Prognostics*.[115]

Its author had opened his treatise with a memorable and all-encompassing definition. Prognosis involved a knowledge of everything that had happened, was happening and would happen to the patient in future. It was indeed foreknowledge, but that depended on what the doctor could perceive in his patient and glean from what had happened earlier (although this past history may not have stretched back much before the initial encounter). It also involved understanding the effects of the seasons, climate and locality, and distinguishing good signs from bad.[116] The purpose of prognosis was to predict whether the patient was likely to recover or not, and thus to allow the doctor to inform the patient or any relatives of the potential outcome. Failure in a case pronounced to be fatal, and even a refusal to treat except to offer palliative care, could thus not be blamed on the doctor, while success would only add to his reputation. A knowledge of the future course of a condition brought two further benefits. It allowed the doctor to plan a long-term therapy and, if made public, it could be checked against the actual outcome. The more accurate the prediction, the greater the confidence that might be placed in the individual doctor, and the higher the chances of professional success.

This credo, supplemented by statements in other Hippocratic treatises such as *Aphorisms, Epidemics* and *Airs, Waters and Places*, became Galen's own. Not only did he write extensive commentaries on all these works, but he emphasised throughout his oeuvre the importance of prognosis both as a guide to therapy and as something that set him aside from all his competitors. How far this claim was true is hard to determine. His great predecessor Rufus of Ephesus had accepted that it might be necessary to enquire about what had happened earlier to the patient, such as changes in sleep or eating patterns, and complained that questioning the patient and his attendants was almost a lost art.[117] But neither he nor another writer in the Hippocratic tradition, Aretaeus of Cappadocia, for all their evident abilities as nosographers and clinicians, extended the remit of prognosis as far as Galen. Indeed, Aretaeus, in a nice foreshadowing of Galen's opponents, describes the general amazement on the part of both physicians and family when the ravings of a feverish patient about what he fears will happen to him turn out to be true, since they were regarded as little different from imagined conversations with the dead or the absent.[118]

That there was a debate about the meaning of prognosis among students of Hippocrates is clear from the opening sections of Galen's commentary on *Prognostics.* Some disputed the relationship of the term 'foreknowledge' to other words used in the same passage such as 'forethought' and 'foretelling' or 'prediction'. 'Forethought', πρόνοια, he concludes is used by Hippocrates in an unusual sense, for its normal meanings include taking care (illustrated by a quotation from Euripides' *Hecuba*), and deliberation, especially when used in a legal context. When applied by philosophers to the governance of the world, it is concerned only with its future well-being, but Galen takes this 'providence' to encompass both good and ill.[119] He also rejects as sophistic and unhelpful the distinction, promoted centuries earlier by Herophilus and his followers, between foreknowledge, prognosis, which was secure and resulted in a sure outcome, and the more speculative and fallible 'foretelling'. He himself acknowledged two types of foreknowledge, both of which he illustrated from astronomy. One can know for certain that spring will follow winter, but the statements of the astronomical poet Aratus that this or that appearance of the moon will be followed by a North or South wind do not always come true.[120] What matters for Galen is that the doctor should endeavour to be as accurate as possible in the conclusions he bases on what he has discovered.[121] Like trainers in the gym who can predict the result in a wrestling bout from the very first moves by analysing the strength of the competitors, so a doctor should be able to forecast swiftly the outcome of the struggle between patient and disease. But medical prognoses are not infallible. Nature can get in the way, and one must always add "if all goes according to plan".[122] Patients, as the Hippocratic author knew, do not always reveal everything: they may not know what particular part of the body is affected or the antecedent cause, and even some of the symptoms they perceive they may omit to mention. Events too may wreck an otherwise sound judgment; a house fire, a leaking roof, a flood, an attack by robbers, a worrying message or even noisy neighbours disturbing a patient's sleep may frustrate the cure.[123] All these things hamper the doctor in a search for a sure prognosis, but if he reveals them to the patient and if external circumstances do not conspire against him, the resulting prognosis and the successful outcome of the case will be a source of amazement as well as of increased confidence in him in the future.[124]

One of the most spectacular of Galen's cases is described at length in Book Five of *Affected Parts,* a long treatise in which Galen explains how to diagnose and treat diseases in various parts of the body (*Fig. 1.2*).[125] As in the *Method of Healing*, Galen illustrates his advice with long descriptions of exemplary cases from his own practice, here on the treatment of liver diseases. After a brief account of his treatment of Stesianus for an abscess deep in the muscles of the abdomen, wrongly diagnosed as a liver abscess, and an attack on Empiricists and Methodists for calling themselves "champions of medical theory" although they neither listen to the patient nor bother to palpate, he describes a case from his first Roman stay that convinced at least one person of the merits of Galenic medicine.[126] I translate the passage in full because its sentiments, as well as the language used, give a remarkable impression of Galen at his best and, one might also argue, his worst in the competition for patients. He uses his remarkable powers of observation not only to discover what was wrong but also to reveal what the patient himself believed was wrong, and what sensations he felt, in order to create an impression of the superiority of Galen to any competitor.

On meeting me in the street the philosopher Glaucon said my appearance was timely. Putting his hand in mine, he went on, "We are near the invalid I have just been to see, and I invite you to come with me and see him. He's the doctor from Sicily whom you saw a few days ago walking with me." "Well, what's the matter with him?", I said. He then gave me a very clear and well-ordered account, for he was incapable of dissimulation or stupidity. "Besides", he said, "Ever since Gorgias and Apelas told me yesterday of your diagnoses and prognoses that seem to be more the result of mantic prophecy than medicine, I have been eager to carry out a test for myself, not so much of you personally but of the medical art, to see whether it can make such diagnoses and prognoses." He was still talking when we reached the sick man's door, so I could not respond verbally to his challenge or explain what you all know I say frequently, namely that definite signs are fortunately sometimes visible, but sometimes everything is ambiguous and we require a second or even a third examination.

Just as we were going in. a servant met us bringing a small chamber pot from the sick room to the toilet which contained a thin, bloody liquid like the watery fluid from a freshly slaughtered beast, an absolutely certain sign of liver disease. Pretending not to notice this, I came with Glaucon to the patient and put my hand on his wrist, wanting to know if there was actually some inflammation or merely a lack of tone. The invalid, as I have said, was a doctor, who said that he had just returned to bed after an evacuation, and so his pulse rate had increased because of standing up. As he was saying this, I discovered an indication of inflammation. Spying a little pot on the windowsill containing hyssop prepared in honey-wine, I concluded that the doctor thought he was suffering from pleurisy since he had a pain underneath the false ribs, which sometimes occurs in liver inflammations. Since this is what he felt and was taking frequent short breaths, as well as being troubled by tiny coughs, I posited that he thought he had pleurisy, and so had prepared some hyssop in honey-wine. Seeing that Fortune had given me a way to impress Glaucon, I put his hand on the right side of the patient's false ribs, and pointing to the spot, said that that was just where he felt pain.[127] When he agreed, Glaucon was clearly amazed since he supposed that my diagnosis of the place affected had been made simply from taking the pulse. To astound him still further, I added, "Since, you have already agreed that it hurts here, tell me also if you have an urge to cough, and if you have little dry coughs at quite long intervals but without expectoration. As I was talking, I chanced to notice him have a similar cough to what I had just described, with the result that Glaucon was greatly amazed, and could not stop himself from emitting a loud paean of praise. "Please don't think", I said, "that our art is capable of making prophecies like this about the sick or about what I'm going to tell you now, which the doctor will confirm." I began to address him again. "When you take a big breath, you feel a pain where I showed you, and it is getting worse, and you also feel as if a heavy weight was lying on top of your lower hypochondrium." At this the patient could no longer keep quiet but joined Glaucon in shouting out his amazement. Realising my good luck, I wanted to comment about the drawing down of his clavicle, but aware that this often followed some substantial inflammation there, as in scirrhus, I had not the confidence to announce this, afraid that it would destroy some of the plaudits I had already gained. So, I decided to make a safe choice of words, and so, looking at the patient, I said, "Very soon you're going to feel your collarbone being drawn downwards a little, unless you already have had this sensation."

> When the patient agreed with this and I saw he was absolutely amazed, "There is just one more prophecy", I said, "to add to what I have already said: I am going to tell you what the patient suspects is the ailment that is troubling him". Glaucon declared that he could not now fail to believe in even this prophecy, while the patient, awestruck at the marvellous nature of my promise, gave me a searching look as he attended to what I was going to say. When I declared that he believed it was pleurisy that was troubling him, he confirmed this, utterly amazed, and not only him, but also the servant who only a little while earlier had applied warm oil to him as if he had pleurisy. Ever since then Glaucon had the highest opinion of me and of the art of medicine, whereas formerly he did not think there was much to it, because he had never previously made the acquaintance of excellent practitioners well trained in the art.

This lengthy case history is not explicitly designed to teach the art of prognosis – the word 'to prognose' appears only twice in the narrative, both times put into the mouth of others – but to instruct his audience, already familiar with the theoretical underpinnings of such cases, how they too can perform successfully in any situation, even one that happens by chance. Nonetheless, Galen here displays to the full his powers of observation, of things as well as people, and fulfils the conditions laid down in the opening section of Hippocrates' *Prognostic*. Not only does he predict the course of the disease, but he convinces both Glaucon and the patient of his ability by revealing things that have occurred earlier or are believed by them to be taking place, even though they are not necessarily true. Only after this elaborate exposition does he reveal to the patient his own diagnosis of liver disease. The link with prognosis is also indicated in the language used by Galen, for throughout he uses words for forecasting that elsewhere he rejects completely: "mantic prophecy", "being a prophet", "miraculous", and several instances of "amazing". In *Prognosis*, for example, he derides those who use these terms for what to him is a rational deduction from observed phenomena on Hippocratic principles.[128] Here he uses the terms in order to go along with the beliefs of Glaucon and the doctor-patient, just as he is willing to accept their false beliefs in the nature of the symptoms and, even more, in the apparent derivation of the diagnosis simply from the taking of the pulse. Both Galen and his intended readership already know that the examination of the pulse is only one element, and not necessarily the crucial one, in reaching a diagnosis of this sort. But whether this is viewed as prognosis or prophecy, the result is the same: the praise and glory of the practitioner.

Galen's understanding of human psychology, evident here, features prominently in other stories of prognosis. As he argued at the end of his life in *The Soul's Behaviour depends on the Mixtures of the Body*, no matter what philosophical position one takes about the soul, whether one is a Platonist, an Aristotelian or a Stoic, it is universally accepted that at times one's behaviour is affected by what one has eaten, drunk or done. Too much wine makes one drunk, too much food sluggish, too much exercise over-tired. Galen turns this truism on its head to argue that conversely one's thoughts and emotions have a direct effect on the body. Standing on a mountain ledge makes one's legs tremble, and any exposure to what we would term stress can have physical consequences. A long section in his commentary on *Epidemics VI* also provides a series of examples of the possible fatal consequences of grief, fear and other emotional stresses.[129] The mother of the lawyer Nasutus died suddenly after hearing of the death of an old friend, a bird diviner Maeandrus was terrified by the omens that he believed he had seen of his own death, and a man fell ill through sleeplessness because he dreamed that he was bearing on his shoulders the weight of the world that Atlas had passed to him.[130] Several cases described in *Prognosis* are similarly designed to show off Galen's skill in understanding the relationship of body and mind: the son of Boethus scared that his forbidden food might be revealed, a slave steward afraid of a mistake in his accounts, and the wife of Justus, wasting away through love for an actor (*Fig. 1.2*).[131] But, contrary to general belief, and despite famous examples in literature and history from Sappho onwards, Galen derides the notion that there are specific pulses associated with love, arguing that changes in the pulse are the result of stress in general, rather than of one type in particular.[132]

Women and the limits of observation

In interpreting his at times remarkable observations, whether of anatomy, patients or the world around him, Galen displays considerable learning, both medical and non-medical, as well as a near-impeccable logic, and it is no wonder that he gained such a great reputation and his high positions. But there is one area of medicine and medical activity about which he says relatively little: women. This is not surprising, for many women in Antiquity would be treated in the first instance by other women with a certain amount of medical experience, *maiai* or *medicae*.[133] Along with children, they form only a small percentage of his cases, often where Galen has been specially called in when others have failed.[134] Social constraints and prejudices also will have played a part in this. Even the most important ancient writer on gynaecology, Soranus of Ephesus, although giving very detailed instructions to the *maiai* and nurses whom he expected to be responsible for almost all aspects of the care of women and very young children, wrote his tract primarily to inform men, anticipating that it would be the male doctor who would intervene when things become difficult.[135] Galen's early (but later revised) tract on the anatomy of the womb, written at the request of a midwife, is unusual in having a female recipient.[136] Although Galen makes some interesting observations, for example about the differences between male and female breasts, his relative lack of experience with female patients means that there are many gaps and errors in his accounts, not least of foetal development, where he displays many uncertainties and changes of mind. His anatomy of a womb with cotyledons is that of a ruminant, and his description of diseases of the uterus is concerned with those of the vagina and cervix rather than with what today would be considered common uterine conditions. On the other hand, he does seem to have altered some of his comments over the years in the light of his dissection of female animals, including some of pregnant goats.[137] It should also be remembered that for centuries after Galen there were always fewer opportunities to dissect female bodies, and that it was not until the seventeenth and eighteenth centuries that accurate description of the internal female body became at all common. He himself shows a fair acquaintance with the earlier literature, but this is an area where his own observations play only a minor role.

In a society where women's roles were largely confined to the home, and where political, economic and social power were almost always in the hands of men, it is hardly surprising that Galen should believe that it was childbirth and the womb that most distinguished women from men. He is clear that they were equally human and, in contradiction to Aristotle, rational beings and capable of acquiring knowledge, but, at the same time, he can dismiss their testimony, like that of the poets, as worthless in philosophical discussion, and their contributions to medicine as 'old wives' tales' or rambling and inconsequential.[138] It is not only individual women who attract Galen's disdain. Their whole somatic economy, to use Rebecca Flemming's term, differed from that of the male.[139] Galenic humoral medicine allowed for a variety of bodily types, but it assumed the male body and the male character to be superior. Nature had adapted the female body for bearing children and to fit the character of the soul that inhabited it. There was thus no need for women to have beards, since they do not possess the august character of men and require less protection from the cold because they usually stay indoors. Their body is also colder and moister, which makes them more susceptible to diseases that are cold and wet, as well as to specifically women's diseases related to their reproductive system.[140] This predisposition also determines the sort of therapy that they should be given. They should be treated gently, but not because they are female *tout court* but because they share the same position on the spectrum of hardness and softness as children, eunuchs and men who are passionately addicted to the baths. They are as far removed from Galen's average man as he is from tough peasants and sailors, and their lifestyle also protects them from the deleterious consequences of such male activities as over-exercise in the gymnasium.[141]

Galen's own prejudices and experiences, and, not least, his debt to the Hippocratic writings and to a long tradition of Hippocratic interpretation, will also have influenced his ideas and his attitude towards his female patients.[142] With one very dubious exception, his references to his association with women are at best neutral and often dismissive.[143] Even if he is prepared to accept information from skilled midwives, they are his subordinates who must follow his orders exactly. He is scathing about the pampered lifestyle of rich Roman women, who cannot stand the smell of a hair pomade made of oil and pitch and, so he claims, if they do try it, may even die because of its powerful chilling effects.[144] But he is still willing to provide suitable cosmetic recipes for the benefit of those who have to attend the court, emperors as well as their female relations.[145] The example of his mother, always angry and emotional, must also have influenced him from his earliest years, and, if she was still alive at the time, this may have further encouraged him to move away from Pergamum for most of his medical education. A quotation ascribed to Galen and preserved in several Arabic writers, if it is genuine, may introduce a further personal element. Galen is said to have compared falling in love to the chance meeting of two individuals on the same highway. Had they not been on the same road, they would not have met. But what woman would have been considered by Galen a worthy traveller along the same intellectual highway?[146] Galen's reflections on women are perhaps the weakest section in all his writings, partly through his ignorance of feminine matters and partly because of preconceptions, both medical and societal, that he shared with many other doctors. But even here, he gives evidence of his powers of observation and, as with his account of foetal development or his account of the womb, his willingness to modify some of his views as a consequence.[147]

Throughout his writings, he reports things that others did not see, or, if they did, their accounts have not come down to us. He is insatiably curious, and he always tries to integrate what he observes into the wider intellectual picture, and to relate it to his medical and philosophical projects. As some of the examples in this chapter also show, he is often capable of an effective rhetorical presentation, whether in writing or in his remembered (or imagined) conversations with others, but it is accurate observation above all, in anatomy and in prognosis, that is his most effective weapon in the power-struggle with his rivals and, at times, with his patients. One can only agree with so many of his interlocutors that it was indeed marvellous.

Notes

1 Friedländer 1862–71.
2 *San.Tu.* III,2: 6,180 K; p. 261 tr. Johnston; *UP* III,16: 3,262 K, cf. I,17: 3,48 K; I, p. 202, p. 91 tr. May, but without the comparison; *Loc.Aff.* VI,3: 8,397 K; p. 176 tr. Siegel, probably the rose-coloured starling, Arnott 2007: 213–4.
3 Respectively, *Purg.Med.Fac.* 4: 11,336 K; *Alim.Fac.* II,1: 6,663 and 666 K; *Subf.Emp.* 10: 75–6 Deichgräber; pp. 39–41 tr. Frede, with the later version at *SMT* XI,1,1: 12,312–3 K.
4 *MM* XIV,16: 14,998–9 K; III, pp. 503–5 tr. Johnston-Horsley; for buyers' responses, *Hipp. Epid. VI*, iii,30: *CMG* V 10,2,2, 168.
5 *Temp.* III,2: 1,657 K; p. 163 tr. Singer PN; for another Pergamene story, *Loc.Aff.* II,10: 8,132 K; p. 69 tr. Siegel.
6 *SMT* IX,3,8; 11; 21; 34: 12,214, 219–20, 226–7, 238–40 K.
7 *MM* V,7: 14,334–5 K; II, p. 45 tr. Johnston-Horsley.
8 *UP* I,24: 3,80 K; I, p. 110 tr. May, with n. 73. The comparison goes back at least to Aristotle, *Parts of Animals* IV,10: 687b17–20.
9 *SMT* IX,1,2: 12,169–75 K; Harig 1987–8; Hasluck and Hasluck 1929: 671–88, report on the continuation of the practice into the early twentieth century. Photos-Jones *et al.* 2017, forthcoming, noting the remarkable precision of his language here and in his account of the Cypriot mines offer a scientific hypothesis for the anti-bacterial properties of the Lemnian earth.
10 Galen implies he arrived by chance at the time of the festival, which would have taken place over several days, but given his expressed wish to see the ceremony, this seems unlikely.
11 Cf. his location of the mines he saw at Ergasteria (the Greek word for 'mines'), "some 450 stades (ninety kilometres) from Pergamum on the road to Cyzicus", *SMT* IX,3,22: 12,230 K; and for a particular type of medicinal water on Lesbos, "forty stades from Mytilene", *MM* XIV,15: 10,996 K; III, p. 501 tr. Johnston-Horsley. For death from fumes, *UP* VII,8: 3,540 K; I, p. 346 tr. May.
12 Martelli 2012: 133; see also 139–42, for Galen's acquaintance with oriental languages, evident in his careful transcription of the words. The Syriac version is translated in Afif *et al.* 2018.
13 *Diff.Puls.* II,5: 8,583–7 K, not necessarily a complaint about Latin; see also Petit 2018: 44–54.
14 Respectively, *Alim.Fac.* I,13: 6,514–6 K; pp. 53–4 tr. Powell; *Ant.* I,10: 14,53 K; *Alim.Fac.* II,68: 6,656–7 K; p. 113 tr. Powell.
15 *Alim.Fac.* II,20: 6,594 K; p. 86 tr. Powell; *San.Tu.* IV,8: 6,287 K; I, p. 417 tr. Johnston; Wilkins in Powell 2003: xvi–xviii. Cf. the long discussion of the length and timing of months around the Mediterranean, *Hipp.Epid.I* 1: 17A,2–4 K; *Hipp.Epid.II*, vi,9: *CMG Suppl.Or.* V 2, 827–31, and the Pergamene name for a locust-eating bird, above, note 2.
16 Until the appearance of the long-promised edition by Gotthard Strohmaier, one must use sections preserved in Oribasius, the Hebrew summary in Wasserstein 1982, and information provided by Dr Strohmaier in Liewert 2015: 89–106.
17 *San.Tu.* V,9: 6,424 K; II, p. 177, tr. Johnston; *CMG* V 4,2, 186. For Allianoi, see above, p. 8; for Lakettoi or Laketta, Jones CP 2012: 407.
18 *SMT* X,5,9: 12,272 K; IV,20: 11,693 K; for the more common cold spring, *Comp.Med.Loc.* II,1: 12,508 K.
19 *Hipp.AWP* G.36: p. 53 Wasserstein, who calls it the Aqua Damnata. Dr. Strohmaier in his forthcoming edition rightly prefers Aqua Domitiana, to be identified with the mineral spring at Vigarello, N. of Rome.
20 *Hipp.Epid.VI*, iv,11: 17B,159 K; *Alim.Fac.* III,29: 6,722–3 K; pp. 140–1 tr. Powell.

21 *Temp.* II,6: 1,630 K; p. 142 tr. Singer PN.
22 *Bon.Mal.Suc.* 1: 6,749–50 K; Petit 2018: 141–5.
23 *Alim.Fac.* II,21: 6,597 K ; p. 87 tr. Powell; I,14: 6,523 K; p. 56 tr. Powell.
24 *SMT* X,2,22: 12,299 K.
25 *Bon.Mal.Suc.* 1: 6,749–50 K.
26 *Nat.Fac.* I,14: 2,55–6 K; p. 87 tr. Brock. Cf. *UP* IV,1–2: 3,267 K; I, p. 204 tr. May, stones, dirt, and foreign seeds should be removed before carriers take it from the tax office to the communal bakery.
27 *Alim.Fac.* I,37: 6,553 K; pp. 69–70 tr. Powell. But cf. *MM* X,2: 10,668 K; III, p. 13 tr. Johnston-Horsley, praise of peasants in the mountains who learn from nature and, when they are on the mend after fever, eat hearty meals; *MM* XII,8: 10,865 K; III, p. 309 tr. Johnston-Horsley, a farmhand observed by Galen with a successful dietary remedy for his colic.
28 *Vict.Att.* 32: p. 64 Marinone; p. 310 tr. Singer PN.
29 *Alim.Fac.* I,13: 6,519 K; p. 55 tr. Powell.
30 *Vict.Att.* 44: p. 70 Marinone; p. 312 tr. Singer PN; *Alim.Fac.* I,13: 6,514 K; p. 53 tr. Powell
31 *Alim.Fac.* I,13: 6,514–6 K; p. 53 tr. Powell.
32 *San.Tu.* IV,7: 6,282 K; II, p. 411, tr. Johnston; *Ant.* I,14: 14,76 K, with the emendation of Jones CP, 2012: 403. For another type of 'parsley' from the Amanus range in Syria, *SMT* VIII,32: 6,128 K; for other exports from the region, *Hipp.Epid. VI*, iv: *CMG* V 10,1, 340.
33 *Alim.Fac.* I,11: 6,507 K; p. 50 tr. Powell.
34 *Ant.* I,4: 14,23–4 K. Jones CP, 2012: 408, noting that Strabo and Pliny call the district Abrettene, suggests that the name should be emended to Abrēttos. For cytisus, André 1985: 85.
35 *Bon.Mal.Suc.* 11: 6,800 K; *Ant.* I,5: 14,28 K; *MM* XII,4: 10,830–6 K; III, pp. 255–61 tr. Johnston-Horsley; *HVA* III,7: 15,645 K, with the readings at *CMG* V 9,1, 228; *Vict.Att.* 102; p. 104 Marinone; pp. 320–1 tr. Singer PN.
36 *Dig.Puls.* I,1: 8,774 K; *Ant.* I,5: 14,28 K.
37 *Hipp.Epid. VI*, iv,11: 17B,164 K; *Ant.* I,4: 14,21 K.
38 *Ant.* I,3: 14,14–18 K; Jacques 1996, 1999.
39 *Ant.* I,2: 14,9 K (possibly from near Cumae, Pliny, *Nat. Hist.* 14,70; Juvenal, Sat. 9,56); *Ant.* I,3: 14,19–20 K; Jacques 1996: 174–7.
40 *SMT* V,6: 11,724 K.
41 See the Introductions to the edition by Wilkins 2013 and the English translations by Grant M 2000 and Powell 2003.
42 *Bon.Mal.Suc.* 1,1–7: 6,749–52 K. These tracts are respectively 6,749–815 K; better text in *CMG* V 4,2, 389–429; 6,816–31 K; better text in *CMG* V 4,2, 455–63; tr. Grant M 2000: 62–7; *CMG* V 4,2, 433–51; better text in Marinone 1963: tr. Singer PN.
43 *Vict.Att.* 114–17; 56–8; 96: pp. 110–2, 76–8, 98 Marinone; pp. 323–4, 315, 320–1 tr. Singer PN.
44 *Vict.Att.* 112, 102: pp. 110, 104, Marinone; pp. 322, 321 tr. Singer PN.
45 *UP* 13,8: 4,114 K; II, p. 605 tr. May.
46 *Hipp.Epid. VI*, vii: *CMG* V 10,2,2, 393.
47 Stern 1956: 93–4; Walzer 1962: 152–3. *Mor.* I: pp. 25–6 Kraus; pp. 136–7 Singer; *Hipp. Epid. VI*, viii: *CMG* V 10,2,2, 465, for a comparison with animals to show different developments between and within species over time.
48 *Mor.* III,1: p. 42 Kraus; p. 160–1 tr. Davies; cf. Plato, *Phaedrus* 253c–254c. But given this is an Arabic version, the breed of animal may have been changed to fit the new context.
49 Stern 1956: 94–5 (not in Singer PN 2013).
50 A similarly detailed description of a falcon building its nest is ascribed to Galen by al-Mas'ūdī, tr. Barbier de Meynard 1861–77: II,33.
51 Von Staden 1989: 158–62. Cf. also Skoda 1987; King H 1998; Wee 2017.
52 Frede 2003; Petit 2018: 170–86, noting religious metaphors in his descriptions of the body as well as his emphasis on the beauty and purpose of divine creation.
53 Lloyd 1983: 149–67. Soranus of Ephesus also wrote a similar work, now lost, entitled *The Etymologies of the Body of the Human Being*, Orion, *Etymology* 34,9.
54 Modern editions of the shorter tracts by Garofalo and Debru 2005, 2008; English versions by Singer C 1952; Goss 1961, 1963, 1966.

55 *Lib.Prop.* 8,4: 19,33 K; p. 158 BM, with her note, p. 209; p. 15 tr. Singer PN. Dissection of a human corpse seems to have stopped within a few years of the death of Herophilus.

56 Ormos 1993 provides a summary of his edition.

57 Celsus, *Medicine, Proem.*, 40–44.

58 Soranus, *Gynaecology*. I,5.

59 Gleason 2009.

60 *AA* I,3 and VII,11: 2,227, 625 K; pp. 6, 189 tr. Singer C; *Lib.Prop.* 3,15 and 40; pp. 144, 154 BM.

61 *Lib.Prop.* 1,7–10: 19,13–4 K; p. 138 BM; pp. 5–6 tr. Singer PN.

62 Nutton 2012d; Petit 2018.

63 *Lib.Prop.* 1,10: 19,14 K; p. 138 BM, with her note, p. 206; p. 5 tr. Singer PN. See also Boudon-Millot 2018: 305–6. For the different circumstances of dissection, *AA* VIII,4: 2,672–3 K; p. 210 tr. Singer C.

64 Craik 2015: 27–9, 53–6, 119–25, 224–30.

65 *Lib.Prop.* 1,8: 19,13 K; p. 138 BM; p. 5 tr. Singer PN.

66 If, as he implies, many of his treatises were taken down from his commentary during his dissections, the context would have added to his apparent egocentricity, for he would have had little opportunity during the actual dissection to refer to the work of others.

67 *AA* I,2: 2,221, 223 K; III,6: 2,385–6 K, also adding the bodies of exposed infants; pp. 4–5, 77 tr. Singer C.

68 *Comp.Med.Gen.* III,2: 13,604 K; *AA* III,6: 2,385 K; p. 77 tr. Singer C.

69 *AA* I,2 and III,6: 2,223–4, 385 K; pp. 4, 77 tr. Singer C; *Comp.Med.Gen.* III,2: 13,609 K. Although implying that such occasions might be frequent, he distances himself from such participation.

70 *AA* IV,2–3 and VI,3: 2,422–30, 548–9 K; pp. 94–8, 151 tr. Singer C, for an Aristotelian *scala naturae*, starting from the "perfect ape".

71 *Mot.Dub.* 11,19–22, with the note at Nutton and Bos 2011: 360–2. At *AA* VI,1: 2,537 K; p. 149 tr. Singer C, Galen claims to have dissected not just mammals, but, birds, fish and things that crawl on legs or on the abdomen, but not ants, gnats, fleas and other tiny creatures, whose internal structures would be too small to be of value in understanding teleology. See also *AA* XV,2: pp. 227 8 Dkw; p. 1090 Garofalo; *PHP* VI,5,9: 5,540 K; *CMG* V 4,1,2, 391. For Praxagoras, fl. 320 BC, Lewis 2017, esp. pp. 215–22.

72 *AA* VII,10: 2,619–20 K; p. 187 tr. Singer C; Hankinson 1988.

73 Plato in the *Republic* and *Timaeus* had located the third part of the soul in the gut or lower abdomen, "near the liver", but by Galen's time it appears that many Platonists had placed it in the liver, see below, p. 95, notes 54–5.Typically, Galen twice raises the possibility that there is a fourth source of power in the testicles, *Ars Med.* 5: 1,319 K; p. 351 tr. Singer PN; *MMG* II,4: 11,97 K; p. 485 tr. Johnston. Trompeter 2018 discusses the interconnections between the three organs, which Galen, *UP* VI,18: 3,501 K; I, p. 326 tr. May, regards as essential if the three organs are to heed and communicate with one another.,

74 For his earlier view, *Sem.* I,8,9–10: 4,541 K; and for the later, *Foet.Form.* 3: 4,662–72 K; pp. 181–6 tr. Singer PN; *Prop.Plac.* 11: *CMG* V 3,2, 90–2, with my commentary on pp. 177–9; pp. 182–3 BMP; pp. 102–9 Garofalo-Lami; pp. 206–9 Vegetti, with Debru 1995b, Rosen 2017: 288–95.

75 Tieleman 1996.

76 *HNH* II,6: 15,145 K. At *Part.Hom.Diff.* 4,4: *CMG Suppl. Or.* II, 60–61, the simile applies also to the veins and nerves; cf. also *UP* IX,7: 3,708 K; I, p. 436 tr. May.

77 *PHP* VI,3,7 and 4,6–12: 5,521, 534–5 K; *CMG* V 4,1,2, 375, 385–7.

78 Harris CRS 1973: 333–8.

79 *Ven.Art.Diss.* 10: 2,828 K; p. 365 tr. Goss; *UP* VI,21: 3,509 K; XV,6: 4,243–6 K; I, p. 331, II, pp. 669–72 tr. May. Galen claims no credit for this discovery, and others, like Lycus, *Lib. Prop.* 4,37: p. 153 BM, had investigated the foetus before him.

80 *Nat.Fac.* II,6: 2,105 K; p. 165 tr. Brock; *UP* VI,10; VII,3; and 8: 3,455, 521, 539 K; I, pp. 303, 337–8, 345 tr. May.

81 Harris CRS 1973: 2–3, 268; Debru 2008a.

82 Debru 2008a: 272, rightly warns that Galen's own tripartition is more hesitant and inconsistent in its details than in later Galenism; cf. his uncertainties discussed in *Problematical Movements.*

83 Both the stomach and the hot heart were perceived by Galen as cooking organs, changing the qualities of the material originally presented to them.
84 *Art.Sang.*: 4,703–36 K; Furley and Wilkie 1984: 144–83.
85 Although the *rete mirabile* is not found in humans, it appears in ungulates, which Galen dissected (Rocca 2002, 2003) and was given its name by Herophilus or one of his followers (T. 121 Von Staden). See also below, note 99.
86 Temkin 1977: 154–63, points out that Galen referred only rarely to a 'zotic *pneuma*' and only once, and very tentatively, to 'nutritive *pneuma*'. Trompeter 2018, argues for an upwards communication via blood, pneuma, and innate heat from the liver to the heart and thence to the brain, allowing changes in the lower organs to influence the behaviour of the rational soul.
87 May 1968: 40–2. See below, pp. 147–9, for Vesalius and his later criticism of Galen.
88 May 1968: 42, a preliminary list.
89 *UP* II,3; III,10: 3,96 and 225 K; I, pp. 117–8, 182–3 tr. May; *Musc.Diss.* 20,7: 18B,953–4 K; *AA* I,9: 2,266 K; p. 24 tr. Singer C.
90 *AA* IX,12–3: pp. 20–4 Dkw; pp. 845–54 Garofalo; *Praec.* 5,18–19: 14,628–9 K; *CMG* V 8,1, 96–9.
91 *PHP* II,445–8: 5,239 K; *CMG* V 4,1,2, 126–9. He also often saw in sacrifices hearts being removed from animals while they were still alive, *MM* II,6: 10,121 K; I, p. 189 tr. Johnston-Horsley.
92 Baumgarten 1962; Nutton, forthcoming 2, gives an improved text of *De voce*, arguing that it represents extracts taken in order from the genuine lost work.
93 *AA* XIV,6: pp. 203–8 Dkw; pp. 1062–8 Garofalo.
94 *AA* IX,1: 2,708–9 K; p. 794 Garofalo; p. 227 tr. Singer C. Rocca 2008: 247–53, discusses the problems of performing such dissections and experiments.
95 *AA* IX,7: p. 5 Dkw; p. 831 Garofalo.
96 *AA* VIII,9: 2,696–7 K; p. 221 tr. Singer C; *PHP* VII,3,23–9: 5,606–8 K; *CMG* V 4,1,2, 445–7. Rocca 2003: 202–9; 2008: 253–6, notes the complexity of the dissection.
97 Harris CRS 1973: 379–88, positing that the experiment was repeated.
98 *AA* XIV,7: pp. 209–10 Dkw; pp. 1069–70 Garofalo; *Us.Puls.* 2: 5,150 K: p. 195 tr. Furley and Wilkie.
99 Rocca 2008: 247–52.
100 *Nat.Fac.* I,13: 2,36–8 K; pp. 57–61 tr. Brock; Temkin 1977: 162–6.
101 *Mot.Dub.* 11,28: p.164–5 Nutton.
102 Siegel 1968: 83–7; Harris CRS 1973: 367–9; and further, below, pp. 105–7.
103 Harris CRS 1973: 410–420.
104 *Diff.Puls.* I,16: 8,537–41 K; *Caus.Puls.* II,6: 9,76–80 K.
105 *Puls.* 12: 8,473–4 K; p. 335 tr. Singer PN. The difficulties of defining rhythms in the manner of Herophilus are discussed at length at *Diff.Puls.* I,2: 8,511–4 K; and *Dig.Puls.* III,3: 8,901–16 K.
106 *Puls.* 9–11: 8,462–73 K; pp. 329–35 tr. Singer PN.
107 *Ibid.* 12: 8,477–92 K; pp. 337–44 tr. Singer PN
108 Mattern 2008: 185. But his own exposition also disguises his debt to others.
109 *Praes.Puls.* I,1: 9,218–20 K.
110 Barton 1994; Van Nuffelen 2014.
111 For his use of claims for precision as a rhetorical weapon, Heilen 2018: 236–40.
112 Lehoux 2017.
113 *MM* XIII,15: 10,915 K; III, pp. 379–81 tr. Johnston-Horsley.
114 *Praec.* 4,2: 14,620 K; *CMG* V 8,1, 88–9, also indicating Galen's doubt that *Prorrhetic* was a genuine work of Hippocrates. The quote is *Prorrhet.* 2,1: IX, p. 8, 2 ed. Littré.
115 *Praec.* 3,7: 1,8; 14,615, 602 K; *CMG* V 8,1, 84–5, 70–1; *Opt.Med.Cogn.* 1: *CMG Suppl. Or.* IV,1, 55; Deichgräber 1976; Van Nuffelen 2014.
116 Jouanna 2013 is the best edition of this Hippocratic text.
117 Rufus, *Medical Questions* 1–10. Gärtner, in his commentary at *CMG Suppl.* IV, p. 48 notes Rufus' general avoidance of 'prognosis' and similar expressions found frequently in Galen.
118 Aretaeus, *Acute Diseases* II,4,4–5; *CMG* II, 24.
119 *Hipp.Prog.* I,4: 18B,6–10 K.

120 *Ibid.* I,4: 18B,12–13 K; *CAM* 17,8–11: 1,292–3 K; p. 160 tr. Johnston, criticising the 'prophet' for undue certainty.
121 *Ibid.* I,4: 18B,14–5 K.
122 *CAM* 17,8–11: 1,292–3 K; p. 160 tr. Johnston.
123 *Di.Dec.* I,11: 9,824 K.
124 Conversely, the more one knows about medicine, one will no longer be surprised at what is not surprising, *MMG* I,16: 11,68 K; p. 443, tr. Johnston.
125 Tr. Siegel 1976: the major edition with German translation and commentary by Florian Gärtner, *CMG* V 6,1,1, so far includes only Books I–II.
126 *Loc.Aff.* V,8: 8,356–8, 361–6 K; pp. 159–63 tr. Siegel, modified.
127 The Latin translator emended the Greek to 'my hand', perhaps correctly.
128 *Praec.* 4,2–3: 14,629 K; *CMG* V 8,1, 98–9 cf. also 3,7 and 17, 5,5, 7,9 and 10,18: 14, 615, 620, 625, 638, 656 K; *CMG* V 8,1, 84–5, 88–91, 94–5, 106–9, 124–5. Galen benefits both from his principled rejection of the notion of prophecy and from the reputation he gained from others' misunderstanding.
129 Cf. also the section in the commentary on *Epidemics II*, later circulating independently, where Galen explains how to tell if a patient is malingering, ed. Deichgräber and Kudlien 1960.
130 *Hipp.Epid. VI*, viii: *CMG* V 10,2,2, 483–7.
131 *Praec.* 7,1–18; 8,10–13; 6,1–10: 14,635–41, 633–4, 631–3 K; *CMG* V 8,1, 104–11, 102–5, 100–3. For Galen's variant versions of the last case, see my notes at *CMG* V 8,1, 194–7.
132 *Praec.* 6,16: 14,635 K; *CMG* V 8,1, 104–5. At *Puls.* 12: 8,473 K, he does not mention this pulse alongside those manifested in fear, grief, pleasure, and anger. Cf. the comic poet Philemon, frag. 106, on grief as the common source of madness and many diseases
133 The Latin equivalent of *maia, obstetrix*, may give too modern an impression. She was a woman attending to concerns of other women about pregnancy and birth.
134 Mattern 2008: 108–14.
135 Soranus, *Gynaecology:* tr. Temkin 1956.
136 *Lib.Prop.* 2,2: 19,16 K: p. 140 BM; p. 7 tr. Singer PN; *Ut.Diss.*: 2,887–98 K; *CMG* V 3,3; tr. Goss 1962. For his possible use of female authors, Parker 2012.
137 Flemming 2000: 296–7
138 *SMT* VI,pr: 11,792 K; *PHP* III,4,15–18; *CMG* V 4,1,2, 194–196.
139 *PHP* IX,23,25–6; *CMG* V 4,12, 556; Flemming 2000: 342; cf. for a wider perspective, Carroll 2018: 51–82.
140 Soranus, *Gynaecology* III,1–5, shows that some doctors even went so far as to deny that there were any female diseases, placing both male and female complaints in the same explanatory category.
141 *Hipp.Epid.I*, i,2: *CMG* V 10,1, 32, noting that those women who do succumb to such diseases will have been younger, hotter, and more energetic. One might compare the satirists' contempt for athletic women at the gymnasium, as well as Galen's complaints about the unhealthy nature of some athletics in his *Exhortation to Medicine*, König 2005: 291–300. For peasants, *SMT* X,2,22: 12,299 K; *Hipp.Epid.I*, 1,3: 17A,210 K; *Comp.Med.Gen.* VII,11: 13,1009 K.
142 In *The Seven-month Child*, ed. Schöne 1933: Walzer 1935, he accepted the popular (and Hippocratic) view that children born at seven months were likely to live, but not those at eight and explained the Hippocratic methods of calculating days. For the Hippocratic tradition of gynaecology, see King 1998; Flemming 2002.
143 The author of *Theriac, for Piso* 2: 14,218 K, refers to a female Platonist philosopher, Arria, as "most dear", but this treatise is unlikely to be by Galen, above, p. 51, note 144.
144 *Comp.Med.Loc.* I,3: 12,443–5 K; *MM* VIII,5: 10,574–5 K; II, p. 413 tr. Johnston-Horsley. Cf. also *Hipp.Prog.* II,11: 18B,129–30 K (rich Roman women sleeping in the day and waking at night for dissipation).
145 *Comp.Med.Loc.* I,2: 12,435 K. For the later legends of his acquaintance with Cleopatra and Mary Magdalene, see below, p. 140.
146 Meisami 1989: 275–6, perhaps a hint, that the highly rational Galen never married: we hear of no relations with members of the opposite sex or of any close friends.
147 For the former, above, pp. 60–1 for the latter, Flemming 2000: 296–7, tracing changes over several treatises.

4 Galen the thinker

The recognition of Galen's importance in the history of ancient philosophy has been one of the most significant developments in Galenic scholarship over the last forty years.[1] It has revealed his enormous debt to Plato, visible not only in his teleology and his theory of the tripartite soul and its three locations in the body, but also in his summaries of the Platonic dialogues and his literary reminiscences throughout his writings.[2] He was similarly steeped in Aristotle, whose logic and works on animals he studied in expert detail, and whose views on the make-up of the universe he adapted to fit his own ideas about the body.[3] He shows a deep and often critical acquaintance with Chrysippus and other Stoics, although he has less time for the Epicureans.[4] Given his substantial early education in philosophy, this familiarity with the doctrines of the major philosophical groupings is hardly surprising, but he is much more than a transmitter of others' ideas. In his debates with contemporary philosophers he asserted his independence, refusing to commit himself to any one school or to take up a definite position on any subject where he felt that such a judgment was unwarranted.[5] It is a stance that has attracted many modern scholars, who have subjected his strengths and weaknesses to critical examination, not always to his advantage. They have shown how his enormous learning and his ability to pounce on the weak points in the arguments of others, verging at times on the unscrupulous, are counterbalanced by errors of his own and by the overwhelming conviction of his own superiority. He moves too easily from proposing something plausible to treating it as certain enough to use as the basis for further discussion, while his reluctance to come down decisively on one side or another of an argument has been condemned as 'fudge'.[6] But such an analysis, valid though it is, risks underestimating Galen's achievement. He was both doctor and philosopher, and to consider either in isolation is to miss their fruitful interaction. Not only did he believe that his medical experience and knowledge could contribute something to philosophical debate by confirming the theories of others or by reducing the range of possible solutions to contentious issues, but he readily applied his analytical skills to the medical problems that he faced and to the phenomena that he investigated.

Defining the philosopher

Towards the very end of his life Galen wrote three treatises, *My Own Books, My Own Opinions*, and *The Best Doctor is also a Philosopher*, that, each in its own way, exemplify his conviction of the supreme importance of philosophy for the practising doctor. 'Philosopher' is for Galen a term of approval that establishes a contrast with the sophists and the charlatans whom he detests, as well as setting him apart from humbler or less theoretically inclined practitioners of medicine.[7] His importance as a philosopher was acknowledged by at least two of his contemporaries, the miscellaneous writer Athenaeus of Naucratis and the Aristotelian philosopher Alexander of Aphrodisias, and some of his philosophical ideas continued to be discussed for centuries.[8] But, conversely, there were those, both then and since, who had little truck with Galen's musings and who applied to him the same opprobrious epithets that he deployed against those who disagreed with him. The Aristotelian Alexander's "mule-head" or, on another translation, "a man of mere definitions", reflected his disdain for Galen's eclecticism, even as he chose to engage with him on a variety of topics.[9]

At first sight, the works that Galen included in the catalogue of his writings under the heading of philosophy fit happily into such modern categories as methodology, logic, philosophy of language, epistemology and psychology.[10] But this is too constricting, for two reasons. For Galen, medicine and philosophy were intertwined as part of an exercise that was useful to both. His anatomical discoveries, for instance, he believed contributed to resolving disputed philosophical issues. Conversely, understanding the basic principles, the philosophy, behind medicine and healing was as much part of the doctor's life as knowing what drug should be applied, and, indeed, involved intellectual challenges that went beyond the realm of theory. Secondly, the remarkable list of titles in *My Own Books* places Galen in a much broader context as someone who literally 'loves wisdom', a public intellectual, capable of thinking deeply about a broad range of questions.

His own sub-divisions of this catalogue make the point clearly. He begins with works on logic and demonstration, excluding those specifically relating to an earlier author. His tracts on Plato's theory of logic and on *Analogical Procedures in the Philebus* are to be found with his summaries of Platonic dialogues and *The Soul's Behaviour depends on Bodily Mixtures* under the heading of *Works concerning the Philosophy of Plato.*[11] A similar but longer list relating to the philosophy of Aristotle includes his commentary on *Interpretation* and seventeen books on the *Analytics* and *Categories*, in addition to discussions of topics in the writings of his Peripatetic successors Theophrastus and Eudemus.[12] His writings on the Stoics dealt exclusively with their logic, those on the Epicureans with their views on pleasure, including attacks on two near contemporaries Celsus and Pudentius, and another dealing with Metrodorus' arguments against the sophists (if the text is correct).[13] To judge from the title of another lost work, Galen would have criticised them for neglecting 'physiology', an understanding of the natural organisation of the body, in their advocacy of a life of pleasurable ease. It would have repeated a message found in *Affections and Errors of the Soul, Avoiding Distress*, and *Character Traits*, which have an obvious link with medicine and psychology because of Galen's views on the complex interrelationship between soul and body. Other titles included by Galen under the heading of "moral philosophy", however, reveal a very different side to his activities, one that appears to go far beyond medicine. Some of their contents cannot now be divined from titles such as *A Discussion with Bacchides and Cyrus at the Villa of Menarchus* or the mysterious *Croniskoi* in seven sections, but others can best be compared with the *Moral Essays* of Plutarch, whose *Homeric Studies* and possibly other books were known to Galen.[14] Some have political connotations, such as *Concord* or *How far should Public Esteem and Opinion be taken into Account?*, others, like *Modesty* or the part-autobiographical *Slander*, fit neatly among topics chosen by professional sophists, as does *Solitary Readers*, but why Galen chose to write on *Making a Will* must remain a mystery.[15] At the very least, this miscellaneous list warns against too close an identification with the modern Anglo-Saxon use of the term philosopher.[16]

In a second tract, *The Best Doctor is also a Philosopher* (which may have been originally entitled *Hippocrates*), Galen spells out more clearly the relationship of philosophy to medicine. In it he complains that despite paying lip-service to Hippocrates, many of his own contemporaries have failed to follow him because, like second-rate athletes, they lack either the necessary capacity or the eagerness to study and practise hard.[17] Those, however, who do live up to this picture of Hippocrates are thereby also philosophers, for like him they know the three parts of philosophy – logic, natural philosophy and ethics. They will have used logic in making discoveries about the body, distinguishing between diseases, and devising appropriate therapies; natural philosophy in understanding the world around them as well as the body's make-up, its elements, mixtures and uniform parts; and ethics in their relationships with patients through exercising self-restraint and moderation and being immune to a desire for money or sex. Besides, if they command one part of philosophy, the others should also follow, since they are all connected as if by a string, an idea that went back to Plato's picture of Socrates and to the ideal sage of the Stoics.[18]

Few historians of ancient Greek medicine today agree with Galen in this characterisation of the historical Hippocrates. The stories of his dealings with patients, including his refusal to serve the King of Persia for money, derive from the so-called Hippocratic letters, fictional creations of the Hellenistic period, while the term 'homoeomerous or uniform parts', at least as a descriptive term for such things as flesh, skin and bone, goes back to Aristotle, and is not found in the so-called Hippocratic Corpus.[19] Even the ascription to Hippocrates of a belief in elements and mixtures also requires the setting aside of most texts in the Corpus. Galen's proof of Hippocrates's skill in logic is equally dependent on some special pleading, although he could rely on Plato's praise in the *Phaedrus* of Hippocrates' ability to perform logical differentiations, *diaireseis.*[20] In short, like Hippocrates the anatomist, Hippocrates the philosopher is very much the creation of Galen himself, reading back into the life of his hero his own interests and abilities, and then, in turn, justifying them by the example of the Father of Medicine. But to acknowledge that this image of Hippocrates is an ahistorical construction is not to downplay its importance in Galen's own life – he was, after all, educated from his youth in philosophy by some of the leading experts of the day – or the validity of his insistence that the best doctor should be also a thinking, learned and moral individual.

Galen's praise of philosophy and the examples selected from within the life of this idealised Hippocrates link with what he says in the opening section of *My Own Opinions.* There Galen makes it clear that his is a practical philosophy, one that looks for achievable solutions, an attitude in which, he says elsewhere, he follows the advice of his father Nicon. He refuses to take sides in many contemporary philosophical debates, on the eternity of the world, the nature of the soul, or the nature of the divine, because he can see no way in which one can reach a secure conclusion. That the world, the soul and the divine (or the Gods) exist, he is certain from his own knowledge and experience, but beyond that he can see no logical way of deciding between opposing views, should one wish to go into further details. None is more plausible than any other, let alone certain.[21] This was a stance that annoyed many later commentators, who dismissed as weak or irrelevant some of the objections he made to positions that they themselves adopted, or could not understand how he could retain his agnosticism while at the same time pointing to data that would support a more definite conclusion. Several Arabic philosophers, for example, argued that his refusal to take sides over the question of the eternity of the world was at variance with a passage in *Demonstration* in which he drew attention to the apparent stability of the universe. If, he suggested, the seas still remained the same after centuries and astronomical observations for thousands of years showed that the sun had not diminished in size, this indicated that the universe was not liable to corruption.[22] But, for Galen, this may not have been enough to counter all objections to a belief in the eternity of the world, and, besides, the question was irrelevant to medical practice. When dealing with matters medical, he could summon the evidence of experience to supplement that of logic to allow the doctor to choose the more plausible option or at least to limit the possibilities.[23] Hence, in *The Soul's Behaviour depends on Bodily Mixtures*, he argues that, contradictory opinions on the nature and incorruptibility of the soul notwithstanding, everyone accepts the proposition that the soul is influenced by changes in the body.[24] But this universal belief does not entail assent to any specific position as to what the soul is, a position Galen maintained throughout his life, while, at the same time, allowing the doctor and physical treatment a role in caring for the mentally ill.

Logic

Central to all Galen's activities was his interest in logic, of which he was a remarkable exponent.[25] In his autobibliography he lists some forty-five tracts on logic, as well as a further twenty-seven dealing specifically with the ideas of Plato, Aristotle and the Stoics.[26] Some were short and focussed on detailed questions, such as *Similarity, The Value of Syllogisms*, *Mixed Premisses*, and *Possibility*, but others ranged more widely.[27] His treatise on *Demonstration* in fifteen books he regarded as fundamental to far more than the practice of medicine, and its disappearance, apart from quotations, allusions and fragments in Arabic, is a major loss.[28] Even these scattered portions show his engagement with all the major writers on logic from Aristotle and his immediate pupils to the Stoics, as well as his awareness of their limitations. So, for example, in his *Introduction to Logic*, he insisted that in addition to Aristotelian categorical and Stoic hypothetical syllogisms, there was a third type, "coming about through a relation", "something very useful for those who do arithmetic and calculations".[29] He argued against the Stoics that not every premiss introduced by 'if' was sufficient to qualify as a conditional, and took issue with the followers of Theophrastus for their interpretation of what is meant in logic by 'necessity'.[30]Arabic logicians claimed that he was the first to discover the fourth figure of the simple categorical syllogism, but this seems to have been a misunderstanding of his discussion of a fourth figure in a compound or 'chained' syllogism such as he encountered in the works of Plato.[31] Nonetheless, the accolade shows the respect in which his argumentation was held by later logicians, even if many of the examples of logic that Galen uses in his writings are open to criticism, and his description of Stoic logic in particular is far from clear.[32] Jonathan Barnes' dismissal of him as simply a bogus inventor of syllogisms (a far cry from his earlier description of him as the third great logician in Antiquity after Aristotle and Chrysippus) would appear to undervalue the considerable interest he took in such reasoning and his acquaintance with sources lost to us.[33]

What cannot be impugned, however, is his insistence on the importance of logical reasoning for medicine, something emphasised in his accounts of his clinical practice in the *Method of Healing*, as well as in his short treatises on causation, and elsewhere.[34] The opening books of the *Method of Healing* serve as a philosophical introduction to understanding what is meant by illness.[35] Demonstration, "the beginning of the road to Truth", was at the very heart of his work, as he sought ways to move from the merely plausible to what he judged 'solid', 'secure' or 'certain' knowledge.[36] His model was geometric reasoning, which proceeded from premisses by means of deduction to demonstrable conclusions, and successful examples of this type of logic can be found throughout his writings, and not only in those on philosophy.[37] These demonstrations must proceed from premisses that are both true and agreed by everybody and are either first principles (axioms) or so evident to sense perception that they need no proof.[38] Discerning what was or was not a viable premiss from a variety of options was the first stage in the process, to be followed by careful logical demonstration.[39] As a tool for separating truth from falsehood, not least in dealing with particular propositions, such as the condition of an individual patient, demonstration was Galen's main weapon against scepticism on the one hand and dogmatism on the other. Its conclusions were also not simply theoretical but open to empirical testing. Just as his grandfather, the land-surveyor, *geometres*, would have seen the truth of his calculations in the accuracy of measurements on the ground, so Galen, the doctor-philosopher, would see the correctness of his diagnosis in the fate of his patient.[40] There was no place here for what Galen termed dialectical, rhetorical or sophistical premisses, let alone the acceptance of statements simply on the word of an authority (although, of course, he was content if weaker brethren simply followed his instructions).

The virtues of this demonstrative, 'scientific' method, and the follies of those who fail to follow it, are proclaimed at length throughout Galen's writings, notably in his attack on Chrysippus and the Stoics in *The Opinions of Hippocrates and Plato.*[41] In his medical practice also, where there were so many variables in any individual case, Galen's diagnostic conclusions followed almost impeccably from the premisses that he selected.[42] He was aware of the dangers of ambiguity in the choice of words and phrases, a topic on which we have a surviving short treatise, but at the same time he was prepared to adopt a more relaxed attitude to a choice of terminology, if he considered that it did not impinge on actual therapy.[43]

But there were also serious flaws in his method that he did not, or would not, recognise. Some of the premisses that seemed evident to him would not be considered valid today, and were not accepted by all his contemporaries. Methodist physicians, for instance, would have rejected the belief in an ensouled body in a connected universe that lies at the heart of his studies of human behaviour. Similarly, his vigorous denunciation of their logical inadequacies in defining illness is only convincing if one starts from the same understanding of the body's constitution and the nature of illness as he did. They had simply no interest in deciding whether to classify something as an illness or a symptom, a constitutional condition or a localised phenomenon, for this was for them a theoretical game of no relevance to the treatment of the patient.[44]

The body in nature

The fact that Plato had mentioned Hippocrates as an example of supreme expertise in medicine and appeared to know something about his ideas and practice, albeit in what modern scholars judge to be the vaguest of outlines, encouraged Galen to believe that some of Plato's ideas about the body derived from, or were at least compatible with, those of the great Coan.[45] Hence, his abiding interest in Plato's *Timaeus*, a treatise that he not only summarised (it is the sole survivor of his abridgements of the Platonic dialogues) but also commented upon for its medical content.[46] In Plato's mathematical universe, four primary bodies, earth, air, fire, and water, made up from triangles, lay at the very foundation of all matter in the world.[47] From these four elements were derived all the parts of the body: flesh, blood, and marrow, the most important of all tissues, whose degeneration into their original constituents was a further cause of illness alongside any imbalance of elements.[48] Others besides Galen considered Plato an important medical thinker: the contemporary author of the Anonymus Londinensis papyrus devoted four columns, XI–XVIII, to the views expressed in the *Timaeus*, more than to those of any doctor – and Galen was unlikely to have been alone in aligning them with the theory of the four humours as expressed in the Hippocratic treatise, *Human Nature*, which, long before Galen, had come to be regarded as quintessentially Hippocratic.[49] That Galen himself believed that some parts of this tract, particularly its anatomical sections, were not by Hippocrates himself, did not matter greatly, for, in his view, the whole book was written in close proximity to Hippocrates, who was himself responsible for its notions of balance and imbalance of the humours, as well as for its ideas on disease and its overall method.[50]

In the *Timaeus* and in the *Republic*, Plato had developed a theory that was crucial to Galen's ideas on body and soul. In the *Republic*, another dialogue summarised by Galen, Plato explained through a series of mutually reinforcing analogies that the health of a city, characterised by justice, depended on an appropriate relationship between its three main constituents, the rulers, the guardians and the great majority of the population, which corresponded to the three parts of the soul, reason, spirit or energy, and desire.[51] In the *Timaeus*, Plato had gone further by locating each part of the soul in a specific part of the body. The highest part of the soul, reason, he placed in the brain, the energetic part in the heart, and the lowest, appetitive part, in the space between the diaphragm and the midriff, near where the liver, stomach and spleen were to be found.[52] This schematic description of the internal body coincided, in Galen's opinion. with the results of his own and of earlier Hellenistic dissections, thus disproving the cardiocentric view of the unitary soul adopted by Plato's pupil Aristotle and by the Stoics. As he argued at length in *The Opinions of Hippocrates and Plato*, they relied on weak arguments and even weaker knowledge of anatomy in asserting the primacy of the heart, although that did not prevent Galen from using some Aristotelian terminology to characterise the parts of the Platonic soul.[53] But he also corrected Plato's anatomy (and that of some contemporary Platonists) by placing the seat of the third part of the soul in the liver itself rather than nearby for, in his view, there was no other organ in that region of the body, except for the liver, that could serve as the seat of the appetitive soul or had such a wide-ranging system of conduits supplying food and drink to the entire body.[54]

Equally significant for Galen was Plato's conviction that the whole construction of the body had been carefully and purposefully organised out of disordered matter by a Craftsman, the Demiurge or Creator, to produce a living being that was itself a participant in an ordered universe (*kosmos*, a word that in Greek can also stand for beauty).[55] Through a 'shaping capacity' flesh, for example, was carefully distributed around the body according to the design of the Creator. Because both solid bone and thick flesh inhibited sensitivity, he had reduced the thickness of the covering of the skull around the brain, the seat of the intellect, its enhanced sensitivity outweighing the loss of protection and the possibility of increased pain. The neck, through which tiny channels go to the head, further protects the brain from any polluting effects of the mortal elements of the soul located lower down in the body.[56] The construction of the body in the *Timaeus*, however, is more than a medical phenomenon. It is an example of teleology throughout the universe, a teleology which is ultimately ethical in that it seeks order for its own sake. A doctor who understands how teleology works in the body is thus guided by a princíple higher than his empirical craft skills.[57]

Plato's pupil Aristotle developed his ideas further. Like him, he rejected mechanistic or chance explanations for phenomena, but he saw no need for a Demiurge, for in his view purposefulness was immanent in everything. Nature (*physis*) itself is a cause that operates for a purpose: it does nothing in vain. Hence, for him, teleology was essential in any critical assessment of the data furnished by experience and provided a methodological component for all scientific enquiry.[58] The studies of living organisms in Aristotle's biological writings, often based on dissection, not only provided Galen with a model for his own enquiries into the human body and human anatomy, notwithstanding some major disagreements, but also further strengthened his conviction of the importance of purpose.[59]

Galen was convinced that Hippocrates too was a firm believer in teleology, citing a variety of texts in support. Particularly striking is a sentence from the opening of *Fractures*, where the author declares that "this Nature (or nature) is most just", which provides some small justification for his claim in *The Use of Parts* that Hippocrates "often used to call Nature just".[60] 'Often' is a typically Galenic exaggeration for, as Elizabeth Craik points out, the conjunction of the two words occurs only in the surgical texts *Fractures* and *Joints*, where it is used to describe the natural and proper position of a limb. Typically, in his commentary on *Fractures* at this point Galen argued that this applied also to shape, colour and size, as well as to the part as a whole.[61] There are also other passages in our Hippocratic Corpus where one can find traces of 'incipient teleology', particularly in works written after 400 BCE, but they occur in books by different authors, none identifiable for certain with the historical Hippocrates or coming close to the position that Galen ascribes to him.

The key to his interpretation of teleology lies in the fluidity of the word *physis*, sometimes with the addition of the definite article, which can be translated into English as 'nature' or 'Nature'. Franjo Kovačič in his study of the use of the word in Galen distinguishes three separate meanings.[62] In its commonest it refers to what is immanent in the individual, its 'nature', but it can also denote the system of rules and organisation that governs the species. Particularly with a definite article it may stand for a transcendental, godlike and providential Demiurge, a Creator deriving from Plato via Aristotle and Stoicism. Nature is almost deified in what Kovačič calls Galen's original theology.[63] It is at one and the same time the means whereby the workings of the divine are mediated in the human world and something that acts autonomously. The limitations of nature impose constraints even on the gods. Hence Galen's repeated criticism of Jews and Christians for their belief in an omnipotent divinity with the power to work miracles. His respectful appreciation of their high morality is more than counterbalanced by their, to him unphilosophical, faith in a god who can, whenever he chooses, suspend or break what might be termed the laws of nature.[64] The acquiescence of God in these laws is for him a further proof of a purposeful universe, even if it might have imperfections.[65]

In his investigations into the human body, Galen, following Aristotle, was particularly keen to establish the function, need or use (all meanings incorporated in the Greek word *chreia*) of each bodily part. In a treatise such as *The Use of Respiration* or, still more, the seventeen books of *The Use of Parts*, his exposition of his own anatomical discoveries for the benefit of Aristotelian philosophers, he explained how the organisation of a particular part served a particular purpose and use.[66] (*Fig. 7.1*) The muscles in the arm were formed with the capacity to expand so that they could function to lift heavy weights; they did not become large, as Erasistratus had argued, simply because of the work that they had done.[67] Similarly, were a part to change from its natural state, some malfunction would certainly occur, leading to illness and even death. The final book of *The Use of Parts* is almost a hymn, Galen calls it an "epode", to the creative power that had so carefully and purposefully organised the human, functioning body.[68]

If Galen's teleology can be traced back to Plato, it was Aristotle who provided the overall theory and vocabulary on which Galen drew for his understanding of the natural world and of the place of the human body within it.[69] It was an interconnected and harmonic universe, far removed from the disconnected world of chance and atoms envisaged by the Epicureans (and his medical enemies, the Methodists). In the treatise *Critical Days* he uses a rare word, *plēmmelein*, 'to play a wrong note', to suggest that a mistake in therapy by a doctor upsets this cosmic harmony by frustrating nature's efforts on behalf of the patient.[70] The Aristotelian theory of the four elements could also be taken easily to mesh with what was described in *Human Nature*, a text which by Galen's day had come to be regarded as one of the most important 'Hippocratic' writings, although perhaps not as central as it became after Galen.[71] For Aristotle the matter that underlies all these elements is without qualities and it is the conjunction of this matter with the four primary qualities – hot, cold, wet, and dry – which engenders the four elements, earth, air, fire and water. In Galen's universe these elements, each the result of a conjunction of a pair of elemental qualities, form the most basic structures of the living organism.[72] In *Elements according to Hippocrates*, Galen reprises at length the arguments already put forward against a variety of opponents, monists as well as atomists, by the author of *Human Nature*, and, although he does not spell this out, also by more recent writers, including Plutarch.[73]

He adds observations from his own medical practice, as well as extending his own criticism to Asclepiades of Bithynia, fl. 100 BCE, and the followers of his pupil Athenaeus of Attaleia. Among them was a man who had wished to explain to the eighteen-year-old Galen why Athenaeus was right but was discomfited in a lively display of forensic analysis by the young man.[74] In the human body the elements come together to form the four humours, blood, phlegm, bile and black bile (or melancholy).[75] In his relatively early treatise on *Elements*, Galen argued that all parts of the body were produced out of matter provided by maternal blood, which was a combination of all four humours and thus capable of engendering a variety of body parts. However, in the later *Seed* he modified this view, arguing that only those that contain blood were formed from humours and that the rest, and in particular the so-called homoeomerous or uniform parts, such as skin, cartilage and bone, were formed from semen.[76] These living tissues, made up from unified combinations of these elemental building blocks, in turn constitute the basis from which organs are formed. This hierarchy, which can be paralleled in Aristotle, is defended not only against Methodists, but also against another group of doctors called Pneumatists, believers in humours who introduced a fifth elemental body, *pneuma* or spirit, which pervaded everything and served to contain and govern it.[77]

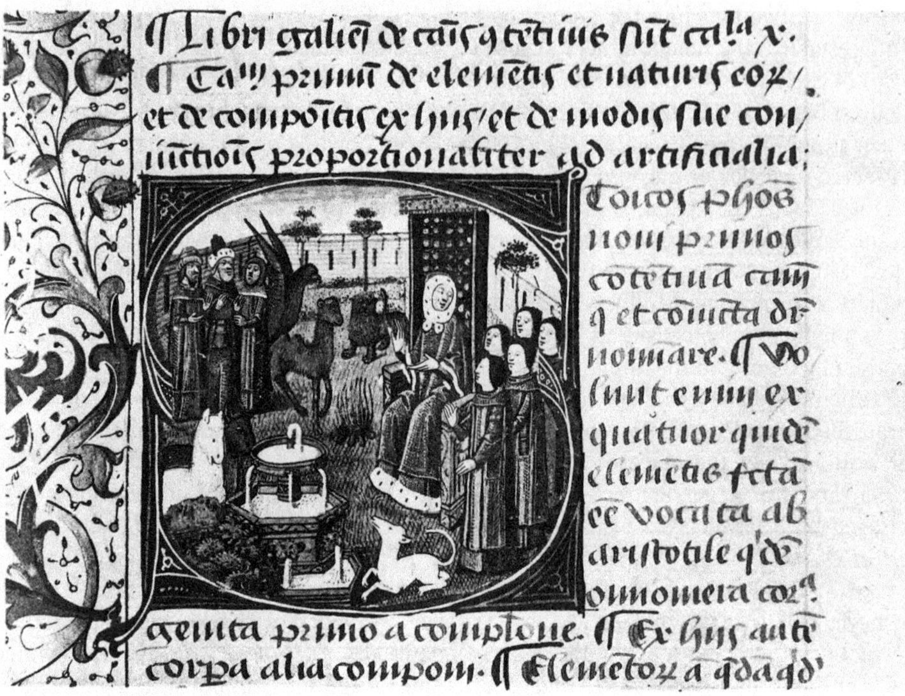

Figure 4.1 Galen explains to his pupils the Hippocratic doctrine of elements in the opening chapter of *Containing Causes.* Erasistratus, Asclepiades and Thessalus glower in the background. Dresden, Sāchsische Landesbibliothek D b 93, fol. 378r.

The relationship between this theoretical understanding of the basis of the natural world and everyday medical practice is explored at length and with considerable subtlety in two further treatises, *Elements* and *Mixtures* (or, to use an older translation, *Temperaments*).[78] All the variations in living beings, including humans and plants, depend on the different degrees and proportions of the elementary qualities, which can be correlated with both the elements and the humours, and, most important for a doctor, can be perceived by the senses, especially by sight and touch. Some of these variations are designed by Nature with its 'shaping capacity', and any departure from their natural perfection may result in a loss of function.[79] (Others may be acquired, and some harmful results mitigated through long-term habituation.)[80] Although Galen can talk of an ideal human form on the model of the so-called *Canon* of the sculptor Polyclitus, he allows for a certain latitude in the healthy individual body and accepts slight variations from an ideal in which all the elements, qualities and humours are in balance.[81] The other eight temperaments, in which a single quality or a combination of two qualities predominates in the natural mixture, are less good, but by no means unhealthy.[82] Indeed, some doctors and philosophers, admittedly in his view wrongly, considered a warm and wet temperament to be best of all, since it was at the opposite pole from the cold and wet characteristic of plants and dead bodies.[83] For Galen, however, this natural imbalance merely indicated a predisposition that a good doctor should be aware of in diagnosis and treatment, and particularly in prophylaxis, where the aim should be to keep this imbalance within the bounds of health. It is a balance that changes according to age: the elderly, like plants, are drier and colder than the young, despite the appearance of more and wetter residues. It explains why the flesh of young lambs or piglets is unpleasant to eat (that of young kids, which are naturally hotter, is less so), just like that of old animals, whose lack of moisture results in meat that is dry and leathery.[84] The effects of climate on this balance, like that of age, are easily detectable. Those who live in hot, dry climates, like the Egyptians, Arabs, and Indians, have dry, curly and brittle black hair, those from the cold damp North, the Illyrians, the Germans, the Sarmatians and the Scythians long, thin, straight tawny hair.[85] Although at times Galen's ideas come close to those of contemporary physiognomists who claimed to divine the overall character of an individual from his or her physical, his approach is more subtle as well as having Hippocratic precedent. Physical appearance is only one factor in the doctor's endeavour to ascertain as precisely as possible the basic humoral balance of his patient in order to restore it by appropriate therapy.[86]

Every part of the body has been created in such a way as to have the capacity to perform the task for which it was formed, and any change has the potential to reduce or weaken that capacity (or, in therapy, to strengthen and restore it). The Greek word that Galen uses, *dynamis*, conveys a variety of meanings. It can indicate some kind of power, potentiality as opposed to actuality, or the capacity of an individual or part to act in a certain way. Galen also uses it almost as a shorthand term to denote a physical cause whose exact essence is unknown; so, there is a blood-making faculty in the heart and a special faculty in every other part corresponding to its activity. This is not, as Renaissance critics alleged, merely multiplying entities unnecessarily, but something essential in his physicalist outlook: a faculty is the result of the organisation and proportion of the elements in any part at the most basic level, invisible as such to the observer but detectable from the macro-phenomena they engender.[87] As in modern genomics, these combinations can be both universal (for example, allowing humans to walk) and individual (walking in a certain way or not at all) at the same time. They are ubiquitous. Every living thing, including plants, has in every part four so-called natural capacities or faculties, without which it would be unable to exist, grow or act; the faculties of attraction, expulsion, digestion (or assimilation) and retention.[88] Through them, each part attracts whatever nutriment is appropriate and discards whatever is inappropriate; in digestion, it alters that nutriment to a state in which it can be assimilated to itself and, through its retention, allows the organism to remain in its natural, healthy state. The crucial organ of the body in this process is the liver, which is continually sending forth the appropriate nutriment to the rest of the body, and which resembles the base of the stem of a plant at its junction with the roots, a comparison that goes back to the Hippocratic *Nutriment*, although, characteristically, Galen makes it more precise by specifying the crucial point at which this transfer of nutriment takes place.[89] Even if a particular shoot or root itself dies, provided the plant as a whole retains this power, it can still live. So, in animals the liver remains a constant source of nutriment, right from the development of the foetus, providing the essential assistance for the faculties that are innate in every part.[90] This differs from the intermittent power sent from the brain via the nerves in sensation and motion and from the so-called innate heat that is produced in the heart and which is responsible for energy and vigour, both physical and mental.[91]

The doctrine of innate heat plays a central role in Galen's understanding of the body, for he was prepared to regard it, if not as the essence of the soul in all living beings, at least as its chief instrument.[92] Galen places a considerable emphasis on the Hippocratic lineage of his doctrine of innate heat, although he never acknowledges that the passage he relies on for Hippocratic authority, *Aphorisms* I,14, is unique in the pre-Hellenistic texts in the Hippocratic Corpus in using the adjective ἔμφυτος and the meaning of the adjective is far from clear.[93] Lycus of Macedon, for example, if Galen's quotation is accurate, argued that this aphorism referred to the amount of heat in the normal body of the young as a whole and not to any specific substance.[94] The innate heat, which is present in all living things from the very first, gradually diminishes over time: the heat of childhood and youth fades away to the chill of old age, and its disappearance marks the end of life.[95] Before then it is sustained by the nutriment passing from the liver to the left ventricle of the heart and cooled by air drawn in from outside in respiration.[96] Too little nutriment or air and the flame of life goes out, but, equally too much, particularly when the body itself becomes further heated as in fever, is dangerous and even fatal, for, as with a fire, too much fuel heaped on at the same time may snuff it out because of its lack of access to air. Likewise, if dangerous sooty superfluities are not removed, as with an unswept chimney, the fire will die because of a lack of ventilation.[97] "Acquired heat" is thus more immediately potent than the innate, and the doctor must always be aware of its dangers.

Mind and body

Galen's vitalist approach and his view of the body as a living universe, responding to changes and actively seeking whatever it needs in order to exist and to function, was not shared by all ancient doctors. Erasistratus and Asclepiades had little time for teleology in its Galenic form, and they put forward a much more mechanistic understanding of the body, in which, for instance, there was no need for innate heat, since acquired heat by itself was sufficient to produce rigor, and the excretion of residues through the kidney and bladder did not require any active participation from the organs themselves but only obedience to the laws of physics.[98] The body is ensouled – that Galen regards as universally true – but what precisely this meant exercised him throughout his life. In *My own Opinions*, despite his assertions that he knows nothing about the *ousia*, the essence or substance of the soul, he reverted time and again to the question of the relationship between soul and body, only to confess his own perplexities or his disagreement with the views of others, as he had done at various points in his earlier writings.[99] Coming to a definite view on this was also unnecessary, for the treatment of disorders involving the soul did not depend on whether one could be precise about just what it was. In a tract written at the very end of his life, he argued that everyone, no matter what philosophical view of the soul they held, be it Platonist, Peripatetic, Stoic or Epicurean, accepted that it was affected in some way by changes within the body. Too much drink, for example, altered the moral behaviour of an individual, and he appealed to the authority of the Hippocratic *Airs, Waters and Places* for evidence that one's environment affected one's mental as well as one's physical state.[100] Galen himself went further in asserting that emotions such as fear, anger or grief could in turn have a deleterious effect on the body, and might even lead to death.[101] His commentary on Book VI of the *Epidemics* includes a series of such cases ranging from a scholar shattered by the loss of his library to a man who was ashamed at breaking wind in public.[102] The earlier treatise *Prognosis* recounts similar stories of individuals whose physical symptoms could be ascribed to what today might be called stress. This can affect the body in the same way as sleeplessness, the heat of the sun, overeating or bathing too long because it affects the body's innate heat, which can be suddenly chilled and even occasionally completely quenched by fear or distress.[103] Conversely, an appropriate reaction to illness and a refusal to be overwhelmed by it could prolong one's life. Galen recalled seeing the famous orator Aelius Aristides during one of his long periods of residence at the shrine of Asclepius at Pergamum and marvelled at how such an obviously enfeebled body could be kept alive for a long while by his mental strength and willpower.[104]

But if restoring the innate heat requires physical remedies, such as emetics, the effects of a stress situation can also be mitigated, and even entirely removed, by an appropriate philosophical training. How this might be achieved, Galen explained in *Avoiding Distress*, a tract ostensibly written to a friend amazed at his apparent equanimity in the face of the loss of his books and much else in the fire of Rome in 192.[105] He had faced this crisis in the same way as he had suffered the death of all his slaves during his first Roman stay, as well as the reign of the murderous emperor Commodus, "the worst in recorded history", when one expected at any moment to be sent to a desert island, like other innocent victims.[106] His advice, buttressed by a quotation from the playwright Euripides, may appear banal: if one always expects the very worst to happen, one can remain unmoved when it does not, even if the situation is dire. This practical approach is mirrored also in his treatise on the *Affections and Errors of the Soul* where he reveals that he read twice a day the *Precepts* attributed to Pythagoras as a way of cultivating an appropriate moral stance, free from outbursts of anger or greed, luxurious idleness and envy.[107]

Affections and Errors, written in response to a friend who had come across his criticism of a work by an otherwise unknown Epicurean, Antonius, falls within a Hellenistic tradition of practical ethics. Contrary to Antonius, Galen distinguishes between errors, which arise out of false belief, and affections, which come from some non-rational capacity that is not amenable to reason.[108] 'Education', in a broad sense of the word, is for him the key to both. Errors are best eliminated by a proper training in logic and in the sort of practical thinking displayed by architects, geometers, lawyers and the like. They are very different, in his view, from modern philosophers, who engage in speculative and inconclusive debate and neglect to explain the importance of making a proper choice of goals in life (a topic which Galen discussed frequently and to which he devoted another treatise, now lost).[109] Rationality plays a smaller part in learning to control one's affections or emotions, which require a combination of natural talent and education. Some children are born naughty, and their undesirable character may appear at once, and certainly by the age of two or three, in their reactions to their nurses or playmates. For them to achieve the proper psychical balance is harder, indeed almost impossible, for they will not set themselves to learn and resist any attempt at character training.[110] In general, those brought up in a moral environment, with examples around them they can follow, are more likely to avoid such excessive displays of emotion as kicking and biting those near them or attacking them with sticks and stones whenever they think they are wronged – Galen here once again refers to the influence of his father.[111] Bad habits, what one eats or drinks, the spectacles one watches, the music one listens to, and the arts as a whole can alter the whole character of the soul. After all, had not Asclepius, his "ancestral god", prescribed songs, music and even theatrical spectacles as a way of treating the mentally disturbed?[112] But over time, even if the road is rough and laborious at first, one can learn to practise self-control, and put aside any insatiable longing for possessions or fame.[113] Wealth is not a function of Virtue but of Fortune, which makes slaves and ex-slaves wealthier than the so-called "well-born", among whom Galen counts himself.[114] His third suggestion is that one should make the acquaintance of someone of good moral character and invite him (and it is always a him) to point out one's failings and advise how best they may be corrected, for, in a famous comparison from Aesop's fables, we always notice the bag strapped to our front and filled with others' wrongdoings while failing to see the one behind filled with our own.[115] But, he admits, anyone who has not been tamed by a good trainer before the age of forty is likely to be beyond the reach of such therapy, rather like bears who may give an occasional impression of being tame but have no such steady disposition, or, even worse, vipers and scorpions which can never be tamed.[116]

That Galen saw himself as ideally suited to be such a moral tutor is illustrated by a story that he often repeated to friends. On his way back to Pergamum from Rome, he was accompanied by a man from Gortyn in Crete who was normally straightforward, friendly, kind and generous, but had one major failing. He was liable to fall into a rage and beat his servants at the slightest failing. On this occasion, when his servants could not immediately locate a piece of luggage, he attacked them with a sharp knife, cutting two of them badly in the head. When he saw the amount of blood, he hurried off to Athens, leaving Galen to patch up the wounded slaves. When the two men met up again in Athens, the remorseful Cretan asked Galen to flog him with a strap as punishment. Galen merely laughed, and instead gave him a very long lecture about how with the proper moral education he might avoid similar incidents in future. According to Galen, he improved greatly over the next year, somewhat faster than might be expected, for progress in such training can be slow at first, and its rewards not always reaped for several years.[117]

Similar moralising can be found in many other writers in Classical Antiquity, including Plutarch, the Stoic Musonius Rufus, and even the satirist Lucian.[118] Galen's distinctive contribution is two-fold. On the one hand, as he argued in his relatively early treatise on *The Opinions of Hippocrates and Plato*, he believed that his anatomical investigations confirmed Plato's belief in a tripartite soul (even if, in his ethical writings, like many other contemporary Platonists, he sometimes elided the distinction between the three parts of the soul in favour of a dichotomy between the rational soul and the two lower parts).[119] On the other, he uses his wide range of observations, especially of animal behaviour, to offer a valuable corrective to the view of Stoics like Chrysippus, who attributed all types of error to false judgment. In Galen's view, natural endowment plays a substantial part in determining how one behaves, especially in establishing the character traits that allow the actions of the soul to be performed automatically without first making a deliberate choice. This explains why animals exhibit different patterns of behaviour: a dog is friendly to people, unlike the wolf, the bee or ant collects food to store, whereas the pigeon acquires it daily, and magpies steal and hide gems, rings and money, a list that impressed a later Arabic zoologist, al-Marwazi.[120] Similarly, humans have different character traits, just as they are born with different physical attributes, a theme explored by Galen elsewhere in *Seed* and *The Formation of the Foetus.*[121] Contrary to Aristotle, he believed that both male and female seed contributed to the genesis of the individual, and this explains why a child can display features shared with either parent.[122] Exactly how the embryo was actually formed, and how it became ensouled, were questions that troubled him throughout his long life. In his early training in anatomy, he had summarised four books by Lycus on this theme; on the uterus before and after conception, and on a living and a dead foetus.[123] Later in life he confessed that the order in which the three major organs of the body were created was the only topic on which he admitted to changing his mind, having at first believed they were formed simultaneously but later accepting that the liver came first.[124] But his anatomical researches could only take him so far. They could show the intelligence and power of the one who made the human body, but he left it to philosophers to show who or what this creator was, whether a wise and powerful god or some other type of soul that was similarly able to carry out a design.[125]

But to focus solely on treatises that he himself categorised as philosophical is to miss the point of what he was trying to achieve. Many of his surviving writings are best described as meditations on the body in health and disease. He is not a nosographer carefully describing all the signs of illness, like his near contemporary Aretaeus, although he includes many precise and accurate observations in his *Affected Parts*, but he tries to go beyond the phenomena to understand how the body works or what differentiates a symptom from an illness.[126] So, for instance, his *Method of Healing*, his largest work on therapy in fourteen books, begins with two books explaining its theoretical basis at some length. Some treatises, like *Elements, Humours* and *Mixtures*, try to explain the workings of the body in terms mainly derived from Aristotelian natural philosophy; others, particularly the four tracts on *Causes and Symptoms*, attack problems familiar to any doctor faced with the need to diagnose and treat but unsure, at least at first, what is really wrong.[127] These essays have been regularly attacked as verbose and irrelevant, criticised for denigrating opponents by distorting their views or by raising objections that they would not recognise therapeutically significant. But in them Galen is also endeavouring to resolve many of the difficulties involved in the encounter with a patient, raising questions that remain relevant and challenging today.[128] For Galen, it was important to distinguish between a symptom, a syndrome and an overall condition, a *diathesis*, and between a cause and its visible manifestation. If as he believed, all illness was primarily something individual, the result of changes in the body that could occur at the deepest level of its organisation, it was incumbent on the doctor to understand the natural processes within the macrocosm in order to appreciate what was occurring in the microcosm of the body. Likewise, even if Galen's ultimate answers are schematic, it remains crucial, if not essential, for the doctor to have some idea of the stages through which a condition or a disease may pass in order to judge the appropriate point for intervention. Such questions can be dealt with empirically (and Galen has great respect for some of the so-called Empiricists as healers), but they are best resolved by the application of thought as well. Repetitive though many of these tracts may be, at the same time they also reveal that Galen was constantly thinking about the medical situation in front of him, something that can be fully comprehended only by those who have been faced with a potential life or death situation depending on the doctor's individual judgment, or who need to decide whether the patient is in fact ill or not.

The medical thinker

Indeed, it is perhaps here in his medical practice that Galen's strength as a philosopher is most evident, as a thinker outside the study or the seminar, responding to facts or ideas that have attracted his attention during his clinical practice. Sometimes, he alights on a question for which he can offer no clear answer. Pain, for instance, is part of the body's response to change, diminishing in as much as the body adjusts to or reverses that change. It is a sensation interpreted in the brain, and, for that reason, an absence of expected pain would be a good indication of damage to the brain. But that does not explain why one might feel greater pain from an injury when tucked up in bed at night rather than during the day. The example of a fellow philosopher encourages Galen to believe that this was simply because the absence of other concerns and activities in the brain let the pain predominate and apparently increase, a suggestion he regards as plausible, and quite possibly true.[129]

On another occasion, he ponders why in a crowded theatre only a handful of individuals develop sunstroke when, presumably, there must be many spectators with similar tendencies in their bodily balance. His solution is to suggest that only a few individuals had the 'seed' of the disease, and hence reacted badly to the hot sun.[130] It was a phrase that he used again in two other tracts written around the same time. In his commentary on *Epidemics* I he talked of 'seeds' of a disease within the body, which, without proper attention to diet, might bring about a recurrence of fever.[131] Elsewhere, in *The Different Types of Fevers*, he posed a hypothetical question as to which of two individuals, one with a healthy body, the other with blocked pores, would fall ill when taking in air containing 'seeds of plague'.[132] Exactly what Galen understood by this metaphor of seeds, one common among Epicurean thinkers whose view of illness was more mechanistic, is not at all clear. In the last example it seems to be something airborne that, so to speak, triggers the harmful changes within the body, whereas in the second, and possibly also in the first, it could be some harmful residue left over within the body which is called back to life as the result of inappropriate diet or exposure to heat. It is, at best, a metaphor thrown out and used briefly before being discarded, and is not developed further, as it was by a sixteenth-century Galenist, Girolamo Fracastoro in his *Contagious Diseases*, into a theory of the specific pathogens of certain diseases.[133] Besides, it is always subservient to Galen's overall theory of disease as a morbid alteration within the individual.

The little tract *Problematical Movements* offers a different example of the way in which Galen can pursue an argument along unusual lines as things strike him. The first half of the treatise attacks the view that assigns voluntary movement to the brain operating via the nerves and muscles, and other movements to the body's own organisation working independently of the brain.[134] This generalisation he attacks in two ways. Firstly he shows that, anatomically, some movements do not depend on muscles pulling in a certain direction, the tongue, for instance, or the penis, and, secondly, that some bodily movements which do involve muscles can hardly be classed as voluntary.[135] When one stands on a cliff, one's legs begin to shake, clearly a muscular movement, but one that is hardly under the conscious control of the brain. Galen's solution is to revise the notion of voluntary, by including in it the notion of imagination, which triggers these movements. He then lists several similar movements including yawning, but he can find no adequate explanation for his final example, contagious laughter, and he confesses himself baffled – a conclusion that led a Renaissance author to conclude that this could not be a genuine work by Galen, who would assuredly have found an answer.[136]

These examples, more perhaps than any more carefully presented theory, show Galen thinking on his feet, reacting to ideas and situations in different ways, sometimes in an oral presentation before an audience and simply dictating to a secretary. He may not always reach a satisfactory conclusion, and sometimes, as with the metaphor of seeds, it is something that he does not follow through, but often one can see Galen's thought processes in action as he responds to questions from a friend or to something he has read or found. As many modern scholars have argued, he was no mean philosopher and he offered his own individual interpretation of many of the most familiar theories of his predecessors, notably Plato and Aristotle. Given the fragmentary state of our knowledge of the ideas of other ancient thinkers, it would be rash to conclude that he never depended on some of their conclusions, but it is also significant that, where comparison is possible, he shows both a detailed acquaintance with the works of his major predecessors and a considerable degree of independence. He is eclectic in his willingness to adopt ideas from across the philosophical spectrum and in the varied uses to which he put them, while being at least occasionally prepared to acknowledge their plausibility or provisionality. But his philosophical writings, including his work on logic and demonstration, cannot be viewed in isolation from his activity as a doctor. One can debate, for example, the extent to which his ideas on psychology derive from his experience with patients or his familiarity with earlier philosophy, as well as their internal consistency, but even the most rebarbative of his medical tracts can be viewed as attempts to instruct others how best to think about their encounter with the sick. Galen strove for clarity, precision and certainty, and enlisted the aid of philosophy to those ends, for, as doctors both ancient and modern all know, certainty, however desirable, is not always possible in medicine, and any diagnosis or therapy must depend on what the doctor decides is the most favourable or the most plausible course of action among a range of choices when at least some of the factors are unknown or unknowable. There is little room for agnosticism when faced with a possible life and death situation.

Galen's philosophical writings have a double purpose. On the one hand, they provide the doctor with ways of logical thinking that will allow him to gain a better understanding and assessment of the immediate medical situation. On the other, the medical information, as well as the sharp criticism, that he has at his disposal is used to demolish or at least modify the conclusions of others and to suggest new approaches. This dual focus is summed up in the words Galen put into the mouth of an emperor-philosopher. Marcus Aurelius' praise of Galen as "first among doctors and unique among philosophers" (a characterisation that invites comparison with the similar phrasing on monuments to champion athletes) certainly corresponds to Galen's own image of himself, but he was far from alone in this period in pursuing both interests.[137]

Some other medical philosophers

The close connection between the two disciplines had long been a commonplace. The author of a collection of aphorisms, preserved in the Vatican Library, quoted Erasistratus for his declaration that medicine and philosophy were sisters: one cured the ills of the body, the other of the soul.[138] Other writers more famous today for their moralising or philosophical writings occasionally commented on matters medical. Plutarch, for example, in his *Table Talk* discussed at length the question of the possibility of new diseases appearing, and began his treatise on *How to Keep Well* with criticism of a doctor who refused to have anything to do with philosophical debate.[139] Medicine also figures in various series of *Natural Questions* from Aristotle down to Galen's own time and beyond. On the other hand, several leading members of other medical sects also gained a reputation for philosophy. The Methodist Soranus of Ephesus wrote a treatise on the soul that was later utilised by the Christian theologian Tertullian, and Sextus the Empiricist is far more famous for his writings on Scepticism than for anything he wrote on medicine, such as his *Medical Notes*, which may or may not be identical with his *Notes on Empiricism*.[140] Inscriptions of Greek doctors also indicate an interest in philosophy. Asclepiades, perhaps a younger contemporary of Galen, who was commemorated on a large, beautifully carved and floridly verbose inscription in Rome, is praised not only for his medicine but also for the writings in which he proclaimed to errant mortals that the soul was imperishable and immortal.[141] Galen would not have approved of this dogmatic assertion, as we have seen. Another Roman, the wife of Hortensinus, set a tombstone in honour of her late husband, "a doctor by profession and admired for his philosophical language and behaviour".[142] His contemporary, Gaius Calpurnius Macedo of Antioch in Pisidia, who died aged thirty already a town councillor, is compared to the ten orators for his rhetoric, and described as a pupil of Plato and Socrates in philosophy who followed Hippocrates in both word and deed.[143] In Athens, Sarapion, poet, doctor and Stoic philosopher, was commemorated by his grandson around 150 CE with a large and complex inscription enumerating the moral duties of the physician in terms that reflect, although they do not entirely match, those of the Hippocratic *Oath*.[144] He was a contemporary of another epigraphically attested medical philosopher, the immensely wealthy Heraclitus of Rhodiapolis, who was honoured by the Epicurean philosophers of Athens for his achievements as a man of letters as well as medicine.[145] Such men as these and the medical friend of Arria, a Roman woman with a passion for Plato, all show that Galen's demands for an alliance between medicine and philosophy would have found wide acceptance from elite doctors in the Greek East and in Rome during the second century. What Galen was doing was not unusual, except in its extent – he includes over 120 relevant titles in *My own Books*, to say nothing of any he forgot to mention there – and perhaps for its range of themes.[146] But, none of the writings of these medical philosophers survives today, save for those of Sextus, and these have not, until recently, been subjected to the same detailed attention as Galen's. That, despite his flaws and his self-centredness, Galen can still withstand the most detailed analysis and criticism and still have something interesting, if not always convincing, to say is a sure testimony to his abilities as a thinking physician.

Notes

1 Frede 1985; Frede and Walzer 1987; Barnes *et al.* 2003; Hankinson 2008; Adamson *et al.* 2014; Boudon-Millot 2019.
2 Singer 1991.
3 Moraux 1984: 607–808 is fundamental for his debt to Aristotle: see also van der Eijk 2009.

4 Tieleman 1996, 2009. His old teacher Eudemus in 162 regarded him as a philosopher and was surprised to find him acting as a doctor, *Praec.* 2,11: 14,608 K; *CMG* V 8,1, 76–7.
5 Chiaradonna, 2009b, 2019, sets out his differences from contemporary Middle Platonism; see also Schiefsky 2012; Rocca 2018.
6 Donini 1992 is very critical; Long 1996: 198–206, is more appreciative of his 'eclecticism', comparing it also as a practical expedient with the ideas of Ptolemy. Cf. also Hankinson 1992.
7 Hahn 1989, 2011; Singer PN 2014: 7–20, notes also that at times Galen could describe philosophers as a group to which he did not belong.
8 See below pp. 183-4; Pietrobelli 2020.
9 Thillet 1984: xxii–xlix; the two original Greek words are indistinguishable in majuscule script as ΟΡΙΚΟΣ. For his pride in his use of definitions, Galen, *Diff. Puls.* IV,16: 8,764 K, with Hood 2010, and for contemporary criticism, *Diff. Puls.* II,1: 8,571 K. The medieval interpretation of 'mulehead' as indicating the strength of his arguments seems unduly favourable.
10 See the chapter headings in Hankinson 2008a.
11 *Lib. Prop.* 16,1–3: 19,46 K; pp. 170–1 BM; p. 21 tr. Singer PN.
12 *Lib. Prop.* 17,1–3: 19,47 K; pp. 171–2 BM; pp. 21–2 tr. Singer PN.
13 *Lib. Prop.* 18,1–19,2: 19,47–8 K; pp. 172–3 BM; p. 22 tr. Singer PN.
14 *Lib. Prop.* 15,1–5: 19,45–6 K; pp. 169–70 BM; p. 21 tr. Singer PN. For Galen's knowledge of Plutarch, Nutton 2009a: 24. Plutarch himself not only wrote a treatise on how to keep well, *Moral Essays* 122B-137E. but also knew several medical texts and discussed medical themes in his miscellaneous *Table Talk*, Grimaudo 2004; Ruffy 2011, 2012.
15 The meaning of the title translated here as *Surreptitious Readers* is disputed. BM, pp. 170 and 192–4, linking it with the previous entry on "*Lecturers' Relationships with their Audience*", translates it as "those who give fraudulent lectures", i.e. using others' works. Other scholars, including Singer, more plausibly relate it to reading by oneself in private or when others are present; cf. Gavrilov 1997; Burnyeat 1997.
16 Fragments remain in Arabic of a work known as *How to Profit from one's Enemies* and containing autobiographical information (Meyerhof 1929: 84): was this a part of *Slander* or a book forgotten by Galen? Today's French and Italian philosophers display similarly wide interests.
17 *Opt. Med.* 2,3: 1,56 K; p. 31 tr. Singer PN. A similar, but not identical, statement is attributed by Ibn 'Abi Usaybi'ah to the [ps] Galenic *Commentary on the Oath* (Alessi 2019: 285). The need for constant training and practice is ubiquitous in *Opt. Med. Cogn.: CMG Suppl. Or.* IV.
18 *Opt. Med.* 3: 1,61 K; p. 33 tr. Singer PN.
19 For the *Letters* see Pinault 1992. Galen's ethics of medical practice in no way depend on the Hippocratic *Oath*, which is cited only in his *Hippocratic Glossary* among his surviving works. Fragments of a commentary on the *Oath* by a contemporary from Pergamum are preserved, but these say more about history or mythology than ethics (Rosenthal 1956, 1990) Another doctor, Sarapion of Athens, above, p. 92, did make some use of the *Oath* in formulating his own medical ethics. For the Aristotelian origin of the term, see Strohmaier's commentary at *CMG Suppl. Or.* III, 87–94. Whether Anaxagoras used the term a century earlier, a much-disputed question, is here irrelevant, as he employed it in a very different meaning and context.
20 Plato, *Phaedrus* 279c–d.
21 *Prop. Plac.* 2,1–2: *CMG* V 3,2, 56–9, with the many parallels given in the apparatus; pp. 172–3 BMP: pp. 60–3 Garofalo-Lami; pp. 186–9 Vegetti; *PHP* IX 7,9–15: *CMG* V 4,2, 588. He accepted both divine providence and divine intervention in human affairs. See also Hankinson 2008c: 178–9; Pietrobelli 2013; and, for the significance of 'plausibility', Chiaradonna 2014. For his father, *Aff. Dig.* 8: 5,42–3 K; pp. 273–4 tr. Singer PN.
22 Quoted by al-Rāzī, *Shūkūk* (Mohaghegh 1971: 241); al-Ghazzālī, *Tahāfut al-Falāsifat* p. 82 ed. Bouyges 1927; Averroes, *Tahāfut al-Tahāfut*, I, p.74; II, p. 56 ed. Van den Bergh 1954.
23 Hankinson 2008c 178–9.
24 Singer PN 2013: 335–59.
25 Moraux 1984: 701–30; Barnes 2003; Morison 2008.

26 *Lib.Prop.* 14,17–23; pp. 167–169 BM, which has a much improved and enlarged text. Only one of them survives for certain, *The Best Type of Teaching, against Favorinus, Opt.Doct.* 1,40–52 K: *CMG* V 1,1, but the *The Constitution of the Art of Medicine* may be one of the three books of *The Constitution of the Arts.* The tract *The Best Sect*, preserved as [*Opt. Sect.*]: 1,106–223 K, is almost certainly spurious.

27 An often unnoticed fragment of *Possibility* is edited and discussed by Rescher and Marmura 1965: 67–69.

28 Although given the abundance of references in a variety of Arabic authors, it is probable that a complete version in Arabic may yet be found, or even in Greek, see below, p. 135. The basic collection of fragments remains that of von Müller 1895, but much more has been added since, see Chiaradonna 2009a, 2014, 2019. Havrda 2015 provides a good overview.

29 *Inst.Log.* 16. For Galen's logic of relations, see Barnes 2002: 400–401, but note his conclusion, 417, that "his great logical invention … was neither admired nor copied".

30 Rescher and Marmura 1965: 69–70; Morison 2008: 94–5.

31 Rescher 1965, 1966; Morison 2008: 85–91. The surviving fragments of Galen's logic, however, are inconclusive.

32 Bobzien 2002.

33 Barnes 2002, 2003; cf. 1991.

34 Barnes 1991; Hankinson 1991a.

35 Hankinson 1991a.

36 *CAM proem.*: 1,224–7 K; *Opt.Med.Cogn.* 5,4–5: *CMG Suppl. Or.* IV, 68–9.

37 *MM* I,4: 10,32–5 K; I, pp. 51–55 tr. Johnston-Horsley; *Aff.Dig.* II,1: 5,59–60 K; pp. 284–5 tr. Singer PN; Barnes 1991; Lloyd 2005; Hankinson 2008c.

38 Barnes 2003; Morison 2008: 70–83; Chiaradonna 2014. The same adjective 'clear' is used to characterise the life-changing divine intervention to Nicon in a "clear dream", above, p. 14.

39 Tieleman 2018.

40 *Aff.Dig.* II,1: 5,59–60 K.

41 Tieleman 1996; Lloyd 1996.

42 Barnes 1991. This is not to say that the reasons he gave for the recovery or death of the patient would be accepted by modern physicians, merely that the steps in his reasoning proceeded logically.

43 *Soph.*: 14,582–98 K; ed. Edlow 1977; Ebbesen 1981; *Nom.Med.*, ed. Meyerhof and Schacht 1933; see also Morison 2008: 129–54.

44 *MM* I,2: 10,1–156 K; I, p. 241, tr. Johnston-Horsley, with Hankinson's commentary (1991a); Frede 1982; Tecusan 2004; Nutton 2013a: 191–206.

45 Plato, *Protagoras* 311b–c; *Phaedrus* 270c–d. Plato may not have been referring to any specific medical theory, as Galen imagined, but solely to Hippocrates' (to him logical) procedure in dealing with a case.

46 *Plat.Tim.Comp.* ed. Kraus and Walzer 1951; *Plat.Tim.: CMG Suppl.* I. Larrain 1992 and Lorusso 2005 add new fragments. See also Nickel 2002; Das 2014, 2019.

47 Plato, *Timaeus* 32b–34a; 81b–e. Galen does not concern himself with these Platonic triangles but follows an Aristotelian view of elements.

48 Plato, *Timaeus* 82a–83a. Philistion, whom Plato knew, is an even more likely source for these ideas, see Anonymus Londinensis 20,25–50.

49 Galen, *HNH I, Proem.: CMG* V 9,1, 8–9, asserts that Plato had incorporated ideas from *Human Nature* into the *Timaeus.*

50 *HNH I, Proem.: CMG* V 9,1, 7–10. Smith (1979: 166–72) notes that not every contemporary Hippocratic believed that this book was written by Hippocrates, and Galen himself thinks of it as made up of several diverse sections.

51 At times, in his psychological and ethical writings, Galen, like most contemporary Platonists, operated on a simple dichotomy between reason and desire, eliding the two lower categories. It was in commenting on the *Republic* that Galen praised the high moral standards he had observed among Christians, Walzer 1949: 15–16, 56–69 (for possible contexts).

52 Plato, *Timaeus* 44d–45b,69d–76e. None of the surviving fragments of Galen's commentary treat these sections.

53 Tieleman 1996; for Aristotelian terminology, Moraux 1984: 773–85.

54 Plato, *Timaeus* 70a–b, 71a–d; on the problem of the third part of the soul see Delacy 1988; Hankinson 1991b; Donini 2008: 187–94; Schiefsky 2012; Trompeter 2018. At *PHP* VIII,9,14: 5,725 K; *CMG* V 4,1,2, 537, he says that the region indicated by Plato contains the stomach, intestines and liver, whereas at *PHP* VI 8,52: 5,576 K; *CMG* V 4,1,2, 419 he is clear that the liver is the seat of the third part of the soul, adducing the evidence of Hippocrates and his own dissections to confirm it. Nonetheless, his failure to comment on the discrepancy in such passages as *Plat.Tim.Comp.* 18,19; p. 74 Kraus and Walzer or *Plat. Tim.* II,2: *CMG Suppl.* I, 12 is striking. Or did he and his teachers follow a tradition as represented in Plutarch, *Moral Virtue*, 450F, and Timaeus Locrus, 46, in emphasising *Timaeus* 71d, that puts this part of the soul 'by the liver'?

55 Frede 2003; Flemming 2009.

56 Plato, *Timaeus* 44d, 69d–74a.

57 Scolnicov 2017: 55.

58 Moraux 1984: 764–73; Rocca 2017: 12–13.

59 Moraux 1984: 731–5; Cosans 1998.

60 Craik 2015; Jouanna 2003: 252–5.

61 *Hipp.Fract.* 1.1: 18B,335 K.

62 Kovačič 2001: 251–2, although much goes back to the Stoics and even earlier.

63 Jouanna 2003 stresses Galen's modifications of others' views on nature.

64 Walzer 1949: 11–16, 23–37; Gero 1990; Barnes 2002; Ramelli 2015. Galen, like most of his contemporaries, had no difficulty in reconciling devotion to an individual god, such as Asclepius, with the notion of a Divine Creator.

65 Tieleman 2013; van der Eijk 2017.

66 *Us.Resp.:* 4,470–511 K; ed. Furley and Wilkie 1984; *UP*: 3,1–4,366 K; ed. Helmreich 1907–9; tr. May 1967.

67 Cf. *UP* II,16: 3,153–9 K; I, pp. 146–8 tr. May, with *Plen.* 6: 7,539 K.

68 *UP* XVII,3: 3,365–6 K; II, p. 733 tr. May. Cf. Frede 2003; Petit 2018.

69 Moraux 1984: 736–44.

70 Cooper 2011a: 137.

71 Although he claims that many commentaries were written upon it, he mentions only one, by Sabinus.

72 Boudon-Millot 2018: 308–9, on Galen's "subtle shift" in moving from a theory of the four humours to one stressing elements and qualities.

73 Kupreeva 2014; Leith 2014, esp. 222–9.

74 *Hipp.Elem.* 6,17–25: *CMG* V 1,2, 106–110. A similar reminiscence of a confrontation with a ninety-year-old follower of Archigenes is reported at *Diff.Puls.* III,3: 8,653–6 K. Both have also a literary purpose, to enliven a lengthy exposition, the latter also adorned with choice quotations from ancient comedy.

75 *Prop.Plac.* 4,1: p. 174 BMP; p. 70 Garofalo-Lami; p. 190 Vegetti. On black bile, see Jouanna 2003; Stewart 2019.

76 *Sem.* I,5,1–3; 11,1: *CMG* V 3,1, 78–81, 102–3.

77 Kupreeva 2014; Leith 2014.

78 *Temp.* I–III: 1,509–694 K; tr. Singer PN 2018.

79 *Temp.* I,9: 1,567 K; p. 93 tr. Singer PN; II,6: 1,635 K; p. 146 tr. Singer PN, with Singer PN 2018: 93–5, giving further examples of the phrase.

80 *Temp.* II,4: 1,604–5 K. Galen also wrote a treatise on *Habituation, Cons.:* ed. Schmutte, *CMG Suppl.* III.

81 *Temp.* I,9: 1,566 K; p. 93 tr. Singer PN, with the reffs. in n. 191.

82 *Temp.* I,2–3 and II,1: 1,510–22, 572–3 K; pp. 51–9, 103 tr. Singer PN; *Prop.Plac.* 5: *CMG* V 3,2, 66; p. 175 BMP; p. 76 Garofalo-Lami; p. 193 Vegetti.

83 *Temp.* I,3: 1,519–34 K; pp. 57–68 tr. Singer PN: *Prop.Plac.* 5: *CMG* V 3,2, 66; p. 175 BMP; p. 76 Garofalo-Lami; p. 193 Vegetti.

84 *Temp.* II,2: 1,578–86 K; pp. 108–14 tr. Singer PN.

85 *Ibid.* II,5–6: 1,618–41 K; pp. 134–41 tr. Singer PN. Galen adds his own examples to those already assembled in the Hippocratic *Airs, Waters, and Places*, 17–20: II,66,4–74,17 L. For the parallels with physiognomy, particularly clear in this treatise, see Barton 1994; Popovič 2007; Swain 2007b.

86 In general, Müller IW (1993).
87 *Nat.Fac.* I,3 and III,7: 2,7–9, 16–7 K; pp. 10–13 tr. Brock.
88 *Prop.Plac.* 3,5–6: *CMG* V 3,2, 62; p. 174 BMP; pp. 68–70 Garofalo-Lami; p. 190 Vegetti; *Nat.Fac.*: 1–204 K; tr. Brock 1916.
89 [Hippocrates], *De alimento* 31: IV,666,8 L.; *CMG* I 1, 82–13.
90 *Prop.Plac.* 11,1–4: *CMG* V 3,2, 90–3; pp. 182–3 BMP ; pp. 102–7 Garofalo-Lami; pp. 206–8 Vegetti.
91 *Mor.* 1: p. 28 Kraus; p. 140 tr. Davies.
92 *SMT* V,9: 11,731 K. In general, Harris CRS 1973: 167–9, 374–8, noting that at least the concept goes back to Aristotle and the Stoics. Cf, also *PHP* VIII,7,18: 5,700 K; *CMG* V 4,1,2, 524, for his claim that Plato in the *Timaeus* should have used 'innate heat' instead of simply 'fire'.
93 *Prop.Plac.* 4,2–5: *CMG* V 3,2, 64–67, with my notes *ad. loc.*; pp. 174–5 BMP; pp. 70–2 Garofalo-Lami; pp. 190–2 Vegetti. The other mention of the word is in the Hellenistic tract *The Heart* 6: IX,84,9 L. Cf. *PHP* VI,8,75: *CMG* V 4,1,2, 424–5 for another attempt to find innate heat in Hippocrates. See also Boudon-Millot 2018: 307–8.
94 *Adv.Lyc*, 6,1: 18B,225, 227 K. The whole tract is an attack on Lycus' interpretations.
95 At *Prop.Plac.* 4,14: *CMG* V 3,2: 64–5; p. 175 BM; p. 72 Garofalo-Lami; p. 192 Vegetti, Galen says cryptically that its essence is blood and semen, from which humans are produced. At *Sem.* I,15,40: 4,578 K: *CMG* V 3,1, 124–5, the loss of a testicle as described as 'like' the loss of a second source of innate heat. His ideas on generation, in which male semen, female semen and menstrual blood have complementary roles, are given at length in *Sem.*: 4,512–651 K: *CMG* V 3,1, and *Foet.Form.*: 4,652–702 K: *CMG* V 3,3; pp. 177–291 tr. Singer PN; Flemming 2018.
96 *UP* VII,9: 3,544 K; p. 349 tr. May; *Hipp.Epid. VI*, 2: 17B,316–17 K.
97 *Us.Resp.* 8–9: 4,491–2 K; pp. 106–9 Furley and Wilkie.
98 *Trem.Palp.* 6: 7,614 K; *Nat.Fac.* I,17: 2,68 K; p. 107 Brock.
99 *Prop.Plac.* 3,1–2; 7,1–3; 13,1–15,5: *CMG* V,3,2, 57–60; pp. 173, 178–9, 185–9 BMP; pp. 64, 86–8, 120–40 Garofalo-Lami; pp. 188, 199, 212–20 Vegetti, along with the parallel passages at *CMG* V,3,2, 58 and the notes on pp. 140–4. The fact that he so often returns to this theme is significant. See also Singer PN 2013: 30–3 and add *Mot.Dub.* 20–24: pp. 138–9 Nutton for his agnosticism about the arrival of the soul in the embryo. Marechal 2019 talks of his 'constitutive materialism' in his complex discussions on the soul.
100 *QAM* 4,767–821 K: tr. Singer PN 2013: 374–409; for dating, *ibid.*: 335–6.
101 Von Staden 2011; Mattern 2013: 250–6, 2016.
102 *Hipp.Epid. VI: CMG* V 10 2,2, 483–7. Cf. above, pp. 68–9 for other cases mentioned here.
103 *Praec.* 7,16: *CMG* V 8,1,110; *Us.Resp.* 4,2: 4,495 K; p. 113 tr. Furley-Wilkie. See also *Mot. Dub.* 4,18–9; pp. 138–9 Nutton.
104 Galen, *Plat.Tim.* IV: *CMG Suppl.* I,33.
105 *Ind.* 3–6: pp. 3–4 BJP; pp. 8 Garofalo-Lami; p. 262 Vegetti; pp. 78–9 tr. Nutton, with pp. 61–8. At *MM* VII,1: 10,456–7 K; II, pp. 237–9 tr. Johnston-Horsley, written after the Fire, he remarks that he was sometimes so affected by pain that he could not bear to open a book.
106 *Ind.* 54–5; p. 18 BJP; p. 38 Garofalo-Lami; p. 276 Vegetti; p. 93 tr. Nutton, with pp. 49–50; Nicholls 2011, 2019.
107 *Aff.Dig.* I,6: 5,30 K; p. 264 tr. Singer PN. These *Precepts* are probably to be identified with the 'Golden Poem', a series of moral precepts in verse attributed to Pythagoras (Thom 1995: 40–3), apparently quoted at 5,26 and 33 K: pp. 260, 267 tr. Singer PN.
108 *Aff.Dig.* I,1: 5,2–3 K; p. 239 tr. Singer PN; *Mor.* I: pp. 141–3 tr. Davies.
109 *Ibid.* II,4–5: 5,76–93 K; pp. 297–307 tr. Singer PN; *Mor.* II: pp. 152–5 tr. Davies. Galen refers also to this tract at *Lib.Prop.* 15: 19,46 K; p. 170 BM; p. 21 tr. Singer PN.
110 *Mor.* I: pp. 141–3 tr. Davies, a much-neglected passage. Cf. Kagan 1994; Kaufman forthcoming.
111 *Aff.Dig.* I,5: 5,14–19 K; pp. 251–6 tr. Singer PN; and for the contrast between his father and the dreadful example of his mother, I,8: 5,40–3 K; pp. 272–4 tr. Singer PN.
112 *San.Tu.* I,8: 6,41–2 K; I, p. 61, tr. Johnston, undoubtedly a reminiscence of theatrical performances at the Asclepieion in Pergamum; those less affected could be prescribed riding or

some form of armed combat. See also *Hipp.Epid.VI*, 8: *CMG* V 10,2,2, 494. The psychological effects of different types of music were also well known.
113 *Aff.Dig.* I,4,5: 5,15, 33 K; pp. 252, 267 tr. Singer PN.
114 *Aff.Dig.* I,9: 5,50 K; p. 278 tr. Singer PN. At *Mor.* Fr. 2,12; p. 181 tr. Davies, Galen cites the example of the slaves of Perennis who refused to incriminate their master under torture as an example of 'natural goodness'.
115 *Aff.Dig.* I,3; 10; 5,8–10; 55 K; pp. 245–7, 281 tr. Singer. For Aesop, *ibid.* I,2: 5,7 K; p. 243 tr. Singer PN.
116 *Ibid.* I,10 and 7: 5,54, 40 K.
117 *Aff.Dig.* I,4: 5,18–20 K; pp. 254–5 tr. Singer PN.
118 The pre-Roman medical background is covered in detail by Thumiger 2017.
119 Gill 2010; Singer PN 2013: 119–34, 205–32.
120 In general, *UP* I,3: 3,6–7 K; I, pp. 69–71 tr. May. He uses many animal comparisons in *Mor.*, to which add Stern 1956: 94–5.
121 *Sem.* 4,512–651 K: *CMG* V 3,1; *Foet.Form.*: 4,652–702 K: *CMG* V 3,3; pp. 177–201 tr. Singer PN.
122 Flemming 2018.
123 *Lib.Prop.* 4,37; p. 153 BM, with a much-improved text. Lycus presumably dissected animals, although one cannot exclude the possibility that he had seen an aborted or a dead human foetus.
124 *Prop.Plac.* 11,1–4: *CMG* V 3,2, 90–3; pp. 182–3 BMP; pp. 102–7 Garofalo-Lami; pp. 326–7 Vegetti. Debru 1995b; Rosen 2017, emphasising Galen's avowed uncertainty in his discussions of embryology; cf. also above, p. 60.
125 Rosen 2017: 195–7, emphasising the dichotomy between anatomist and philosopher at *Foet.Form.* 1 and 6: 4,651, 696 K; pp. 177, 198 tr. Singer PN. Galen is probably thinking here of the Cosmic Soul, *ibid.* 6: 467–8, 701 K; pp. 194, 201 tr. Singer PN.
126 Oberhelman 1994.
127 See the Introductions to Hankinson 1991a; Singer and van der Eijk 2018; Johnston 2006.
128 Kräupl Taylor 1979: 17–20, 111–3; Georges Canguilhem in Caplan *et al.* 2004: 40–42, 65–90.
129 *Mot.Dub.* 8,21–9, with Nutton 2011: 343–7. See also Roby 2016; King D 2018, neither of whom notes this passage or the fragments ascribed to his *Timaeus* commentary, Larrain 1992: 163–75; Nickel 2002; Das 2014, 2019. For Galen's theories of pain, Harris WV 2018: 36–54, 72–6.
130 *Caus.Proc.* 8,100 8, 126: pp. 104–7, 114–5 Hankinson.
131 *Hipp.Epid.I*, iii,7: 17A,239 K; *CMG* V 10,1, 119–20.
132 *Diff.Feb.* I,3: 7,279 K.
133 Nutton 1983; Pastore and Peruzzi 2006.
134 *Mot.Dub.* 1–8; pp.122–63 Nutton-Bos, with Trompeter 2018.
135 *Ibid.* 4–5: pp. 136–47 Nutton-Bos, He does not consider the tongue as a muscle in itself or discover the distal ligament in the penis.
136 *Ibid.* 8,15–6; 10,5: pp. 158–9, 164–5 Nutton-Bos; Joubert 1579: 11.
137 *Praec.* 11,8: 14,660 K; *CMG* V 8,1, 128–9.
138 Anon., *The Vatican Gnomologium, Sent.* 289, ed. Sternberg. Tertullian, *On the Soul* 2,6, takes it as a commonplace. Agnellus of Ravenna, *Commentary on Sects*, p. 44 ed. Westerink, ascribes it to Plato.
139 Plutarch, *Table Talk* VIII,9: 731A–4C; *Keeping Well* 1: 122B–E. See also the literature cited above, Note 14.
140 Polito 1994; Podolak 2010; Deichgräber 1965; Bailey 2002: 86–99.
141 Samama 2003, 525–527, no. 481.
142 Samama 2003, 522–3, no. 478.
143 Samama 2003, 432–434, nos. 334–335, although not all of Samama's supplements are secure. Gaius died in his twentieth year.
144 Samama 2003, 128–130, no. 022.
145 Above, p. 11.
146 *Lib.Prop.* 14–19: 19,40–48 K; pp. 164–173 BM; pp. 17–22 tr. Singer PN for losses, *ibid.* 9: 19,41 K; p. 166 BM; p. 19, tr. Singer PN.

5 Galen the doctor

The good doctor

Around the year 178 Galen wrote a treatise offering advice on how to choose a physician. He believed this to be necessary because Rome was filled with charlatans and fortune-hunters, eager for gain and ignorant of the Hippocratic principles of proper medicine. Patients, too, unless they were in such pain as to choose the first healer available, were liable to be swayed by fashion, flattery and unscrupulous promises. Some of this was the fault of the wealthy sufferers themselves, addicted to pleasure and frivolity rather than sober philosophical learning, but much could be laid at the feet of the doctors too. In Rome, an anonymous metropolis where medical failure could easily pass unnoticed, choosing a doctor or a surgeon might be literally a matter of life and death.[1]

Galen delivered his advice in the first instance to an audience or readership that already knew him personally or at least had heard of some of his achievements, and he emphasised his own successes as a criterion for judging others. It was an elite audience, literate, well-educated and with the leisure to spend time observing doctors at work and, if necessary, questioning them. Indeed, some of these "medical amateurs" might know far more than most doctors. In the plague, when doctors regularly failed, these laymen were experienced enough to decide simply from smelling a person's breath whether they should expect the worst.[2] Besides, Rome, with its abundance of healers, was very different from a small or isolated town where one was forced to rely on local assistance or wait for a visit from a travelling druggist or the fortuitous arrival of a doctor.[3] The aim of this tract was less to instruct a potential patient where someone might be found to provide healing than to show how to discriminate between a range of practitioners, if friends, family, or past experience failed to provide a guide.[4]

Galen's first requirement was that the physician should be a Hippocratic, not only because through the art of prognosis one could predict the course of an illness and prepare for it by having to hand the appropriate drugs and instruments, increasing the likelihood of success, but also because a detailed knowledge of the Hippocratic writings would suggest many sound therapies that might otherwise be forgotten.[5] A long series of examples of treatment by diet, drugs, emesis, purgation and so on emphasises Galen's infallibility as a follower of Hippocrates. Reliance on a passage from *Aphorisms* VI on treating pains in the eyes by drinking neat wine and bathing, advice never acted upon by his teachers or any contemporary, had resulted in years of unfailing success. A Hippocratic method of treating a prolapsed uvea with a series of different lotions gave him the reputation of a wonder-worker or a prophet (something he always denied vigorously, pointing to Hippocratic precedents).[6] Above all, the accomplished doctor who wished to follow Hippocrates must also be constantly aware of the individuality of the patient, adapting treatment to fit the particular case, for the development of a crisis, and all that follows from it, depends very much on the strength of the patient. It was by such means, Galen boasts, that "not a single day has passed without me showing skill in the art in cases of such dimensions or in similar ways".[7]

But, of course, Galen was not ubiquitous, and the prospective patient might not be able to call on him. Instead, he recommended two ways in which he (and Galen always addresses himself to men rather than women) can discover by himself who is a good or accomplished physician.[8] The first is simply by observing the practitioner at work and noting how well or how badly he treats his patient. Prognosis is again the key, for it allows for a check on any prediction: if a crisis occurs as has been predicted, this is a sign of competence.[9] But the second makes demands on both parties. Patient and doctor alike must be learned: a doctor without book-learning should be instantly dismissed, and a patient well trained in philosophy and logic may be able to make a sound judgment without further questioning simply on the basis of what the doctor says or does.[10] Although a knowledge of the Hippocratic writings is a prerequisite, the good doctor should be able to answer a range of questions about the opinions of a group of physicians Galen calls the "ancients" – Diocles, Pleistonicus, Phylotimus, Praxagoras, Dieuches, Herophilus, Erasistratus and Asclepiades. Except for the last, who lived around 100 BCE, all were active between 350 and 250 BCE and all were later characterised as 'dogmatics' or 'rationalists', not least because of their belief in the importance of reasoning in identifying, and eliminating, the causes of disease. They thus differed from the Empiricists, who rejected a search for hidden causes, and the Methodists, whose ideas on causation Galen derided as simplistic at best. This classification, Asclepiades apart, seems to go back to Hellenistic Alexandria, and continued to be repeated for millennia.[11]

Galen himself certainly owned copies of some of these "ancient" writings, which he deployed to great effect in his debates over venesection with the Erasistrateans in Rome, and he expected his candidate doctor to be able to indicate examples of places where Erasistratus, for example, disagreed with Hippocrates, either in argument or in his recommendations for therapy.[12] But it is doubtful if many, or even most, of his contemporaries, could have amassed such a library. They could, however, obtain digests of such information, some of which have survived, listing the major beliefs of these famous men, and setting out their descriptions of diseases and some appropriate treatments. Whether such handbooks were ever owned or used by the laymen who had the task of selecting civic physicians or granting physicians and specialists tax immunity is impossible to say.[13]

Choosing a doctor requires effort on both sides, from the doctor who should devote all his time and energy, like Galen, to improving his skills, and from the patient, who needs to have a basic understanding of medicine to accompany what is even more important – a mind trained in demonstrative philosophy that can cut through verbiage and surface flummery. Both parties must accept that Hippocratic prognosis is the only sure way to proceed, and that this is an art that requires an appropriate method of gaining information about the body in both sickness and health, as well as constant practice. If a great orator like Herodes Atticus felt the need to apologise for delivering a speech below his usual standard because he had been engaged in other business over the previous three days, how much more important was it for a doctor to eschew dinners and outings in favour of study and sound learning?[14] Anatomical knowledge takes pride of place among the criteria of excellence, followed by the proper use of dialectic in diagnosis and therapy. A knowledge of a physician's previous cases will help a potential patient, especially if he has succeeded in difficult cases where others have failed or given up. Doctors should be particularly praised who can cure by drugs conditions that would otherwise have had to be treated surgically, including a variety of swellings, tumours, eye problems, ulcers, and fistulae. A further list of conditions that the competent physician should be able to treat by diet and drugs includes epilepsy, migraine, madness, asthma and spitting blood.[15]

How far this advice indicates the level of competence of the average healer in Rome is not easy to determine. On the one hand, Galen includes many examples of his own practice where he goes beyond what others have done or prescribed. On the other, he follows this list immediately with a reference to what the "really complete" physician can do, which implies that he has previously been describing conditions that many physicians in Rome would at least expect to treat successfully, even if their performance fell short of his own high standards.[16]

This preference for diet and drugs is not an attack on surgery, but, rather, an awareness of the obvious dangers that any surgical intervention might bring. Galen presumes that his physician will be able to know when and when not to bleed, and he concludes his book with a similar list of conditions that the surgeon should be able to treat. But, as with the physician, the surgeon's judgment is needed to identify which conditions are serious and avoid being misled by appearances. The seriousness of a hernia, for example, does not depend on its size but on its location: a large hydrocele is far less dangerous than a smaller strangulated hernia. But, above all, what distinguishes the good practitioner from the bad is judgment, something that the potential patient in search of healing needs as much as the therapist himself.[17]

But sound therapy, Galen knew well, is not just a question of providing physical treatment or mastery of the very different skills that make up the art of medicine.[18] It also requires what Pedro Laín Entralgo famously called the therapy of the word, persuading the patient to place his trust in the healer and ensuring the best possible environment for the healing process.[19] The Hippocratic *Prognostic*, the treatise on which Galen most depends, opens with a plea for the co-operation of doctor and patient in the struggle against diseases, for without it there will be less chance of a favourable outcome. Galen in his commentary, typically, talks more in terms of the patient's obedience than of his co-operation, and extends his gaze to include family and servants, whose actions, however well meant, might be harmful.[20] The good intentions of a mother in supplying her son with surreptitious food delayed his recovery, and her stratagem baffled Galen, but only for a time, while the intervention of Annia Faustina, a supporter of Methodist doctors, in the case of the young Commodus, her nephew, he regarded as extremely unhelpful.[21]

The (fictitious) stories about Hippocrates treating famous patients such as the King of Macedon or the philosopher Democritus, as well as the equally ahistorical reports of his successful intervention in the Plague of Athens, gave Galen ample opportunity to model his own practice on that of his predecessor.[22] In a lengthy passage in his commentary on *Epidemics* VI he explained an obscure aphorism, "Entrances, conversations, position, clothing, for the sick, hair, nails, odour", as the great Coan's shorthand note to the doctor on how he should present himself at the bedside.[23]

Galen's long exposition combines sound sense with amusing anecdotes about those who failed to follow these injunctions. Some of his advice is banal: one should not arrive at the bedside making a loud noise or shouting, one should dress appropriately, neither flaunting one's wealth nor arriving in shabby clothes, and one should attend carefully to one's nails. The doctor's hair should indicate his good health rather than his taste in fashion. Galen's example of an inappropriate hairstyle is the close-cropped cut that was in vogue in the early 160s until the emperor Lucius Verus jokingly characterised its bearers as mime actors (a low form of entertainer), after which men began growing their hair longer again. Some of Galen's advice remains valuable even today. A doctor who smells of garlic, onions or wine or even has naturally malodorous armpits does not give a good impression to his patients. Still less, if, like Quintus, he retorts that the patient smells far worse. How one speaks to the sick person is also crucial. Inappropriate witticisms or too oily a subservience do not impress, and one should always be careful about choosing the correct tone and volume of voice. An educated patient will think little of a doctor who hectors or whose speech is peppered with solecisms or weird words. Elsewhere, he shows himself aware of the problems of carrying out examination and treatment when surrounded by any number of onlookers, for many of his cases take place either in public or in a crowded room, filled with noisy argument and interruptions.[24] The true doctor must put his point clearly and firmly and be aware of the social as well as the medical situation. One must take care not to reveal parts of the body unnecessarily, especially the buttocks and genitals, and thereby embarrass the patient, and always be ready to assuage the patient's fears, even employing subterfuge, if necessary.[25] Proper attention to these rules will create an impression of authority and make the doctor a god-like figure in whom patients can be expected to put their trust.[26]

The Greek word σεμνότης, which is here translated as authority, indicates something majestic and awe-inspiring, a characteristic of rulers and gods. It conveys a high ideal of the art of medicine, akin to that put forward by Galen's Pergamene contemporary, the author of a commentary on the Hippocratic *Oath*, who explained the qualities of the ideal doctor by the attributes of Asclepius on his cult statue at his shrine at Pergamum. Maturity, mental power, stability of judgment, continuous awareness, foresight were all represented on the statue as contributing to the doctor's power to heal and to preserve the fragile life of mankind, depicted as an egg in the hand of the god.[27] Galen, of course, as he instances time and again in his stories of his relations with patients, claims to possess all these qualities, and he would have increased the authority of his therapy by his learning, his arguments, his rhetoric, and by setting himself up alongside the greatest of his predecessors, Hippocrates and, in therapy, Erasistratus among others. His tale of his treatment of the woman in love with Pylades the actor (*Fig 1.2*) placed him in a line of similar success stories from Hippocrates' cure of Perdiccas, King of Macedon, to the story of Seleucus' love of his stepmother Stratonice that was widely circulated and featured a variety of different protagonists, including Erasistratus.[28] His learned patients and their friends would have immediately recognised Galen's claim for inclusion in the pantheon of famous doctors.

Behind the rhetoric: Galen at the bedside

Penetrating to the reality behind Galen's rhetoric of success is not easy.[29] However, if only half of the mentions of his encounters with patients listed by Susan Mattern turned out to have been successful, their range and complexity would establish Galen's credibility as a healer, even if modern explanations of both the condition and the therapy might differ from his.[30] The variety of testimonials and witness he adduces, and the undoubted fact of his long relationship with the imperial court, add weight to his claims for superiority, even if we factor in his complaints about the tendency of wealthy Romans to be swayed by quacks and fashionable incompetents. For the most part, too, his notions of how best to carry out treatment are far from foolish and stand comparison with those of any other pre-modern practitioner and, *experto credite*, even some of today's physicians.

At the basis of his therapeutics lie the individual patient and individual treatment, and even the individual organ and bodily part. Galen's main criticism of the Methodists rests on this credo:

> They are in the habit of saying that their knowledge is a craft of 'communities' and not of specifics, just as if they were treating a 'common' and generic person and not a series of individuals. Thus, just as they stumble in everything else right from the outset, so too they stumbled here, for it is not the 'common' and generic person that is treated but each one of us, having clearly a different mixture and nature. They think, however, there is one treatment for all people. If I knew how to discover precisely the nature of each person, as I think Asclepius did, I would myself be like him. But since this is impossible, I have decided to approach this ideal as closely as is humanly possible and to exhort others to follow my example.[31]

A generalised approach to the sick was not enough, for, to take one example, age alone was no sound guarantee of how a patient might be feeling or react to treatment. Galen had seen people in their sixties as dry and shrivelled as the very elderly, and others in their nineties or even centenarians still hale and hearty.[32] But identifying this individuality was far from easy. Ideally, one should be acquainted with the patient before any illness, so that one might know in advance his or her natural constitution and be able to use it as a benchmark to aim for in any attempt to restore health. The doctor should also be able to learn about the normal lifestyle of the patient, for this indicated not only the humoral and qualitative balance or imbalance, but also the habits, likes and dislikes that most affected the body. Habit, on which Galen wrote a short treatise, might determine reaction to certain drugs or foods, and a doctor's ignorance of the normal lifestyle of his patient might lead to disaster.[33] But even knowing the patient very well on occasions presented an unexpected problem. When the Aristotelian philosopher Aristotle of Mytilene fell ill, his doctors would have prescribed drinks of cold water, had they not been assured by him that he had fallen ill on every occasion he had previously drunk it. Faced with a dilemma as to what to do, they followed his wishes, with the inevitable result – death. When Galen was asked what he would have done, he declared that he would have said that without cold water, death was inevitable; whereas with it, there was at least the possibility of recovery.[34]

But only the wealthy were able to have a permanent doctor among their retainers, and often Galen had to rely on the patient or friends and family for essential background information that would help towards a diagnosis. His great predecessor, Rufus of Ephesus, wrote a small tract on how to question the patient that provides an excellent introduction to Hippocratic bedside medicine, and particularly to how the doctor should try to find out what is wrong.[35] How Galen interviewed the patient, however, can only be surmised from what he says in his case descriptions or in passing comments. Sleep patterns, eating and drinking, the surroundings of the patient, normal or abnormal excretions, sensations of pain, and any unusual symptoms such as headaches, tinnitus or paralysis can all be discovered by a dialogue with the patient.[36] But there are times when this is impossible, particularly if the situation is serious or cannot be easily described by the sufferer. Here Galen has to rely on what others tell him. Often, he participates in consultations with several other doctors (almost always correcting their initial surmises) or receives at least his initial guidance from members of the family, usually male.[37] But for many of his female patients he has to base his judgment on what *maiai* or midwives can tell him, some of whom he accepts as experts in dealing with pregnancy and gynaecological problems.[38] On some occasions he never meets the patient at all. He reports receiving letters seeking advice from as far afield as Gaul and Spain, and we have, in a letter to the father of an epileptic boy, an example of a reply.[39] Caecilianus, who had approached Galen for advice, was almost certainly a wealthy Italian preparing to accompany his son to study in Athens. Galen's reply is cautious. Since he has never met the boy, he can do no more than speak in general terms. As the author of a monumental *Method of Healing* called in to advise on a specific case, he confesses to feeling a little like the sculptor Phidias, who, having completed his famous statue of Athena, was asked to produces carvings of each individual body part separately.[40] But he knows that doctor Dionysius, who has already communicated with him, will be able to follow his instructions, and supervise the lad on the journey and in the first few weeks of his Athenian stay before returning home.[41]

Galen gives his prescription in the broadest of terms. The first task is to avoid, as far as possible, anything that will trigger an epileptic attack: intense heat or cold, high winds, harmful baths, bad food, the motion of chariot wheels, thunder, lightning, lack of sleep, distress, tiredness and so on.[42] But these things are difficult to avoid on a journey, and apart from staying inside whenever possible and eating sparingly, there is little that can be done immediately in the way of prevention. But after an attack, one can purge moderately, take gentle exercise before lessons with an experienced trainer (but not just anyone) chosen by Dionysius who knows how to prescribe appropriately.[43] Galen then describes suitable massages, before passing on to questions of diet. The overall aim is to avoid rich food that generates sticky humours and especially phlegm. He warns against seasonal fruits in particular, cautioning against assuming that the apples that Caecilianus' wife had picked for the journey will all be ripe.[44] But if the lad wants occasionally to eat fruit, that is fine (although he himself would not do so), for he is not laying out a regimen for philosophers, but for life in general.[45] He recommends drinking oxymel, a mixture of honey, vinegar and water, especially a type produced in Greece and the islands using honey straight from the honeycomb, highly suitable for an Athenian summer.[46]

But even in this letter, Galen cannot resist adding personal touches – his successful cures of chronic ulcers and eye problems by following Hippocratic precepts demonstrate a method that his competitors are too stupid to follow, and meat should be roasted in an oven that keeps in any odour "as you have seen in my house".[47] He ends with his technique for producing a sort of thin jam from the juice of the scilla in a jar formerly containing honey. The scilla flowers are plucked apart by hand, the jar is sealed, covered with skin, and placed in the sun out of the North wind, preferably at the height of summer. The jar is turned around regularly so that it is evenly heated. After a certain period, the jar is opened, to reveal something that resembles scilla when it is stewed. This can then be mixed with first-class honey, and a spoonful taken daily as a prophylactic. Other methods are much inferior. Simply stewing the scilla in water removes all its active properties, and using vinegar makes the concoction more powerful, but "not unharmful" to the nerves.[48]

This patient was known to Galen at second hand, although he was acquainted with Dionysius and perhaps Caecilianus, if only vaguely, and it was the doctor who had described to him his epileptic symptoms. But if, as must have happened often, the patient was previously entirely unknown to Galen, he needed to exercise all his senses and reasoning powers to discover what was wrong and what its cause was.[49] The Galenic art of prognosis was far more complex and required much more thought than the simple correlations between the phenomena and the commonalities proclaimed by the Methodists. We have already noted some of Galen's remarkable powers of visual observation, as well as his insistence on an understanding of anatomy as a prerequisite for therapy. But yet more was needed. As he explained in his long commentary on the opening passages of the Hippocratic *Surgery*, Nature has given us our senses in order that we may recognise the true character of things, and particularly indications that provide cogent and easily recognisable information.[50]

In practice Galen makes relatively little use of some of the senses. He mentions from time to time the odours of urine, sputum, faeces, ulcers and bad breath as important diagnostic guides, but they are insufficiently subdivided to specify exactly what is wrong. Indeed, on one occasion he rightly expresses grave doubts about distinctions made purely from smell. Lawyers would agree with him: bad breath alone was no proof that a slave was suffering from a serious illness.[51]

Taste is involved a little more often than smell. It can differentiate between different kinds of diabetic urine, and the taste of sweat may be equally indicative of the patient's condition.[52] The doctor should lick any that has collected on his fingers during a physical examination, for this might help to identify a disease – jaundice, for instance produces a bitter-tasting sweat – but quality is less significant than quantity and temperature.[53]

Hearing is also largely restricted to interpreting communication or non-communication from the patient, but their content is more significant than changes in vocal quality.[54] Auscultation is used rarely, although it is recommended to distinguish tympanites, caused by an accumulation of gas in a swollen abdomen, from ascites, the result of a build-up of fluid, the former producing a much hollower sound.[55]

Galen employed touch much more frequently. Not only did it indicate the patient's temperature, preferably if the doctor used the palm of the hand, an instrument wisely constructed by the Creator to respond to the slightest of stimuli and the smallest of changes, but palpation was also essential to differentiate between the softness and hardness of the abdomen, something widely practised and even represented on medical tomb reliefs.[56] It was something that required to be learned largely by constant practice with a large number of similar bodies in identical situations – the old, the young, before and after bathing, or in hot or cold weather, for instance – in order to gain an appropriate basis for comparison.[57] But, above all, Galen made much of his expertise in taking and interpreting the pulse, explaining in qualitative terms phenomena that, until the development of technological aids in the late nineteenth century, depended on the diagnostic skill and touch of the individual doctor.[58]

Although Galen himself believed that sphygmology, the diagnosis of illness by means of the pulse, had been practised by Hippocrates, this was a typically Galenic conclusion on the basis of scattered comments in different Hippocratic treatises, for it was not until the late fourth century BC, with another Coan physician, Praxagoras, that one can detect any detailed and systematic interest in the pulse. Praxagoras was the first doctor to distinguish veins and arteries, and to consider pulsation as a natural movement rather than something appearing only when the body was in some way disturbed.[59] His pupil, the anatomist Herophilus, extended Praxagoras' ideas on the pulse, arguing for its crucial importance in diagnosis and even inventing a mechanism for timing it.[60] Between them they laid the foundations for what was to become a major feature of medicine in the Hellenistic and Roman periods, not least in the creation of a vocabulary to identify different patterns of arterial beats. By Galen's day taking the pulse seems to have been common, particularly among the so-called Pneumatists such as Archigenes of Apamea in Syria, active around 100 CE, and his teacher Agathinus, who saw *pneuma* as the prime regulatory substance in the body and one that was manifested in pulsation.[61] The fortunate survival of some contemporary or near-contemporary discussions of pulsation within the Galenic Corpus, such as the treatise on pulses dedicated to Antonius, and of others later ascribed to Soranus and Rufus, as well as one by the otherwise unknown Marcellinus that circulated independently, not only reveal a vigorous debate about the pulse, but also provide a means of assessing Galen's ideas.[62] Sometimes they are all in general agreement. Galen would happily have concurred with the pseudo-Galenic author of *Medical Definitions* who described the pulse as "the truthful messenger of things hidden in the body, a foreteller of things invisible and a proof of things unclear", although he would have taken issue with his further claim that it foretold an unseen condition by its "mantic" beat.[63] For Galen there was nothing mantic or prophetic about interpreting natural signs. At the very least these unfamiliar texts reveal that, as we might expect, Galen's treatises on pulsation were composed in a context of competition equally as polemical as those on anatomy, and also involving a power-struggle for patients.[64]

Galen had been fascinated by the whole art of pulse since childhood, and devoted a considerable portion of his writing to the subject.[65] As well as a commentary in eight books on the pulse doctrines of Archigenes, now lost, and comments throughout his writings on therapy, he wrote a large work in sixteen books on the pulse, which he later summarised in a double volume, as well as in a single shorter book for beginners, and in another short book on the *Use of Pulses*.[66] The sixteen books are divided into four blocks, each consisting of four books: *The Causes of the Pulse, The Distinct Types of Pulse, Pulse Diagnosis*, and *Prognosis from the Pulse*, which are among the most forbidding as well as the least studied of all his works, for several reasons.[67] They are drily technical, often given over to polemics over definitions and inappropriate or unintelligible new-fangled terminology, and embody an idea of pulsation that is vastly different from today's. It is not only that Galen believed that both heart and arteries contract and expand simultaneously, but he also supposed that the function of the arteries was to act as a kind of bellows, drawing in air at diastole and expelling it, along with waste products of combustion, at systole, as well as transporting arterial blood around the body to where it was needed.[68] In order for this to happen Nature had made the arteries elastic compared with the veins, and had endowed their walls with the power to expand and contract, stimulated in some way by the heartbeat. Systole and diastole were thus distinct movements, unrelated to one another: after expansion, there was a tiny moment before the artery contracted to its normal size in systole and then began a longer period of inactivity before the diastolic expansion recommenced again.[69] This rhythmic action was enough to propel the arterial blood forwards, for in Galen's view the take-up of arterial blood as it passed to periphery of the body was slow and the small suction effect that was involved removed any need to posit any strong pumping action from the left ventricle of the heart.

This contrast between a modern (and Erasistratean) mechanistic explanation of the pulse and Galen's vitalist one hampers any understanding of what Galen was trying to do, and more than one scholar, from the sixteenth century onwards, has pointed out the contradictions and contortions in his complex arguments about the relationships between the heart, lungs and arteries.[70] While one can approve of his frequent complaints about the novel, often inconsistent, and always confusing terminology of recent doctors, and his desire to begin with simple agreed definitions, much in his discussion of the different kinds of pulse is simply Galenic logic-chopping.[71] He rejects Archigenes' distinctions between the pulses as being qualitative rather than showing essentially different types but one becomes tired of his insistence on this point, which is passed over briefly in the treatises of the other writers. Similarly, although he, like them, provides advice as to how and where best in the body to take the pulse, he spends far less time on this practical point in his big books than on the complicated theoretical question of whether there is a minute period of rest between the diastole and systole, and how best to identify any systolic movement.[72] Galen was at first unsure about any break between the movements, but it became evident once he had trained himself to observe this through his "most sensitive" touch, something that, in his view, could be gained only by constant practice.[73] Sculptors, painters, wine-tasters, cooks, perfumiers and musicians need many years, not just days or months, to acquire their skill even when they have unlimited time and resources, and doctors, being more constrained in their regular practice, require even longer to acquire this essential expertise.[74]

But, despite the amount of words Galen devoted to sphygmology, it is what can be observed by sight that is most significant, whether this is some change in the patient or in the ambience of the sick room. Galen himself was a remarkable observer, as we have already seen. His exposition of the so-called Hippocratic face, a clear sign of impending death, in his *Prognostic* commentary shows how much he owed to Hippocrates as well as his ability to develop this familiar description for his own purposes, not least by supplying an explanation for the phenomena. Having warned against mistaking a simply thin face for one with a shrivelled nose or sunken eyes, he explains how the latter may be the result of some flesh-eating condition or of the diminution in one's natural heat, particularly in bodily extremities, whereby the fleshy parts contract together because of the cold. The moist flesh of the nose thus shrivels whereas the bony structures remain intact for longer.[75]

His insistence on the need for the use of all the senses and for an overall physical examination rather than a concentration on any one particular affected area may also explain one major difference between his diagnoses and those of later, medieval Galenists: he devotes relatively little space to urine. He does note changes in its colour, consistency, taste and temperature, and draws some valuable conclusions from them, but he never produced a specific tract on urine diagnosis, a source of complaint from some of his successors.[76] Urine is for him just one important sign among many.

Having amassed as much information as possible about his patient, and preferably also possessing previous knowledge of his or her natural state, Galen would proceed to a diagnosis, and usually a differential diagnosis, following the method of division ascribed by Plato to the great Hippocrates in the *Phaedrus*, 270c–d.[77] Many of his observations and diagnoses agree with those of modern doctors. His precise description of the aura that precedes an attack of epilepsy allows it to be identified as a case of Jacksonian epilepsy.[78] Similarly, his characterisation of the age distribution and severity of apoplexy or stroke coincides with modern data: rare but serious in those under forty, and carrying a decreasing likelihood of recovery with each successive attack.[79] However, these are not necessarily his own discoveries, for he indicates his own debts to others (save Hippocrates) far less often than his disagreements. It is only through a casual remark that we learn that his master Pelops had described the epileptic aura earlier, comparing it to the result of a scorpion bite or the sting of a deadly spider.[80] But frequently the details that are given by Galen do not allow for more than a general identification of the condition, particularly when dealing with fevers or skin conditions.[81]

Galen set out the theoretical underpinnings of his therapy at length in the fourteen books of his *Method of Healing*, although later generations found the shorter version that he dedicated to Glaucon far more useful.[82] In both works diseases are classified into three categories (although a patient might be suffering from more than one at the same time).[83] The first is a disturbance of the elemental and qualitative mixture of a part or of the body as a whole. The most important of these disturbances is fever, a particular form of hot distemper or incorrect mixture that takes on various forms depending on their periodicity. They might be ephemeral, lasting a mere day, recur at regular intervals, or be continuous, the last group being the result of putrefaction of the humours.[84] These diseases essentially attack what Galen calls the homoeomerous parts of the body, an Aristotelian term indicating consistently uniform structures, including veins, nerves, bone, cartilages, membranes, ligaments and flesh, all formed from the primary elements and serving as components of the larger and more complex organic bodies such as the liver or stomach.[85] These organic bodies are particularly subject to Galen's second category of diseases, what he calls abnormalities of magnitude, number, position and conformation.[86] These can include inflammations of various kinds, erysipelas, pustules, warts, cataract or simply obesity, and diseases of deficiency such as missing digits, atrophy and baldness. The third category, dissolution of continuity, applies to both uniform and organic parts alike. This can be the result of something external, as in wounds and fractures, or of internal changes, as in ulcers and tissue loss, whether chronic, malignant, or relatively benign.[87] This schema encompasses all disease conditions, and a practitioner who fully understands this will be able to devise suitable treatments from first principles. It also helps to explain why Galen wrote so little about individual diseases or conditions (marasmus, 'wasting fever', and coma being exceptions), and preferred in another long book on therapy, *Affected Parts*, to discuss them topically rather than in individual listings.[88]

These categories allow the doctor to organise his observations and to identify, where possible, the cause of the condition in the individual and eliminate it. Galen is particularly concerned to distinguish between different types of cause, not only because he regards their proper identification as essential but also in part because of his deep acquaintance (and disagreement) with the categories of Stoic logic, to say nothing of the mistakes and misunderstandings he detects in the methodologies of his

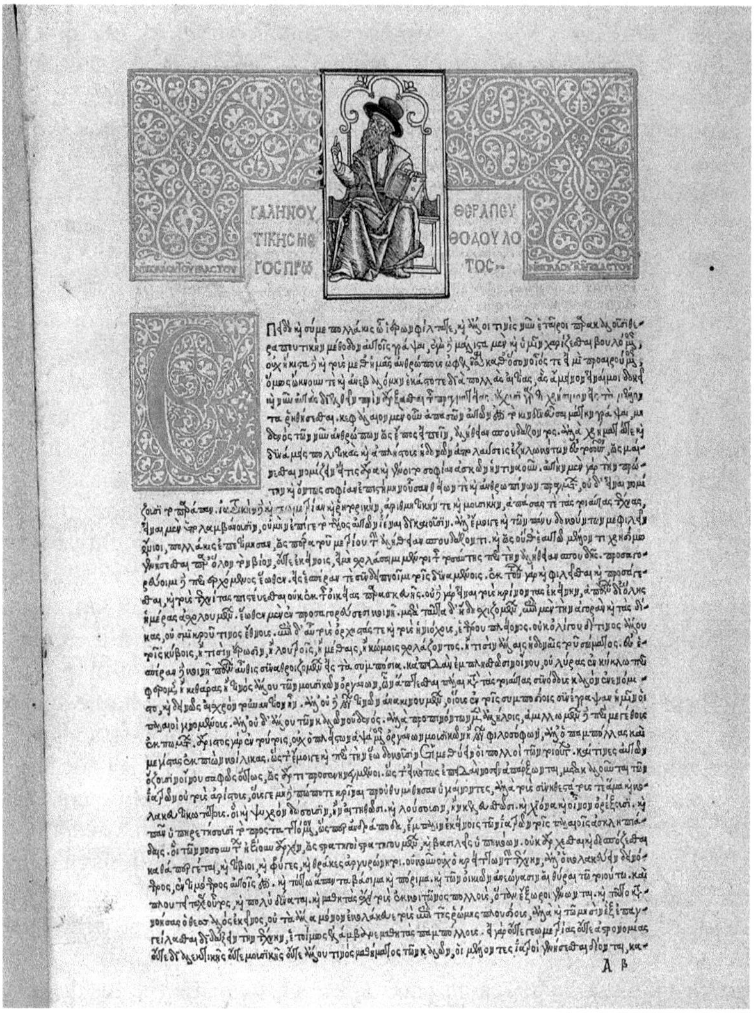
ΓΑΛΗΝΟΥ ΘΕΡΑΠΕΥ
ΤΙΚΗΣ ΜΕ ΘΟΔΟΥ ΛΟ
ΓΟΣ ΠΡΩ ΤΟΣ.

Figure 5.1 Galen, *Method of Healing*, Venice, Z. Kallierges for N. Blastos, 1500, fol. 1r. The first printing of a genuine work by Galen in the original Greek.

competitors.[89] He follows a threefold classification, distinguishing between antecedent, preceding and cohesive causes, which he attributes to the Pneumatist Athenaeus of Attaleia around 100 CE and which is traceable in part to the philosopher Posidonius in the first century BCE and to other even earlier Stoics in the Hellenistic period.[90]

Antecedent or 'procatarctic' causes are external and produce changes within the body, the preceding causes, which in turn are responsible for the cohesive causes of the effects that are under consideration by the therapist. Cohesive causes are co-temporal with effects whose manifestations vary according to variations in the cause itself. A man may be bitten by a dog, the procatarctic cause, which sets up changes within the body, the preceding cause, which may result in rabies or a fever, depending on the nature of the cohesive cause.[91] This is a somewhat crude heuristic schema that Galen defends at length in his treatises on these causes. It justifies his individualist approach to therapy in that he can then explain why not everyone bitten falls ill in the same way, or even at all, or responds similarly to treatment. His opponents could find equally good reasons for their objections to it. The Methodists could claim that it was over-elaborate and Galen's actual practice inconsistent, the Empiricists that investigating causes was time-consuming and unnecessary for successful therapy. But, in context, it is a laudable attempt to provide a clear structure that enables the doctor and the patient to answer, however fallibly, a universal question: how and why do I fall ill?

Defining disease

There is a further consideration to be taken into account when deciding upon treatment – the development of the condition itself. Galen follows a long tradition in arguing for four stages of disease that the doctor should be aware of: its genesis, development, acme, and decline – or, alternatively, the death of the patient.[92] For the first, some understanding of causation is useful, if only to distinguish between long-term and short-term causes, while a different type of therapy may be required if the doctor decides that the disease is on the decline from when it is rising to a climax. Similarly, knowing precisely when to intervene may well prevent any exacerbation, and an inappropriate intervention may only make matters worse. Above all, what matters is to know when and how the critical point, the crisis, is reached, and to prepare accordingly.

The doctrine of crisis is a key feature in Hippocratic medicine.[93] On the one hand, it corresponds to a common feature in many conditions, particular in acute diseases; on the other hand, the case histories in the *Epidemics* are often structured around specific numbers of days on which a crisis or a series of crises occurs, not all of which can be identified with, for example, the periodicity of attacks of malaria. Indeed, many seem to involve number mysticism (or mystification) rather than clinical judgment.[94] Galen devoted one long tract to explaining the significance of crises and how to understand and manipulate them to a successful end, and many of his case descriptions emphasise his sound management of a crisis, often to the amazement of his audience[95] (*Fig 1.2*). Before the advent of modern technology, crisis management was the supreme skill of the clinician, described in many case histories as well as in literature as anxious relatives wait for the crisis to arrive, with subsequent rejoicing or mourning depending on the outcome. In his similarly lengthy exposition of critical days, Galen shows his mastery of the technicalities of mathematics and astrology in his attempts to justify and explain what Hippocratics believed about periodicity.[96] His first two books are devoted to refuting those sceptics who denied that there were any such things as critical days, an approach which Galen rebuts by combing through the Hippocratic *Epidemics* for evidence to the contrary.[97]

There is a natural pattern, for a crisis, he concludes, is likely to fall on certain days more than on others. Some days are "obviously" more dangerous than others, the sixth in particular, "a sadistic tyrant that enjoys most torturing its patients", followed by the thirteenth. By contrast the clearest and most favourable crises are likely to occur on the seventh, fourteenth and twentieth days.[98] The fact that the twenty-first is not a good day presents a problem that he had tried to answer ever since his youth. His conclusion, if it is his alone, is ingenious.[99] A straightforward counting of whole days cannot be sustained, and instead there is a shorter 'medical week' of $6^{35/48}$ days.[100] This he links to the lunar cycle, which in turn has an influence on the climate and weather. Those who believe in patterns of sevens and who argue from the seven stars of the Pleiades, the Great Bear or even the seven mouths of the Nile and the fabled seven gates of Thebes are just talking nonsense, as well as showing their ignorance of astronomy. Farmers and sailors know far better than these sophists.[101] Galen is not here rejecting astrology as such, for he shows elsewhere that he can cast a horoscope with the best of them, but he views the moon and the heavens simply as climatic factors that may influence the course of an illness.[102] Knowing this, the true doctor can thus introduce his understanding of the heavens into his judgment of the case in front of him and prognose accordingly.

The art of prognostic can only take the physician so far. It can warn when death is likely to occur and hence that the most that can be offered is palliative care: refusal to intervene where death is likely is far better than any painful treatment.[103] But, more often than not, the healer is still left with a decision on how to treat and needs to make the best choice from among the traditional trinity of diet, drugs and surgery, all of which Galen expects his accomplished practitioner to be able to use appropriately and effectively.

Galen the surgeon

To discuss Galen's practice as a surgeon is no easy task. It is difficult to put into words the essence of a craft skill, or for a non-surgeon to appreciate the significance of the choice of this or that procedure or instrument. Although Galen had planned to include surgery in his *Method of Healing*, and possibly even in a separate work, he did not fulfil his plan, unless one believes that all he wrote was the hurried and bitty account of abnormal swellings and some minor procedures in its final two books.[104] This is unfortunate since it was his surgical skill that won him his first important job at Pergamum, and we can catch only glimpses of his subsequent activity as a surgeon after his time there.[105]. He was certainly respected enough to be called in by trainers and others to treat sprains and dislocations suffered in gymnasia at Rome and Ostia, and his account of a confrontation with a Syrian quack dentist who claimed to be his pupil suggests that his authority as a surgeon was widely accepted.[106] He was particularly proud of his treatment of the slave of Marullus the mime-writer, who was suffering from an infected sternum after a heavy blow while training in the palaestra. Inflammation and suppuration had set in and cicatrizing the wound had failed to work. Thanks to his knowledge of anatomy, Galen excised the breastbone and the infected tissue, and, somewhat to his surprise, for he had been uncertain of the outcome, the slave recovered and lived for some time.[107] It is likely, too, that he would have been able to perform all the operations described in a contemporary *Introduction to Medicine* that goes under his name as well as those he listed as within the capacity of any competent practitioner – the ability to treat hernia, bladder stone, cataracts, scrofulous glands, trichiasis, tumours and the like.[108] He continued this kind of work until the 190s at least, for he bemoaned the loss of his surgical instruments, many of which he had devised himself, in the Fire of Rome. He had made wax models of what he required, which he then passed on to a professional instrument maker to cast using the finest metal from the mines of Noricum (modern Styria).[109] But he also admitted that he had less opportunity to practise complex surgery in Rome than would have been the case had he stayed in Asia, and that he left it to more practised local surgeons.[110]

But even if, with one exception that will be discussed shortly, we have little detailed information on his surgical practice, it is possible to discover some of the general principles that lay behind it. Depending on the amount, bleeding could be stopped by finger pressure, bandaging, a tourniquet, cauterising, or styptics. Ulcers and tumours required a combination of drugs and, if necessary, surgery as well, something Galen explored at length in his book on unnatural swellings and in Books III–VI of the *Method of Healing*.[111] Above all, Galen demanded a sound knowledge of anatomy, for not only was that essential for any invasive surgery but it could explain, in advance or in retrospect, the difficulties and even failure of the operation. Incompetence in anatomy led inevitably to failure. An artery cut in mistake for a vein would be fatal, a muscle cut transversally instead longitudinally would produce paralysis.[112] Stitching with the wrong sort of thread, or in the wrong place or direction, inevitably weakened the suture when any strain was placed on it.[113] In all these types of case, the principles behind Galen's recommendations are generally sound, and are often followed today.

One invasive procedure that we can be sure was often used by Galen was bloodletting.[114] It was a technique that he advocated vigorously in the face of considerable opposition. Although he was convinced that he could trace it back to Hippocrates himself, it is mentioned only occasionally in the Hippocratic Corpus, but seems to have become popular in the late Hellenistic period.[115] Near-contemporary Hippocratics such as Antyllus and Aretaeus knew and used it, but Galen seems to have relied on it more often and to have provided a lengthier and more codified explanation for it than any other physician.[116] According to Galen, the body was kept alive in part through its natural heat, which gradually diminished over a lifetime. This heat, fed by foodstuffs processed in the liver and the portal system, helped to "cook" them to produce nutriment. Too much heat resulted in fevers, often caused by inflammation or putrefaction produced by residues, the surplus products of digestion.[117] This superfluity might be the result of a weakness in what Galen called the excretory faculty, the body's capacity to get rid of excess, or of too great an intake of food, *plethos*, distending and even rupturing the vessels. Hence the need to keep the body free from residues, or to evacuate them efficiently.[118] The belief in the importance of keeping the bowels open or in the danger of suppressed menstruation goes back a very long way. Bleeding was considered to be a good way of removing these dangerous residues, since it could be seen as assisting the body in its evacuations. Galen advocated it particularly in fever, where it would, at least temporarily, produce a slight drop in body temperature.[119] He also supported its use to draw blood away from a place where there was already some bleeding or a swelling, and he provided a complicated list of appropriate veins from where blood might be let.[120] He also advocated prophylactic bleeding. In spring, for example, when, according to the by now familiar Hippocratic schema, blood predominated in the body, it would make sense for those liable to an excess of blood to be bled to prevent any dangerous condition from developing.

But, although Galen was an enthusiastic advocate of bleeding, proudly mentioning an occasion where he let blood from himself in accordance with instructions from the god Asclepius, and strongly attacking Erasistratus and his Roman followers for their reluctance to bleed, he hedged his advice about with many caveats.[121] Some patients were not to be bled – pregnant women, for this might harm the foetus, and usually the old and the young, for their constitutions might not stand it. Above all, the decision to bleed or not to bleed depended on the severity and intensity of the condition. In a short-lived ephemeral fever, bleeding was very rarely necessary, whereas it was more often to be recommended in what Galen called continuous fevers.[122] But wholesale and indiscriminate bleeding was as dangerous as a refusal to bleed, as he pointed out in a second missive to the Erasistrateans in Rome who had been so convinced by his first one that they had performed a complete volte-face from outright opposition to being in favour of bleeding at all times.[123] Whether venesection would have worked is a difficult question to answer. Peter Brain, himself a haematologist, noted a few conditions for which it might be appropriate, and, thirty years ago, an orthopaedic surgeon in an American audience told me how he been taught how to bleed a heavily muscled American footballer to prostration if a luxation could not be reduced in any other way.[124] Galen records one such case where he let blood until the patient fainted (and was then difficult to awaken).[125] One might add also the obvious linkage (and not only in Galenic theory) between an inflamed swelling and its possible cause in an excess of bad blood, as well as the placebo effect when some action is taken to cure a long-standing condition. But in his belief in prophylactic bleeding as well as in his listing of appropriate places in the body at which to bleed, Galen paved the way for others, particularly in the Middle Ages and down to the nineteenth century, to practice venesection on a frequent and even a heroic scale.[126]

Galenic pharmacology

Surgery was a last resort, and always fraught with the danger of infection or an incomplete recovery.[127] Not surprisingly, Galen regarded it as the mark of a good doctor to be able to treat surgical conditions successfully with drugs rather than the knife.[128] He should know how drugs work – or indeed fail to work – which was not true of several notable physicians he knew who were perplexed when they applied purgatives with no apparent effect. This does not mean that they were utter failures, only that they fell below Galen's own high standards.[129] He proposed two tests for a doctor's knowledge of drugs. He should have a method for ascertaining what was required, especially in the countryside, when he might not have access to the range of substances available in a city base. He would then need a sound knowledge of simple drugs that might be obtained from flowers, fruits, trees and the like. His second test was the ability to suggest a simple drug that might treat a whole range of conditions.[130] One surviving treatise by an anonymous contemporary praises the remarkable property of the plant (or plants) he called centaury to cure almost anything from bruises to menstrual complaints, and from poisoning to depression.[131] Galen himself recommended a drug like litharge (lead monoxide) for a variety of different uses according to whether it was mixed with fresh or sea water, oil of roses or vinegar, as well as with various kinds of sap.[132]

The importance ascribed to drugs by Galen is clear from the extent and number of the writings he devoted to the topic, equalled only by his commentaries on Hippocrates. Leaving aside the pseudonymous works in Kühn's edition, they include four substantial treatises, *The Properties of Simples, Antidotes* and two dealing with compound drugs.[133] The earlier of the pair is organised according to the type of remedy, beginning with plasters in Books I and II and wound treatments in Book III, and ending in Book VII with recipes for removing indurations or reducing tiredness. The second lists his compound remedies topographically. Book I for instance deals with topics such as baldness and dandruff (with recipes taken from a *Beauty Book* ascribed to Cleopatra as well as from a poem by Rufus of Ephesus), Book VIII with the liver, stomach and spleen.[134] All his drug handbooks are compilations of sorts, with most of their recipes drawn often verbatim from a relatively small number of pharmacologists who had lived in the previous century, principally Heras of Cappadocia, Andromachus the Elder and his like-named son, Asclepiades the pharmacist, Archigenes and Statilius Crito, who had served as doctor to Trajan.[135] In addition to these books, Galen claims to have possessed before the Fire of Rome more remarkable recipes than anyone else in the world, some obtained by swaps with colleagues, but others which he acquired via two remarkable collections. The first of these, passed on to him by a friend, had been inherited from rich man in Asia Minor with a passion for drugs, who had paid large sums of money for some special recipes which he then preserved in two parchment volumes.[136] The other had been bequeathed to Galen by his friend and fellow-pupil Teuthras, who had obtained them from an old Pergamene doctor who had collected them in his travels around the world before settling in Rome. All these were lost in the Fire along with Galen's own writings on drugs, which he was forced to reconstruct at even greater length from copies provided by his friends.[137]

In addition to a great collection of drug recipes, Galen also had access to a huge selection of ingredients simply through living in Rome as an imperial doctor, and it was his expertise in pharmacology that led to his appointment under Marcus Aurelius as maker of the emperor's theriac in succession to Demetrius and to other distinguished pharmacologists.[138] He had the run of the imperial stores, which housed items of great rarity or age, some collected specially on Crete by imperial servants and sent back to Rome in wicker baskets.[139] He could also take advantage of officials and governors, as well as friends, travelling to lands where one could obtain plants and minerals of the best quality. He was aware of his advantages, hence his willingness to provide others with information on the costs of some drugs and their various possible substitutes as well as on remedies that might be easily to hand even in the remote countryside.[140] How much of a Greek text on this theme under his name goes back to Galen himself is unclear, although a few fragments of the original are preserved in Syriac translation, but he would certainly have agreed with the sentiments in its preface.[141] Its author explains that country dwellers suffer from extremes of heat and cold as well as ordinary illnesses, yet lack access to many drugs or to therapists competent to use them.[142] Not for them the complex recipes against poisons to which Galen devoted one of his last treatises.[143] Some of these antidotes, whose multiple ingredients might come from all over the known world, were already famous, particularly those associated with kings and emperors. One recipe is headed "The ambrosia of Philip of Macedon", and another, against snake bite, was allegedly devised by Zopyrus for Mithridates himself.[144] Galen prefaces this recipe with a version of the famous story of Mithridates testing his antidote on humans (related at greater length in the pseudo-Galenic *Theriac for Piso*). In Galen's account it is the doctor, Zopyrus, who sends along with his recipe a condemned criminal whom he advises the king to use as a guinea pig.[145]

The sources of the individual recipes collected by Galen in his drug books range from famous doctors and pharmacologists, like Apollonius Mys, and Andromachus the Elder, one of Nero's doctors, to a variety of lesser healers such as Axius, doctor in the British fleet, a masseur, a groom, a Persian mountebank, or a school master.[146] Some, like the Olympic victor's ointment for battered and damaged eyes, carry a hint of advertising, others appear to be domestic remedies.[147] Some can be characterised as folk medicine, others are complex polypharmacy written out in elegant verse.[148] Their authors did this not only to avoid any mistakes in their preparation, for, they claimed, any numbers would be harder to miscopy or misunderstand in verse than as individual letters (the Greek method of writing numerals) but also because it provided proof of their literary ability and social standing.[149] Galen cites as an example of pharmacological poetry the florid opening of a poem on poisons by Heliodorus, an Athenian dramatist of unknown date, though condemning its content because, like Orpheus the so-called Theologian, the younger (H)orus of Mende, and Aratus, its irresponsible author had refused to include in it any antidotes on the spurious grounds that they would already be well known.[150] By contrast, Galen quotes in full the poem on theriac by Andromachus as well as the many other recipes in verse for antidotes by Servilius Damocrates (who lived around 40 CE).[151] One of these, dubbed a "prognostic antidote", was intended to be swallowed immediately one suspected that one had ingested something poisonous, causing anything dangerous to be vomited up; but should the suspicion prove unfounded, the drug would not provoke even the slightest sensation of nausea. It also had the advantage of being effective against pains in the side, back, kidneys and bladder, and was capable of stemming a flow of blood, even from the lungs.

Although possessing a substantial amount of literature about remedies does not of itself imply expertise in using them, Galen demonstrates how he obtained, prepared and employed his remedies, as well as expounding his theoretical understanding of how they worked. Time and again he insists on the importance of securing the best ingredients and of having a sufficient knowledge about herbs to frustrate the wiles of salesmen keen to disguise their substandard wares. He records with pride, and no little detail, his visit to the mines of Soloi on Cyprus, facilitated by a friend's acquaintance with the imperial official in charge of them.[152] He likewise travelled to Palestine to obtain supplies of its famous balsam as well as minerals from the Eastern shores of the Dead Sea, and, while there, he also snapped up the entire cargo of a caravan crossing to Egypt with rare substances that he sent home to Pergamum.[153] But it is the range of personal comments throughout his drug books and particularly in *The Properties of Simples* that best shows his deep interest. Some list alternative names, and not only in Greek – in a learned discussion of the names for Armenian Earth in a recently discovered section of that work, he gives it in both Armenian and Syriac.[154] He explains how some pastilles will remain useful for a long time even if they are old, provided that they are properly stored from the start and occasionally wiped with a clean cloth to remove any dust that might have settled on them and begun to penetrate below the surface.[155] While most healers use only the shell of nuts – in this they are just like dyers – Galen has found that the nuts themselves can be crushed to produce a juice like that of mulberries or blackberries which, when boiled with honey, makes a similarly useful concoction for the stomach.[156] Above all, Galen insists that he never trusted the recipes he had inherited without in some way testing them first.[157] So for instance, he rejected the common idea in his sources that a dead torpedo fish in its entirety would cure headaches as well as an anal prolapse, for he had found that neither of these was true. However, applying it to the head while it was still alive did work for a headache since it dulled the pain like other types of pain-killer.[158] But when he had only the transmitted information to rely on, his expectations were lower and depended on the number and veracity of the writers, and he frequently corrected a recipe or introduced an alternative which he thought superior, either from another source or of his own invention.[159] His so-called *Hiera* ('Holy Drug'), a bitter purgative recommended for almost anything from headache to period pains, was far more familiar to doctors in early mediaeval Europe than any of his medical treatises.[160]

The pharmacological method that Galen wished to impart to his students and colleagues demanded more than empiricism. He had great respect for experience, and at times it might serve as well as a reasoned choice, but for him it was not enough. One needed always to remember that every part of the body, and *a fortiori* every patient, was different.[161] What he called a 'qualified' empiricism was essential in all therapy: this required an understanding of what might be described as drug chemistry – an understanding of how individual ingredients worked together and what their effect was on the body.[162] In *My own Opinions*, one of his very last works, Galen explained in two different ways how drugs worked. Changes in the body are brought about either through one or a pair of a substance's active qualities, the hot, the cold, the wet and the dry, or through the specific property of the whole of its substance, as with laxatives or poisons. Poisons differ from merely dangerous drugs in that the latter can provide occasional benefit when they are taken in small amounts alongside other drugs that are beneficial – his example is opium, a common ingredient in analgesics.[163] Treatment by drugs thus works by contraries, allopathy, restoring the body to its natural state by inducing changes that will eliminate any qualitative excess. That general statement, however, must be qualified by a variety of distinctions and explanations, not all of which are entirely consistent, but which reflect Galen's difficulties both in investigating the actions of drugs and in using the imprecise language of metaphor in his explanations.[164] So, in *My own Opinions*, he argues that some drugs, such as purgatives and emetics, have a specific property that attracts one type of humour. which it then expels from the body: a cholagogue, for instance, removes the excess of yellow bile that is the cause of jaundice, a hydragogue the watery fluid that accumulates in dropsy.[165] They do not, as Julian and other Methodists supposed, simply attract mixed blood, which is then changed into an individual humour during the process of evacuation.[166] Those that work through the property of their total substance, something particularly true of certain compound drugs, may be observed empirically, but cannot easily be linked with qualities or humours.[167] Elsewhere, he makes a distinction between medicines that have a 'thick' or a 'fine' substance, the latter being capable of being broken down into tiny particles without losing their organic unity. Drugs of this type are easily altered, often by heating, as with resin or oil, and they are more active because they can pass more easily into the interior of the body. This type of explanation fits neatly into the tradition of earlier philosophical explanations of the natural world, and particularly that of Aristotle and his school, but it is also one that can be substantiated from everyday experience.[168]

The boundaries between what Galen was prepared to accept or reject from such experience do not always coincide with our own, and also change over time.[169] On the whole he rejected remedies from excreta, although he knew that a learned pharmacologist like Asclepiades the Pharmacist (fl. 90 CE) could write a great deal on the therapeutic virtues of dung.[170] He devoted some of his more exuberant denunciations to writers such as Xenocrates of Aphrodisias (fl. 70 CE) or his slightly earlier contemporary Pamphilus of Alexandria for employing a raft of dubious remedies ranging from human bones and flesh to horoscopic herbs.[171] Pamphilus, a school teacher, he compared to a herald reading out a list of runaway slaves, but unable to recognise them even if they were in front of him.[172] But later on, he was prepared to modify his views on the value of charms, incantations and amulets, all widely used as instanced by surviving papyri and gems, although he still remained cautious about accepting testimony about their efficacy even from an otherwise reliable informant. A report of a cure of snakebite with an amulet made from grape-stone Galen placed in the same category as using a red hawk-stone to treat bleeding piles: neither can be advocated scientifically.[173] His criticism of Archigenes, whom he elsewhere mentions with respect, for writing a great deal about amulets is far milder than his strictures on Pamphilus, and he was prepared to experiment with such remedies himself.[174] A medical book ascribed to the legendary Egyptian pharaoh and magician Nechepso had recommended for stomach problems placing an amulet of green jasper carved with the image of a snake with the sun's rays over the patient's belly.[175] This Galen thought an unnecessary refinement: he had found that it worked equally well uncarved. On another occasion, he observed that a small boy never had an epileptic seizure when wearing a peony amulet but relapsed when the amulet was removed, only to recover when it was replaced.[176] He could not decide whether this was because the patient inhaled effluences from parts of the peony root, or whether the root in some way modified the surrounding air: whichever explanation one adopted confirmed the validity of the empirical observation. In his (lost) treatise *Medicine in Homer* he similarly admitted that he had for a long while doubted the value of incantations in healing, but now acknowledged from his own observations that they might be occasionally helpful.[177]

But pharmacology, as Galen was well aware, was an inexact science, particularly as applied to the individual patient, yet it was a science nonetheless and it had a method that could be learned and was more than simple empiricism. Time and again he insisted that what he was doing was bringing an appropriate 'method', 'argument' or 'reasoning' to a familiar subject that had for too long been handled only empirically. Part of the reason for the imprecision lay in the absence of any clear classification of drug action. He was dissatisfied with a model which, like that used by the great medical botanist Dioscorides, categorised the working of drugs solely in terms of their principal physiological effects on the body. In his view, this formulation was both ambiguous and unhelpful, for it was not precise enough to account for the different results that might be obtained by giving, for instance, one purgative rather than another, and it appeared to take little account of the patient to whom it was given. A Hippocratic doctor wishing to choose a treatment appropriate to the individual sufferer required a more profound understanding of drug action than the bald statement that, for instance, scammony removes bile.[178] Galen had even less time for the

Methodists, with their belief in atoms and pores, for their discussions were both prolix and incoherent.[179]

Instead, he adopted what to him was a much simpler classification that could fit alongside the distinction just mentioned between the different qualities of the drugs. In its most schematic form, he divided their actions into four main grades of intensity, weak, obvious, strong and massive, each of which was subdivided further into three: small, moderate and substantial.[180] At one end of the spectrum were substances so powerful that the slightest of applications resulted in the immediate destruction of the part or the death of the patient – some caustics and poisons, for example. At the other were simple herbs whose action was almost totally imperceptible, to be used in cases where extreme delicacy or precision of treatment was required. These were also valuable adjuncts to the doctor's medicine chest for a different reason: they could be mixed in with other easily available herbs to bolster the price of remedies that might otherwise be rejected by rich patients who judged the potential efficacy of a drug solely by its price.[181] Other substances could be located along this spectrum according to the intensity of their qualitative action, and one could then choose what to use in a particular case and understand how quantities of different herbs or minerals could be mixed together into a compound remedy. How this might be done one can discover from reading Galen's long lists of recipes and from modern research into surviving drugs, some of them pastilles or face creams, and many containing pharmacologically active ingredients.[182]

But to categorise in this graded grid the properties of all, or even most, drugs was no small task, as Galen himself admitted. The eleven books of his revised treatise on the properties of simples constitute a remarkable achievement, listing them in alphabetical order and combining substantial book learning with information drawn from his own experiences.[183] But it goes only part of the way to providing the precision that he would like. In his investigation of 475 botanical simples, he provided detailed grades for only one-third, 161.[184] Correlating the intensity of drug action with the patient's condition was even harder. There was no instrumentation that would allow even the rough categorisation demanded by Galen's schema for classifying drugs, let alone patients. Not surprisingly perhaps, Galen put forward over the years a variety of apparently conflicting suggestions. Writing in the 160s, in the first part of the *Method of Healing*, he suggested that there might be fifteen different degrees of a dry distemper, each requiring one of fifteen different degrees of moistening.[185] Thirty years later, in his *Art of Medicine*, he proposed that if a particular part was ten times hotter than normal and seven times drier it should require a remedy ten times colder and seven times moister than the norm.[186] It is not easy to see how either formulation fits with the twelve categories of drug action that he adopted in his studies of simples and which formed the basis for later Galenic pharmacology, particularly in the Islamic world. These discrepancies, however, reflect Galen's commitment to thinking and rethinking about the wider questions raised in his medical practice.

Galen's dietetics

The third element in Galen's armoury against illness was diet. Diet, for Galen as for earlier writers from the fifth century BC onwards, meant more than just food and drink: it encompassed one's whole lifestyle. It could be used both therapeutically and as prophylaxis to strengthen the body to resist harmful changes in the future.[187] It was a proper understanding of the principles of dietetics in the broadest sense of the term that allowed Galen from his mid-twenties onwards to remain extremely healthy, despite his busy life and in contrast to the many times he fell ill during his childhood and adolescence.[188] While it was in one sense true that one was what one ate – those who consumed the flesh of asses, lions or even camels became like them – it was diet in the wider sense that determined whether one's healthy state developed into the preternatural one of illness.[189] It was only to be expected that wealthy Roman women fell ill and were unable to stand even the slightest of restraints, since their life was entirely one of luxury.[190] The airless crowded city was another obvious source of danger, although the sensible recommendations of Galen and some of his teachers for the layout of a healthy city were impossible to implement in the absence of any effective civic organisation or interest.[191] The countryside also had its own dangers. Galen saw nothing incongruous in both writing sympathetically of peasants in Asia Minor forced for lack of anything better to eat horse and donkey meat and, in more than one passage, dismissing them as asses, thoroughly brutish in their nature.[192] As Galen himself remembered from a youthful excursion into the backwoods of modern Turkey, the rough porridge that was the only food available at the time brought on flatulence, constipation and headaches, and even the natives admitted that it was hard to digest.[193] Famine brought even greater hardship: forced to eat grass and shrubs, and the bulbs and roots of inedible plants, the peasants developed ulcers, many of which proved fatal.[194] One had only to look at the hard skin of the scrawny Egyptians to realise the consequences of a diet of salt fish, snails, beans, lentils and pulses, supplemented by the flesh of vipers, camels and donkeys and washed down with thin wine and barley beer. By contrast, there were few cases of skin disease among the Germans or the Mysians, and almost none at all among the milk-drinking Scythians.[195]

If eating the wrong sort of food produced illness, it was also true that health could be maintained, and often restored, by an appropriate eating plan. As Hippocrates was believed to have said, medication is in alimentation. Others preferred a sharper distinction, like the author of the pseudo-Aristotelian *Problems*, Book I, who saw the two as opposed.[196] Galen accepted a distinction between the two at least in theory. Drugs alter the nature of the body and its qualities, food increases its substance; food is taken over and dominated by the part being nourished, drugs, by contrast, triumph over what is there.[197] But, in practice, both foodstuffs and drugs lay on the same spectrum, and could be viewed in the same way. Galen devoted several large treatises to foodstuffs and their role in health, and hence it is not surprising to find him as one of the interlocutors in Athenaeus' *Sophists at Dinner*. But whereas Athenaeus' speakers are interested mainly in the history of food, capping each other's learned quotations from Attic comedy or oratory, Galen, while not disdaining the occasional learned citation, looked more to the medical value of what is eaten.[198] In his writings he offers a comprehensive survey of the foods available in his time, adding many details from his own observations: the quince tarts exported from Syria to Rome, the ingenious ways in which Egyptian peasants clarified and kept cool the water they had taken from the Nile, and the morning honeydew, "Zeus' rain", that covered shrubs and trees in the hills behind Pergamum in summer.[199] He provides a veritable catalogue of Mediterranean wines, although he himself typically preferred those from nearer to his original home.[200] One should not forget that his father had owned a vineyard and experimented to see how best the life of a vintage could be prolonged.[201]

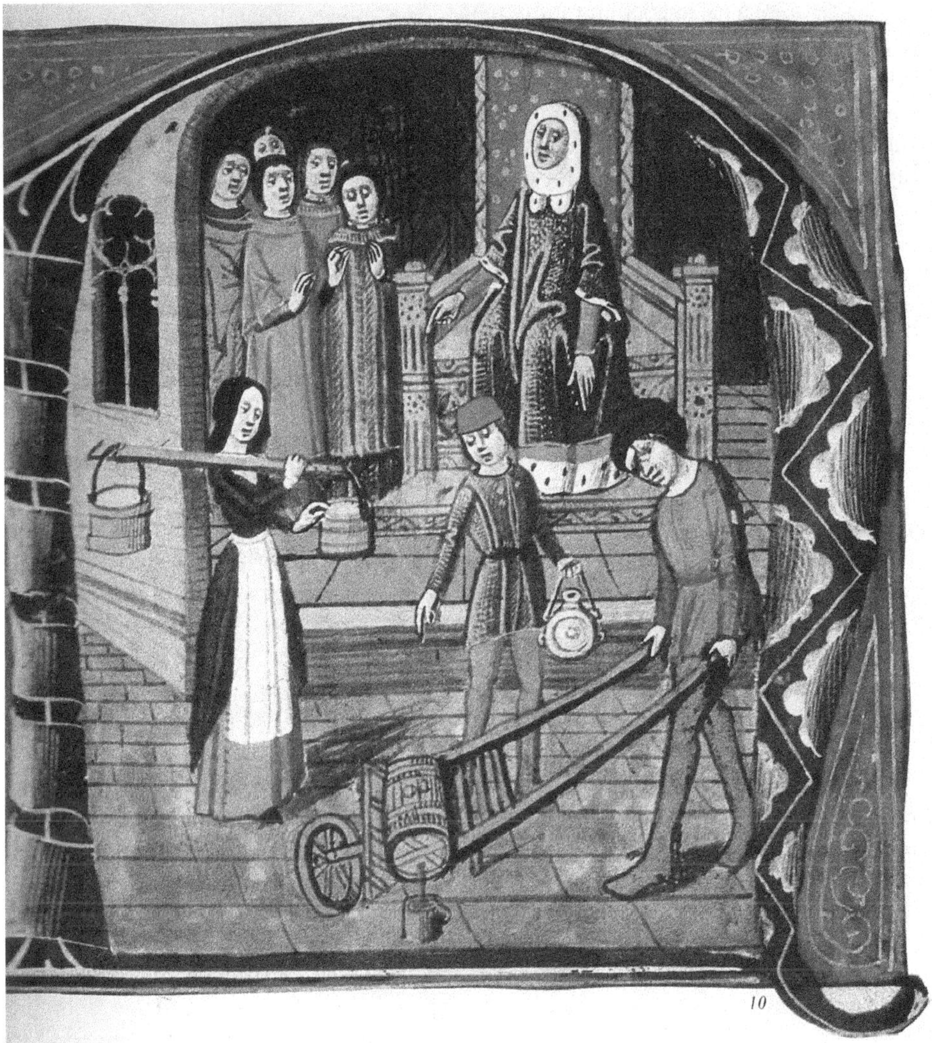

Figure 5.2 Galen gives instructions for food and drink. A chapter illustration from a late medieval Latin manuscript of Galen Dresden, Sächsische Landesbibliothek D b 93, fol. 378r.

Galen tried to relate the properties of foods to the four humours and their various constituent qualities. Some foods were heating, others cooling, moistening or drying; some thickened the humours, others thinned them, making them easier to excrete and thus acting as a remedy for constipation as well as a sort of slimming aid. Galen's listings and his placing of foods according to their digestibility, strength and suitability for human beings differ little from those of other ancient writers on food. White meat, poultry and fish were far easier to digest than red meat; white wines more suitable for the sick than strong red. Pork was the meat most easily digested, since it was most like human flesh, witness the habit of rascally innkeepers in serving up human flesh as part of a pork stew.[202] The sick should initially be given soups, especially barley broth, and gradually returned to their normal diet.[203] Most of Galen's recommendations would meet with the approval of a modern dietician, with one major exception. He placed an almost total ban on fresh fruit, which he considered a frequent cause of illness. His father had warned him of the dangers of eating such fruit, but he had once been led astray by his friends into eating a lot of fresh fruit in autumn. The result was an acute illness. The next year, taking fruit only in moderation, he remained free from illness, but after his father's death the pains returned, until, aged 28, he decided to abandon all fruit save for small amounts of figs and grapes.[204] Others, like his fellow citizen Protas, who fell ill after eating unripe apples and pears, had similar stories to tell, and the difficulties of keeping fruit in a warm climate should not be underestimated. It thus came as no surprise to Galen that Asian peasants fed apples to their pigs.[205]

In his advocacy of physical exercise, Galen followed the same policy of moderation. His heroes were Telephus the grammarian, who lived almost to 100, and Dr Antiochus, who daily walked the kilometre or so from his house to the Roman forum and continued to visit his patients on foot or, if they resided further off, in a litter or chariot, until he was well past 80. He also went in the afternoons to the public baths where he had a massage and indulged in exercises appropriate for his age.[206] Their example showed what benefits could be gained by an active lifestyle, in moderation. For professional athletes Galen had little but contempt, convinced that their passion for training in order to attain peak fitness was counterproductive.[207] How much better to indulge in intellectual pursuits than sweat and struggle in the gymnasium! Galen's quotations from the Athenian playwright Euripides shows that the contempt of the intellectual for the hearty has very ancient roots.[208] But some exercise was essential for a healthy life style: indeed, Galen's ideal of a perfect constitution is that of the 'gymnastic youth', a wealthy man with the leisure to go to the gymnasium to exercise with a trainer or by himself.[209] His *Thrasybulus* is a plea for the medical oversight of all exercise, for only in this way can one avoid the harm inflicted upon the unwary by over-enthusiastic but ignorant trainers.[210]

He must have been a familiar figure in Roman gymnasia, always keen to see what valuable information he might gain for his medicine. An experience in the palaestra with a wrestler even suggested the correct meaning of an obscure passage in the Hippocratic *Epidemics* VI.[211] In an attempt to measure how long it took for food to pass through the stomach, he interviewed boxers and wrestlers, who told him that they felt it took about fifteen hours. This Galen concluded was true of a meal of pork, but the data he obtained were, he concluded, too variable to be of much use.[212] Other observations were more directly relevant to the patient's health. In his *Hygiene*, he gives a long list of appropriate gymnastic exercises including running, shadow-boxing, wrestling, and playing ball games.[213] He particularly recommended using a small ball to tone up the body, writing a short treatise specifically to promote this idea.[214] Exercise shaded off into work: at one end were aristocratic pastimes such as hunting, fishing and military training, at the other activities that provided most people with a living, such as metal-working or house-building. Once when forced to stay in the countryside Galen had to chop wood and crush and grind barley in a mortar for exercise, something country peasants did every day for work.[215] Galen says remarkably little about the public bathing that was traditionally part of the life-style of every Roman, although he was clearly familiar with it, mentioning particularly the Baths or Gymnasium of Trajan.[216] Moralists might denounce the evils of bathing, and even its partisans acknowledged that, along with wine and sex, "bathing ruins our bodies". But it also made life worth living, as both literary texts and the archaeological remains of large thermal complexes from all over the ancient world abundantly attest.[217] Galen regularly bathed and massaged his patients, sometimes within the great public baths, as part of the therapeutic process, and occasionally recommended bathing for the sick in hot springs, especially those with nitre, sulphur and asphalt, like the Aquae Albulae or the Aquae Domitianae near Rome, with its traces of iron and copper but he is very cautious about their possible side-effects.[218] Too much bathing renders the flesh soft, white and flabby, and produces the sort of moist diseases that are typically found in women. Drinking mineral waters over a long time also leads to problems, while some waters are not for the weak and unhealthy, and one of Rome's water supplies (probably the Aqua Alsietina) is best avoided as it causes diarrhoea.[219] Moderation is again his watchword.

Careful attention to diet and exercise, no matter what one's age, was the best defence against ill health, even if, after the age of fifty, one could no longer be as strong or as healthy as Hercules.[220] Nor should one neglect the simple pleasures of talking with a friend or reading a book.[221] All these contributed to what Galen acknowledged was his own long life, sound in both body and mind.[222]

Curing the mind

As we have already seen, Galen regarded himself as an expert in mental conditions.[223] Sometimes, as with the slave steward worried to death about having to submit an incomplete financial account, reassurance alone might prove effective, and, best of all, a proper philosophical training would help to maintain the equilibrium necessary to avoid distress or anger and its physical consequences.[224] Alternatively, one might find ways of distracting the patient, taking him to the theatre or a musical performance or to watch wrestling or cockfighting. One might release one's anger by boxing or pitting oneself against an opponent. Distraction was also his advice when consulted by those who were afraid of the emperor's wrath or of being killed. But passionate love might resist this therapy and become hard to treat.[225] Galen claimed divine precedent for this psychotherapy, for had not his "ancestral god" Asclepius prescribed music, poetry and drama for those of a hot disposition (a reference perhaps to the performances in the small theatre within the Asclepieion of Pergamum) and hunting and riding for those of a cold?[226]

But sometimes the cause of mental disorder was something physical, the result of some damage and harmful change to the heart, in the case of anger, or to the regent faculty in the brain, whether arising specifically there or from 'sympathy' with some other part of the body. It thus differed from mental deficiency or dementia, in which the faculty was removed entirely.[227] Diagnosis was not always easy. Misinterpretation of sense perceptions, *phantasmata*, could be the result of a failure of reason or evidence of some damaging changes within the sensory organs or the brain. But where there was a physical cause, it was important to distinguish mental disorders that were accompanied by fever, frenzies, from those without, which he terms manias, although both were likely to be the result of a hot humour, and principally yellow bile, which could produce hot, acrid vapours that affected the brain.[228] One major exception to this rule was melancholic madness, a favourite theme ever since the fourth century BCE.[229] Galen claimed to identify potential sufferers from both their physiognomy (they were lean, dark and hairy with large veins) and their behaviour, being particularly prone to fear and depression. This might be the result of an excess of black bile, a humour whose existence, Galen alleges, was perversely denied by Erasistratus in the face of universal evidence from legendary times onwards.[230] But in some fevers, the increasing heat might cook the yellow bile within the brain, so that it became ever more dangerous as it changed colour until it ended in the potentially deadly 'adust' or 'burnt' melancholy.[231]

Most of Galen's cases of mental illness relate to his first category, those involving fever. Such sufferers were particularly likely to suffer from hallucinations and delirium, and common signs like plucking at bedclothes (carphology) or chasing imaginary flies had been recognised at least since the fifth century BCE as indicating a potentially serious illness.[232] Galen himself had once struggled, while in an ardent fever, to remove black bits from his bedclothes and similar flecks from his clothing, striving all the harder when he found nothing under his fingers.[233] Only when he overheard two friends saying that he was hallucinating, did he realise that this was what he was doing and that it was a symptom of his phrenitis, which had temporarily robbed him of his reason. Likewise, another doctor, Theophilus, was able to conduct a sensible conversation with those around him while under the impression that some flute players had moved into his house, and were wandering around, making loud noises and playing their music all night long in defiance of his shouts for them to be removed. When his illness went away, he could recall everything including the appearance of the imaginary musicians.[234] In another case from Rome, a man suffering from phrenitis had been left at home with a slave making wool while everyone else went off to the games. Locking the door, he invited passers-by to name household items they would like him to throw from the upstairs window.[235] They thought it was a game and laughed as one object after another was hurled into the street. But things became dangerous when he asked them if they wished to see his slave (in one version of the story Galen gives his actual name), and then threw him also down into the street. Luckily, the crowd realised what was happening and managed to break his fall. Galen uses this example to show that the man had still retained his reason to the extent that he was able to respond to the crowd and correctly identify whatever they asked him to eject, and, in one of his versions of the story, he implies that the patient eventually recovered from his phrenitis. He records similar stories of patients driven mad by phrenitis from Pergamum and Kyme in Asia Minor where they challenged their doctors to a sword fight or a wrestling match.[236]

What is striking in Galen's ideas of therapy in such disorders is that, while he believed that the physical cause needed to be addressed first, with such remedies as bathing, diet and even bleeding, he rejected harsh remedies such as flogging or ice-cold baths.[237] Nor was there much point in attempting to convince patients immediately of the falsity of their hallucinations. Some of them would pass away quickly with the ending of the phrenetic fever, others, as in mania. would take much longer.[238] It was thus important to get alongside the patient and accept the truth in their eyes of what they saw. Sometimes this allowed a speedy cure: a woman who believed she had swallowed a snake recovered quickly after Galen showed her a snake in the bowl into which she had just vomited, being convinced by his sleight of hand that the snake was no longer inside her.[239] In other cases, particularly among the well-to-do, he prescribed a change of scenery, as well as participation in whatever was their enthusiasm; going to the theatre, music, watching the games, reading or simply discussions. In this way the individual could be gradually restored to normal life and forget whatever had been the trigger for the mental disturbance.[240] Simple physical treatments do not work: one needs to cultivate patience, perseverance, determination, ingenuity, and generosity, in addition to attempting to remove these *idées fixes*.[241] Such long-term and non-pharmacological therapies, however, would not have been available to all Galen's patients – and similar differentiation on economic grounds in the provision of treatment for the mentally ill is still with us today – but they show a caring side to Galen the healer that unites all his diverse interests and abilities.[242]

Evaluating Galen's therapeutic methods is far from easy. One may approve in general of his observational skills and his demand for constant thought about the problems in front of the doctor, but we are not dealing with careful case notes dependent on an agreed vocabulary and appropriate clinical data that can be checked against the records of others. Instead we have perceptions and reminiscences redacted over time and embellished to fit a specific context. Galen frequently tells a good story in his case-histories, altering details as the account is repeated over the years as well as changing the focus slightly to make different points about this or that procedure.[243] A throw-away reference may be more informative than an extensive description of exemplary cases, precisely because its presentation is less elaborate and gives the impression of a spontaneous recall. But it is not always obvious whether a case that he reports is one that he knew at first hand. Some certainly are, but others may have been reported to him or gleaned from his own wide reading. One has also to allow for the passage of time and the new context in which a story is repeated. So, for instance, in a brief later reference in his commentary on the Hippocratic *Prognosticon* to his cure of a woman in love with an actor, described at length in *Prognosis*, it is a man, not a woman, who is being treated.[244] A similar confusion can be found in Galen's almost *verbatim* copying in the late revision of *The Properties of Simples* of a series of cures of 'elephantiasis' (probably leprosy) using viper flesh first recorded in the early *Sketch of Empiricism*.[245] Four of the five cases, and possibly even the fifth, come from Pergamum and the neighbouring regions. In the earlier version Galen expressly notes his involvement only in the third and fourth, but in *The Properties of Simples* he includes them all under the heading of "things I have experienced". That he may have had nothing directly to do with the first two cases is suggested by Aretaeus' similar account of the first one, which may have been known to Galen at second hand.[246] The final story, of the cure by Asclepius of a man from central Thrace who had come to the shrine of Pergamum, absent from the earlier version, may also have reached him at second hand, and was perhaps included only accidentally with the others as coming from his time as a young man. But over forty years, as the different focus to the preface to this passage demonstrates, it is easy to see how Galen could have made the transition from describing a local incident that was well known to him in his youth to claiming that he had in some way participated in it. Galen's memory, particularly when he was originally speaking or dictating, was not infallible.

Nonetheless, these few exceptions apart, and even allowing for the fact that our information comes almost entirely from the mouth of Galen himself and that, particularly in the longer case-histories, the piling up of tiny details is a rhetorical device to carry conviction of the truth and authority of what can be read, we have a remarkable record of one ancient doctor's practice, more informative in many ways that the more celebrated Hippocratic *Epidemics*.[247] This is not to say that one should always trust Galen's claims for success and his blaming of others for failure: our information and our ideas of medicine are now so different as to make any identification of either the condition or Galen's therapies problematic, if not impossible. But such constraints apply equally to all ancient writings on medicine, whether by doctors, patients or historians.[248] One may tire of his assertions of his uniqueness through his denigration of others and the constant employment of 'I', and wonder whether this constant self-assertion is not in some way a cover for failure and indecision.[249]

But it should also be remembered that many of his writings were written for friends and colleagues who were already acquainted with Galen and that some of them, like Glaucon or Peitholaus, the imperial servant, may even have participated in the actual case being described. They would have been able to check any large pretentious claims on Galen's part, and, in his accounts, it is they who characterise a procedure or an outcome as 'marvellous'.[250] They would not have balked at his frequent citation of his own cases in his advice on what the accomplished doctor should be able to do, for they were able to see him in action. Despite his own complaints about the ignorance and frivolity of the Roman upper classes in choosing their physician, emperors, consuls, senators and the like entrusted themselves to his care for perhaps half a century, and his reputation was Mediterranean-wide.[251] The best testimonial to his achievements, however, comes from an opponent, Alexander of Aphrodisias, possibly the son of the Alexander of Damascus who had criticised Galen at one of his early Roman demonstrations. The younger Alexander disagreed strongly with Galen on many philosophical points, and, even without naming Galen specifically, took aim at many of the theories that he professed. Nonetheless, despite his low view of Galen the philosopher, Alexander still acknowledged him as greatly celebrated, the equivalent of Plato and Aristotle in his proper field of medicine.[252] Such praise tells us far more about Galen the doctor that many a page of Galenic autobiography.

Notes

1 *Opt.Med.Cogn.* 1,5–13; 5,16–17; 8,9–10, 13,1–4: *CMG Suppl. Or.* IV, 42–6, 76–8, 228–30.
2 *Praes.Puls.* III,4: 9,357 K, written when the plague was still raging.
3 Nutton 2013a: 254–79; Harris WV 2016: 35–5, 98–100.
4 Nutton 1990a. But a recommendation from a friend or a cured patient was always preferable.
5 *Opt.Med.Cogn.* 2,1–6: *CMG Suppl. Or.* IV, 46–50.
6 *Ibid.* 3,4–4,2: *CMG Suppl. Or.* IV, 52–64; for other examples, above, p. 103.
7 *Ibid.* 3,17: *CMG Suppl. Or.* IV, 60. Cf. also *Sect.* 3: 1,69–72 K: pp. 5–6 tr. Frede.
8 Except for the very early *Anatomy of the Womb*, for a midwife, *Lib.Prop.* 2,2: 19,16 K; p. 140 BM.
9 *Opt.Med.Cogn.* 2,1–2; 5,6–15; 6,8–7,4; *CMG Suppl. Or.* IV, 46–8, 70–76, 84–88.
10 *Ibid.* 5,1–5; 9,1: *CMG Suppl. Or.* IV, 68–70, 100.
11 *Ibid.* 5,2–3: *CMG Suppl. Or.* IV, 68; van der Eijk 1999: 295–332, 453–472. For a late example of this list, see Nutton 2012d. As Antoine Pietrobelli reminded me, Galen, when he wanted, could include both Herophilus and Erasistratus among the 'moderns'.
12 *Ven.Sect.Er.* 3–5, 7: 11,155, 160–1, 175–6 K; pp. 20, 22–3, 31–2 tr. Brain; *Ven.Sect.Er. Rom.* 3–5, 8: 11, 200–1, 206, 214, 220–1, 236–40 K; pp. 44–5, 47, 51, 53–4, 60–63 tr. Brain. For his similar use of historiographical material in other texts, van der Eijk 1999: 359–96.
13 van der Eijk 1999: 295–332; Debru 1999.
14 *Opt.Med.Cogn.* 9,18–22: *CMG Suppl. Or.* IV, 112–4.
15 *Ibid.* 9,23–10,5: *CMG Suppl. Or.* IV, 114–8.
16 *Ibid.* 11,1–8: *CMG Suppl. Or.* IV, 118–22.
17 *Ibid.* 14,1–3: *CMG Suppl. Or.* IV, 136–7. For Galen's expectations of a doctor's knowledge of drugs, *ibid.* 12,3–8: *CMG Suppl. Or.* IV, 124–8.

18 Von Staden 2002. The unity of medicine is discussed in *Part.Art.Med.: CMG Suppl.Or.* II, and in *CAM: CMG* V 1,3.
19 Laín Entralgo 1970. The environment extends also to the physical surroundings, *Hipp.Epid. VI*, ii,47: 17A,1000 K.
20 Jouanna 1997.
21 *Praec.* 7,1–18; 12,1–10: 14,635–41, 661–5 K; *CMG* V 8,1, 104–11, 130–5.
22 Pinault 1992; Jouanna 1997.
23 *Hipp.Epid. VI*, iv,10: 17B,144–52 K = *CMG* V 10,2,2, 202–7, commenting on *Epidemics* VI,4,7: V,308,15–16 L. The meaning would have been even more unclear in Antiquity in the absence of punctuation.
24 *Nom.Med.*: p. 21 Meyerhof-Schacht.
25 *Hipp.Off.Med.* I,13: 18B,686–8 K; *Hipp.Prog.* I,12: 18B,59 K.
26 For other 'Hippocratic' ideas on the doctor's behaviour towards the patient, see Deichgräber 1970.
27 [Galen], [*Hipp.Jus.*] pp. 67–72 tr. Rosenthal, with Strohmaier 1970; Nutton 2012b; Van Nuffelen 2014. The author implies an ongoing debate over the meaning of the god's attributes.
28 Hillgruber 2010; Ogden 2017: 207–46. The cases that open *Ven.Sect.Er.Rom.* 1: 11,187–91 K; pp. 38–40 tr. Brain, also use Erasistratus as an exemplar.
29 García Ballester 1994; Nutton 1993c; Mattern 2008; van der Eijk 2008; Petit 2018.
30 Mattern 2008.
31 *MM* III,7: 10,206–7 K; I, pp. 315–7 tr. Johnston-Horsley; cf. also *Sect.* 6: 1,12–15 K; pp. 10–12 tr. Frede.
32 *Hipp.Epid. VI*, v: *CMG* V 10,2,2, 465.
33 *Cons.: CMG Suppl.* III (not in Kühn).
34 *Ibid.* 11–2: *CMG Suppl.* III, pp. 4–6. Galen's description makes it unclear whether he was involved in the treatment of Aristotle, or, more likely, was merely asked his opinion later. For the possibility that Aristotle was the teacher of Alexander of Aphrodisias, see Moraux 1984: 399–425. If Galen was at the time on or near Mytilene (which is not at all clear), either Aristotle's death must predate late 168, which makes Moraux's identification difficult, or, since *Habits* appears to be a tract from the mid-170s at the earliest, any direct involvement of Galen must come from a later and unrecorded visit to Pergamum. (The cross-reference at *MM* VII,6: 10,492,16 K; II, pp. 290–1 Johnston-Horsley is an obviously later addition.)
35 Rufus, *Questions*: pp. 195–218 DR; partial translation in Brock 1929: 113–24.
36 Mattern 2008 is less informative on this than might be expected.
37 *Ibid.* pp. 84–92.
38 *Ibid.* pp. 112–4, 145. Woman and children (*ibid.* pp. 107–9; Gourevitch 2001) form only a small percentage of his reported cases. Whether this is a deliberate choice of examples or indicates that they were likely to be treated by female healers is unclear. But both groups were treated by Galen using the same methodology as for males, making allowances for the slightly different humoral balance.
39 *Loc.Aff.* IV,2: 8,224 K; p. 107 tr. Siegel. The alternative translation of Galatia and Iberia as areas in Central and Eastern Asia Minor is unlikely. The letter, *Puer.Epil.*: 11,357–78 K, is translated in Temkin 1934.
40 *Ibid.* 1: 11,358–9 K; p. 180 tr. Temkin. Dionysius is already "well trained in therapeutic method" and operates logically.
41 *Ibid.* 3: 11,361–2 K; p. 181 tr. Temkin. Presumably Dionysius had been engaged for a period of time and expected to be similarly engaged by a wealthy returning traveller, for the perils of falling ill when alone on a journey were well known.
42 *Ibid.* 2: 11,360 K; p. 181 tr. Temkin.
43 *Ibid.* 3: 11,362–5 K; pp. 181–3 tr. Temkin.
44 *Ibid.* 4: 11,365–7 K; pp. 183–5 tr. Temkin.
45 *Ibid.* 5: 11,371 K; p. 186 tr. Temkin. Galen's dislike of fruit goes back to his youth and his father's advice, above, p. 120.
46 *Ibid.* 4 and 6: 11,368–70, 374–7 K; pp. 186, 188–9 tr. Temkin.

47 *Ibid.* 6: 11,376 K; 5: 11,373 K; pp. 189, 186–7 tr. Temkin. Unless the 'you' is assumed to be Dionysius, Caecilianus will have met Galen at least once.
48 *Ibid.* 6: 11,376–7 K; p. 189 tr. Temkin.
49 Mattern 2008: 52–3.
50 *Hipp.Off.Med.* I,3: 18B,632–57 K (quotation, from I,4: 18B,657 K); Siegel 1970.
51 *SMT* IV,23: 11,700 K (applying to more than drugs); Justinian, *Digest* 21,1,12,4.
52 *SMT* I,37: 11,445 K, cf. *Loc.Aff.* II,6: 8,87 K; p. 50 tr. Siegel; *Hipp.Off.* I,3: 18B,653 K.
53 *Loc.Aff.* VI,3: 8,394–6 K; p. 175 tr. Siegel; *Cris.* I,12: 9,597 K.
54 E.g. at *Praec.* 6,3: 14,631 K; *CMG* V 8,1, 100–3.
55 *Dig.Puls.* IV,3: 8,951 K. At *Hipp.Off.Med.* I,3: 18B,653 K Galen is tempted to interpret a Hippocratic comment on the importance of hearing as that of the patient, not the doctor.
56 *UP* II,6: 3,110–1 K; I, p.125 tr. May; Hillert 1990: 125–7, *Fig. 23*.
57 *Temp.* II,2: 1,592 K; p. 118 tr. Singer PN.
58 Harris CRS 1973: 396–411. A good example of Victorian sphygmology is Broadbent 1890.
59 Lewis 2017: 112–5. He may have been preceded in his notion of the importance of the pulse by a slightly early Aegimius of Elis, who used a different vocabulary, *Diff.Puls.* I,2: 8,497–8 K.
60 Marcellinus, *On Pulses* 11 = Herophilus, T.182 Von Staden, with his comments, 1989: 267–88.
61 Harris CRS 1973: 235–57.
62 [*Puls.Ant.*]: 19,629–42 K; [Rufus], *De pulsibus*: pp. 219–32 DR; Harris CRS 1973: 249–51, 257–66; Lewis 2015.
63 [*Def.Med.*] 110: 19,375–6 K.
64 Barton 1994: 133–168; cf. also Deichgräber 1957; Asper 2005; Lewis 2016.
65 *Dign.Puls.* I,1: 8,770 K; Harris CRS 1973: 396–431.
66 *Diff.Puls.* IV,11: 8,753 K; the summaries are *Puls.*: 8,453–92 K; *Syn.Puls.*: 9,431–549 K; *Us.Puls.*: 5,149–80 K; ed. Furley and Wilkie 1984: 194–227.
67 Deichgräber 1957 remains essential.
68 *Us.Puls.* 7: 5,172–3 K; p. 221 tr. Furley-Wilkie; *Caus.Puls.* I,1–8: 9,1–26 K; Siegel 1968: 83–7, 91–6; Harris CRS 1973: 367, 374.
69 *Diff.Puls.* I,3: 8,500 K; *Dig.Puls.* I,8: 8,806–7 K; *Syn.Puls.* 5: 9,443–4 K.
70 Harris CRS 1973: 430 discusses how close Galen came to anticipating the discovery of the circulation by William Harvey (1628), himself a vitalist and Aristotelian teleologist.
71 He says much less on this in his *Synopsis*, 9,431–549 K, and in the shorter *Pulses for Beginners*, 8,453–92 K.
72 *Dign.Puls.* I,4–10: 8,790–818 K. For the systolic gap, above, note 70.
73 *Praec.* 11,9: 14,661 K; *CMG* V 8, 130–1.
74 *Dign.Puls.* I,1: 8,768–9 K.
75 *Hipp.Prog.* I,6–7: 18B,25–32 K: cf. Hippocrates, *Progn.* 2: II, 112,12–118,6 L.
76 Theophilus, *De urinis, pref.* For later developments, Stolberg 2015.
77 Barnes 1991: 65–8.
78 *Loc.Aff.* III,11: 8,194–5 K; pp. 94–5 tr. Siegel; Temkin 1971: 61–4.
79 *Temp.* II,2: 1,582 K; p. 111 tr. Singer PN; *PHP* VIII,6,29: 5,695 K; *CMG* V 4,1,2, 519; *Loc.Aff.* IV,3: 8,230–2 K; pp. 109–10 tr. Siegel; *Hipp.Aph.* II,42 and III,31: 17B,541–3, 648–50 K; *Hipp.Epid.VI*, viii: *CMG* V 10,2,2,462–4.
80 *Loc.Aff.* III,11: 8,196 K; p. 95 tr. Siegel.
81 Mattern 2008: 119–25, 155–9.
82 *MM*: 10,1–1021 K; tr. Johnston and Horsley 2011; *MMG*: 11,1–146 K; pp. 337–559 tr. Johnston.
83 *MM* II,6: 10,117–8, 126 K; I,183–5, 197, tr. Johnston and Horsley with the commentary in Hankinson 1991a; Johnston 2006: 69–80
84 Unlike in modern medicine, where it is a symptom of a specific disease, fever was regarded as a class of diseases, even if some of its manifestations can now be given labels such as typhoid or malaria. That did not, of course, prevent Galen from treating each type of fever as something different, hence the title of his big book on fevers, *Diff.Feb.*: 7,273–405 K. In counting, Galen counted the day of an illness as day one, hence a tertian (three day) fever occurs on days 1 and 3, a quartan on days 1 and 4.

85 Strohmaier 1970: 88–94. *Part.Hom.Diff. CMG Suppl.*
86 *Diff.Morb.* 4,3 and 5,2: 6,845, 849–50 K.
87 *Ibid.* 11,1: 6,871–2 K.
88 *Marc.*: 7,666–704 K; tr. Theoharides 1971; *Hipp.Com.*: 7,643–65 K; *Loc.Aff.*: 8,1–452 K; tr. Siegel 1975. Aretaeus, for instance, had divided them up into acute and chronic diseases.
89 Hankinson 1998b: 373–402; Johnston 2006.
90 *Caus.Cont.* 2,1–3: *CMG Suppl. Or.* II, 54–5.
91 Hankinson 1998b: 377–8, citing *Caus.Puls.* I,1: 9,2–3 K for an example.
92 *Morb.Temp.*: 7,406–39 K; *Tot.Morb.Temp.*: 7,440–62 K.
93 In general, Pigeaud 2006.
94 Cf. the pseudo-Galenic tract [*Prog.Dec.*], which defines the outcome of a disease from the moment the patient took to his or her bed, and which is heavily astrological in orientation, 19,529–73 K. For Hippocratic arithmology, see Jouanna 1999: 338–41.
95 *Cris.*: 9,550–760 K; ed. Alexanderson 1967.
96 *Di.Dec.*: 9,761–941 K; tr. Cooper 2011b; Miller 2018; see also Cooper 2011a; Heilen 2018.
97 For a probably later attempt by a doctor to gather together Hippocratic material on critical days, Craik 2015: 141–4; Patterson 2017.
98 *Di Dec.* I,1: 9,786–7 K; I,5: 9,791–2 K.
99 He claims it as his own discovery at *Hipp.Prog.* III,4: 18B,240–1 K.
100 *Di.Dec.* III,9: 9,931–4 K, with the revised text and detailed mathematical discussion in Heilen 2018. For his lifelong interest, *ibid.* I,2: 9,775 K; I,3: 9,780 K; *Med.Exp.* 21; p. 127 tr. Walzer and Frede; *Sept.Part.* pp. 346, 353, 355–6 Walzer.
101 *Di.Dec.* III.11: 9,935–7 K.
102 Toomer 1985 (and more can be expected from the *Commentary on Airs, Waters, and Places*); Heilen 2018. Cf. also the remarkable comparison of the working of the body to an astronomical mechanism, *UP* XIV,5: 4,156–7 K; II, p. 627 tr. May, with Jones A 2017: 96, 113, 240, 245.
103 Galen expects his readers not to blame him for not intervening in the case of Theagenes, *MM* XIII,15: 10,909–16 K; III, pp. 371–81 tr. Johnston-Horsley, even although he says he knew that the therapies of his colleagues would prove fatal.
104 As well as abnormal swellings, *MM* XIII–XIV: 10,874–1021 K; III pp. 319–537 tr. Johnston-Horsley, cover a wide range of conditions from priapism and missing digits to warts, alopecia and cataract but without going into details of how, where and when to cut.
105 Above, p. 23.
106 *Hipp.Art.* I,22: 18A,347–8 K; Meyerhof 1929: 83.
107 *AA* VII,13: 2,632–33 K; pp. 192–3 tr. Singer C; *PHP* I,5,1–3: 5,181 K; *CMG* V 4,1,2, 75; Gourevitch 2001: 56 60. Cf. for cases involving the removal of bone from the forehead. *MM* VI,6: 10,452–4 K; II, pp. 231–3 tr. Johnston-Horsley.
108 [*Int.*] 19–20: 14,780–97 K; pp. 90–105 Petit; English summary by Toledo-Pereyra 1973: 366–75, unfortunately under the misapprehension that this treatise was by Galen; *Opt.Med. Cogn.* 12–3: *CMG Suppl. Or.* IV, 134–7. Cf. also the operations recorded on papyri (Marganne 1994, 1998); and the recently published Oxyrhynchus papyri 5232 and 5240.
109 *Ind.* 5: p. 3 BJP; p. 79 tr. Nutton; *AA* VIII,6: 2,682 K; p. 214 tr. Singer C; for other instruments, cf. *Sem.* II,1,10–11: *CMG* V 3,1, 146–7. In general, Jackson 2018.
110 *MM* VI,6: 10,455–6 K; II, p. 235 tr. Johnston-Horsley. He claims to have observed 'vast numbers' of cases of trepanation in Rome, *SMT* X,2,3: 12,256 K.
111 Toledo-Pereyra 1973; Mani 1991. He made also various recommendations for treating abnormal swellings in the late *MM* XIII–XIV; III pp. 319–537 tr. Johnston-Horsley.
112 *MM* V,7: 10,334–5 K; II, pp. 43–7 tr. Johnston-Horsley. At *AA* III,9: 2,396 K; p. 82 tr. Singer C, Galen defends certain well-known doctors for severing a vein by showing that its position in the patient was abnormal.
113 *MM* XIII,22: 10,942 K; III, p. 421 tr. Johnston-Horsley. Majno 1975: 403–5.
114 Brain 1986 is fundamental.
115 Bloodletting in spring was also a common practice at Pergamum, *MM* V,7: 10,334 K; II, p. 45 tr. Johnston-Horsley. For Galen's debates on venesection with the Erasistrateans, see above, pp. 42–3.
116 Brain 1986: 112–21, 147–9.

117 *Cur.Rat.Ven.Sect.* 5: 11,262–3 K; p. 73 tr. Brain.
118 *Ibid.*: 11,266 K; p. 74 tr. Brain; *Plen:* 7,513–83 K; ed. Otte 2001.
119 Brain 1986: 13; Mattern 2008: 141–2; Boudon-Millot 2012: 271–3.
120 Brain 1986: 130, 135–44.
121 *Cur.Rat.Ven.Sect.* 23: 11,314–5 K; p. 98 tr. Brain; *Prop.Plac.* 2,2: *CMG* V 3,2, 58–9; p. 173 BMP; pp. 62–3 Garofalo-Lami; p. 188 Vegetti.
122 Brain 1986: 128–32.
123 *Ven.Sect.Er.Rom.* 1: 11,187–96 K.
124 Brain 1986: 158–72.
125 *MM* IX,4: 10,612–3 K; II, pp. 469–71 tr. Johnston-Horsley.
126 Carter 2017.
127 Majno 1975: 365–9. His claim, p. 415, that Galen would not have known about Roman surgery because Celsus wrote in Latin founders on the fact that Celsus was transmitting Greek Alexandrian surgery.
128 *Opt.Med.Cogn.* 14,3: *CMG Suppl. Or.* IV, 136–7.
129 *Ibid.* 11,7: *CMG Suppl. Or.* IV, 122–3.
130 *Ibid.* 11,7–8; 12,3–5: *CMG Suppl. Or.* IV, 122–5. Galen unusually distinguishes these doctors with a lesser knowledge of drugs and herbs from charlatans and incompetents who know nothing.
131 Nutton 2015b; and for theriac, above, pp. 113–4.
132 *Opt.Med.Cogn* 12,6–7: *CMG Suppl. Or.* IV, 124–7.
133 Fabricius 1972; Debru 1997; Vogt 2008.
134 For Cleopatra, probably copied from Crito, *Comp.Med.Loc.* I,2: 12,403–4 K; for Rufus, *ibid.*: 12,425 K.
135 Fabricius 1972: 183–98; Touwaide 2014.
136 *Ind.* 32–3; pp. 11–12 BJP; tr. Nutton 2013: 87–8. The heir was probably Claudianus, a doctor friend, the intermediate source of a recipe against early baldness, *Comp.Med.Loc.* I,2: 12,423 K.
137 *Ind.* 34–6; p. 12 BJP; tr. Nutton 2013e: 87–8. For the problems with the text and identification, see Nutton 2013e: 88–9. At *Comp.Med.Gen.* II,1: 13,459 K he mentions two colleagues whose recipe collections had similarly been burnt; one died of grief, the other gave up practising.
138 *Ant.* I,1 and 10: 14,4–5, 51 K.
139 *Ibid.* I,1 and 12: 14,9–10, 59–61 K; cf. [*Ther.Pis.*] 1: 14,211 K; Chaniotis 1999: 209–10, 219–20.
140 *MM* XIV,12: 10,986 K; III, p. 485 tr. Johnston-Horsley, for the costs of different sorts of theriac, that made with vipers being the most expensive; his own cheaper version was made from Cretan catmint.
141 [*Rem.*] Pref.: 14,311–4 K. Oribasius, *Summary for Eunapius*, pref. 5: *CMG* VI,6,3, 317–8, regrets that the original no longer existed in his day.
142 The text under Galen's name on substitute drugs, [*Suc.*]: 19,721–47 K, is also suspect: Kessel 2019.
143 King H 2018.
144 *Ant.* II,8: 14,149–50 K.
145 Watson 1966; Totelin 2004. The story in the pseudo-Galenic *Theriac, for Piso* is told from a very Roman perspective: [*Ther.Pis.*]: 16:14,283–4 K; ed. Boudon-Millot 2016a: 84.
146 For the first two, Fabricius 1972: 181–2, 201; *Comp.Med.Loc.* IV,7: 12,786 K; II,5: 13,104 K; *Comp.Med.Gen.* VII,13: 13,1038 K; *Ant.* II,13: 14,190 and 182 K; *Comp.Med.Gen.* VII,13: 13,1036 K.
147 *Comp.Med.Loc.* IV,8: 12,753 K. The ingredients of this remedy, including opium, egg whites, and styptics, would make a simple and probably effective ointment for use in boxing matches: Bartels *et al.* 2006. For analgesics, Harris WV 2018: 62–6, 73–79.
148 Gourevitch 2016; Nutton 2016; Fausti 2017.
149 *Ant.* I,5 and 9: 14,31–32, 52 K; Von Staden 1997b: 67–68; Vogt 2005. The author of *Theriac, for Piso* also copied out the verse recipe of Andromachus for his dedicatee because he would appreciate its literary elegance, 5: 14,232 K; p. 21 Boudon-Millot. The poem was not printed in Kühn. For a fragment in verse by Rufus of Ephesus, *Comp.Med.Loc.* I:1: 12,425 K = Rufus, frag. 3, p. 292 DR.
150 *Ant.* II,7: 14,144–6 K: Kudlien 1974 suggests he lived around 30 CE.

151 Andromachus, fl. 60 CE, Heitsch 1964: 7–15; Cassia 2012; an edition of the poems of Servilius is promised by Sabine Vogt. The prognostic antidote is given at *Ant.* II,5: 14,134 K.
152 *SMT* IX,3,8,11 and 21: 12,214–6, 220, 226–7 K. For Lemnian earth, see above, pp. 53–4.
153 *SMT* IX,2,5–9 and 3,8: 12,199–203, 216 K; cf. Pliny, *Natural History* 12,65, a reference I owe to Nicholas Purcell: *Ant.* I,2: 14,7 K.
154 Martelli 2012.
155 *Ant.* I,8: 14,49 K.
156 *SMT* VII,12: 12,13–14 K; *Comp.Med.Loc.* VI,2: 12,905 K, discovered on a visit to the countryside immediately on his return home from Alexandria.
157 *Comp.Med.Loc.* VIII,6: 13,188 K.
158 *SMT* XI,48: 12,365 K: cf. Scribonius Largus, *Recipes* 1 (headache), 152 (gout), with Debru 2008.
159 *Subf.Emp.* 10: p. 75 Deichgraber; p. 39 tr. Frede.
160 *Comp.Med.Loc.* VIII,2: 13,126–36 K; Goltz 1976: 29–30.
161 *MM* XIV,5: 10,962–3 K; III, pp. 449–51 tr. Johnston-Horsley.
162 Debru 1997; Jacques 1997; van der Eijk 1997.
163 *Prop.Plac.* 9,1–3: *CMG* V 3,2, 84–9; pp. 83–7 BMP; pp.96–8 Garofalo-Lami; p. 204 Vegetti; *SMT* I,8: 11,397 K.
164 Barnes 1997; Von Staden 1997b.
165 *Prop.Plac* 12,1–4: *CMG* V 3,2, 94–9; pp. 183–4 BMP; pp. 108–11 Garofalo-Lami; p. 108 Vegetti; [*Hipp.Hum.*] I.12: 16,124–5, based on Oribasius, *Medical Collections* VII,23,22–4: *CMG* VI 1,1, 223,18–30; *Purg.Med.Fac.* 1–3: 11,324–35 K: this erroneous view is ascribed to Asclepiades and his followers and to Erasistratus and the Erasistrateans, all of whom either disregarded or played down the role of humours.
166 *Adv.Jul.* 8,1–16: *CMG* V 10,3, 62–67. In the small and fragmentary tract on purgatives, *Purg.Med.Fac.*: 11,323–42 K, he gives several examples of his own successful use of purgatives in “this most populous city” and challenges his opponents to do likewise.
167 Röhr 1923: 96–133; Touwaide 1994.
168 Debru 1997: 85–102. Cf. Röhr 1923 for the overlap with ‘occult properties’.
169 Keyser 1997; Jouanna 2011; Gourevitch 2016; Nutton 2016.
170 Gourevitch 2016: 256–9.
171 I.e. herbs whose properties and their prescription are determined by zodiacal prediction, *SMT* X,1: 12,249 K.
172 *SMT* VI,Pr.: 11,792–8 K, a masterpiece of rhetorical denunciation.
173 *SMT* IX,2,19: 12,207 K. Literally, “without methodical usage”.
174 *Comp.Med.Loc.* II,1: 12,533–5 K; II,2: 12,573 K; Jouanna 2011: 69; Van Nuffelen 2014; Petit 2017.
175 *SMT* IX,2,19: 12,207 K; Ryholt 2011; Jouanna 2011: 63–5.
176 *SMT* VI,3,10: 11,859–60 K; cf. *Comp.Med.Loc.* II,2: 12,573 K; Lloyd 1979: 42; Jouanna 2011: Gourevitch 2016: 264–9.
177 Jouanna 2011: 77–8.
178 *SMT* VI,Pr.: 11,792–8 K. For Dioscorides, *Materia medica, Pref.* 5, with Riddle 1985: 21–2, 96–8.
179 *MM* VI,2: 10,400–1 K; II, p. 143 tr. Johnston-Horsley; cf. Tecusan 2004: 96.
180 Harig 1974.
181 *MM* VIII,4: 10,574 K; II, p. 413 tr. Johnston-Horsley; *Comp.Med.Loc.* I,5: 12,425 K; *Comp.Med.Gen.* III,8: 13,636 K.
182 Evershed 2004; Bartels *et al.* 2006; Touwaide 2010; Photos-Jones *et al.*, forthcoming.
183 A team headed by Caroline Petit is working on many aspects of this long treatise.
184 Harig 1974: 195–212.
185 *MM* III,7–9: 10,209–17 K; I, pp. 319–31 tr. Johnston-Horsley.
186 *Ars Med.* 28: 1,383 K; p. 382 tr. Singer PN.
187 Grimaudo 2008; Grant M 2000: 4–10 gives a short summary. For the later canonisation of the six non-naturals as a guiding principle of dietetics, see below, p. 138.
188 *San.Tu.* V,1: 6,308–9 K; II, pp. 7–9 tr. Johnston.

189 *Alim.Fac.* III,1: 6,664 K ; p. 116 tr. Powell; *Vict.Att.* 66; pp. 82–4 Marinone; p. 315 tr. Singer PN.
190 *Comp.Med.Loc.*VI,6: 12,948 K; I,3: 12,443–5 K.
191 Nutton 2000.
192 *Alim.Fac.* I,2 and III,1: 6,486, 664 K; pp. 41, 116 tr. Powell; *Vict.Att.* 66; p. 69 Marinone; p. 315 tr. Singer PN.
193 *Alim.Fac.* I,7: 6,499 K; cf. I,14–5: 6,523 K; pp. 46, 56–7 tr. Powell; *Vict.Att.* 40–1; pp. 82–4 Marinone; p. 310 tr. Singer PN.
194 *Bon.Mal.Suc.* 1: 6,49–50 K. Garnsey 1988 gives the wider background.
195 *Alim.Fac.* I,2; 25–6; III,2: 6,486, 539–40, 669 K; pp. 41, 63–4, 119 tr. Powell; *MMG* II,12: 11,142 K; p. 555 tr. Johnston.
196 *Nat.Fac.* I,11: 2,26 K; p. 43 tr. Brock; *Alim.Fac.* I,1: 6,467 K; p. 34 tr. Powell, citing [Hippocrates], *Nutriment* 19: IX,104,11 L.; p. 142 ed. Jouanna; [Aristotle] *Problems* I,42: 864b.
197 *SMT* I,1; III,3; V,1: 11,380, 545, 705 K.
198 Below, p. 134.
199 Respectively *Alim.Fac.* II,23: 6,603 K (with the reading at Wilkins 2013: 127); p. 90 tr. Powell; *SMT* I,1: 1,387–390 K; *Hipp.Epid.VI*, iv: 17B,155, 161, 163, 182 K; *Alim.Fac.* III,38: 6,738–40 K; p. 48 tr. Powell.
200 *San.Tu.* V,5: 6,334–9 K; II, pp. 35–41 tr. Johnston; *Bon.Mal.Suc.* 11: 6,800–6 K; *MM* XIII,4: 10,830–7 K; III, pp. 255–63 tr. Johnston-Horsley, with Robert 1980: 319–37.
201 *Ant.* I,3: 14,17–19 K; *SMT* IV,14: 11,663 K.
202 *Alim.Fac.* III,1: 6,663 K ; p. 115 tr. Powell
203 *Ptis.*: 6,815–31 K; pp. 62–7 tr. Grant M.
204 *Alim.Fac.* II,20–2: 6,596–602 K ; pp. 86–9 tr. Powell.
205 *Alim.Fac.* II,22: 6,598–9 K; pp. 88–9 tr. Powell.
206 *San.Tu.* V,4: 6,332–3 K; II, pp. 31–3 tr. Johnston.
207 König 2005: 274–300.
208 *Protr.* 10: 1,23–7 K; pp. 45–7 tr. Singer PN; *Thras.* 9, 36, 46: 5,820, 874–5, 894 K; pp. 59, 86–7, 96–7 tr. Singer PN; *Parv.Pil.* 5: 5,910 K; p. 304 tr. Singer PN; *Hipp.Aph.* I,3: 17B,361 K.
209 *San.Tu.* I,12: 6,62–3 K; I, p. 91 tr. Johnston; *MM* IX,4: 10,608 K; II, p. 463 tr. Johnston-Horsley.
210 *Thras.*: 5,806–98 K; tr. Johnston 2018. Cf. *Puer.Epil.* 3: 11,362 K; p. 182 tr. Temkin, Dr. Dionysius is expected to choose a gymnastic trainer for his patient in accordance with Galen's ideas.
211 *Hipp.Epid.VI*, viii: *CMG* V 10,2,2, 502–3.
212 Von Müller 1895: 475.
213 *San.Tu.* II,8: 6,133–4 K; I, pp. 195–6 tr. Johnston.
214 *Parv.Pil.* 5,899–910 K; II, pp. 378–97 ed. Johnston 2018; König 2005: 285–90; Boudon-Millot 2015.
215 Cf. *Alim.Fac.* III,32: 6,661 K, comparing gymnastic activity with the vigorous work of digging; *Thras.* 41: 6,885–6 K, adds rowing, digging, reaping, and ploughing.
216 *MM* XIII,15: 10,909–10 K; III, p. 371 tr. Johnston-Horsley.
217 Fagan 1999; Yegül 2010.
218 *San.Tu.* III,3–4: 6,181–9 K; I, pp. 263–75 tr. Johnston; *Trem.Palp.* 5: 7,601 K; *MM* VIII,2: 10,536–7 K; II, p. 355 tr. Johnston-Horsley; and *SMT* I,7: 11,393 K (Aquae Albulae); *Hipp.AWP* G.36: p. 53 Wasserstein (for the reading, above, p. 71, note 15). Mattern 2008: 40–3, gives examples of bathing therapy.
219 *SMT* I,7: 11,393 K; *Hipp.AWP* G36–75: pp. 54–7 Wasserstein.
220 *Aff.Dig.* 4,1: 5,14 K; p. 251 tr. Singer.
221 *Ind.* 78: p. 24 BJP; p. 97 tr. Nutton, with note 118.
222 *Ibid.* 76: pp. 22–3 BJP; p. 97 tr. Nutton.
223 Above, pp. 86–7. Good discussions of Galenic madness and psychotherapy, from a variety of perspectives, are given by Dols 1992; and by the chapters by Nutton, Boudon-Millot, Gourevitch, Holmes and Gill in Harris WV 2013; Kaufman 2015; Mattern 2016; Stewart 2019.
224 *Praec.* 6,10–13: 14,633–4 K; *CMG* V 8, 1,102–5; *Caus.Puls.* IV,1–5: 9,156–61 K; Gill 2013.
225 *Hipp.Epid.VI*, viii: *CMG* V 10,2,2, 494.

226 *San.Tu.* I,8,19–21: 6,41 K; cf. Edelstein and Edelstein 1945: 206 for Aristides being told by Asclepius to go riding.
227 *Caus.Symp.* III,7: 7,200–4 K; *MM* XIII,21: 10,929–30 K; III, p. 403 tr. Johnston-Horsley; *Loc.Aff.* III,6–7: 8,160–8 K; pp. 81–4 tr. Siegel.
228 Pigeaud 2008; Stewart 2019.
229 *Loc.Aff.* III,10: 8,182–3 K; p. 90 tr. Siegel.
230 *At.Bil.* 7: 5,132 K, citing the (legendary) cure of the daughters of Proteus with hellebore by the shaman-seer Melampus. Curiously, as Michael Dols noted (1992: 37), when compared with frenzy Galen says very little about *mania* and not much more about melancholia.
231 *Loc.Aff.* III,9: 8,178 K; p. 88 tr. Siegel.
232 Thumiger 2017: 151–5.
233 *Loc.Aff.* IV,1: 8,226–7 K; p. 108 tr. Siegel; cf. *Hipp.Prorrh.* I.27: 16,564–5 K.
234 *Symp.Diff.* 3: 7,60–62 K.
235 *Ibid.*; other versions of this story are given at *Loc.Aff.* IV,1: 8,226 K; p. 108 tr. Siegel; and *Hipp.Epid. VI*, v: *CMG* V 10,2,2, 461. The last is a good example of how Galen expands his story over time.
236 *Hipp.Epid. VI*, v: CMG V 10,2,2, 461–2. These stories may date from before 169, although in neither of them is it entirely clear that Galen was himself involved.
237 Pigeaud 1987: 217–8, notes the objections of the Methodist Caelius Aurelianus to such harsh therapies, including bleeding to exhaustion, which might lead to death.
238 Cf. also cases of episodes of coherence and incoherence, *Hipp.Prorrh.* I,27: 16,566–7 K.
239 *Hipp.Epid.II*, viii: *CMG* V 10,1, 207–8; *Hipp.Epid. VI*, viii: *CMG* V 10,2,2, 487.
240 *Hipp.Epid. VI*, viii: *CMG* V 10,2,2, 494; *Hipp.Epid.II*, viii: *CMG* V 10,1, 212.
241 *Hipp.Epid. VI*, viii: *CMG* V 10,2,2, 487. The doctor must set an example to the patient.
242 Some of these psychological treatments were not solely Galenic but were recommended by some Methodists (Pigeaud 1987: 162, 168–73, noting the link in the Pseudo-Aristotelian *Problems* XXX between a medical and an intellectual view of tragic catharsis).
243 Mattern 2008: 43–7.
244 Contrast *Hipp.Prog.* I,8: 18B,40 K, with *Praec.* 6,2–10: 14,631–3 K; *CMG* V 8,1, 100–3.
245 *Subf.Emp.* 10: pp. 75–79 Deichgräber; pp. 39–41 tr. Frede = *SMT* XI,1: 12,312–6 K.
246 Aretaeus, *Chron.* IV 19,19–20: *CMG* II, 89–90.
247 Gourevitch 2001; Mattern 2008; Lloyd 2009; Petit 2018: 124–46.
248 David Wootton's 2007 argument that pre-modern therapy was likely to harm as much as cure applies equally to Galen's competitors and predecessors.
249 His use of the first person, whether as a pronoun or within the verb, is many times more frequent than that of Rufus or Aretaeus, Nutton 2009c; Singer and van der Eijk 2018: 37–38.
250 Cf. the similar expressions in [Galen] *Virt.Cent.* 1: p.161 Nutton: 'incredibilia', 'miratus fui'.
251 One should also be wary of assuming, as he implies, that he was their only physician. There were certainly others who treated the imperial family, and the rich would equally have had a choice; the author of *Theriac, for Piso* also enjoyed a career as long and as successful as Galen's at court and among the upper classes, Boudon-Millot 2016a: LXXIV–LXXX.
252 Nutton 1984b: 320–1; Pietrobelli 2019a: 19–22.

6 Galen the ghost

Around 1501, the Riminese physician Hieronymus Surianus, tired after his editorial labours on medical and philosophical texts, was dozing at his desk when he received an unexpected visitor.[1] This was none other than Galen himself, wearing Greek dress and complaining that previous editors had inflicted such indignities on his writings that they were now almost unintelligible. He had come to invite Surianus to take up the task of preparing a new edition of his writings and had brought with him his own copy of them, a massive volume "a cubit high". He opened this "archetype" so quickly that at first Surianus could make out only one of the many corrections Galen claimed he had made. He then opened the volume "at about two fingerbreadths from the beginning" to show him a page headed with the title *De motibus liquidis*. Surianus counted there sixteen errors marked in capitals, which he could read easily, but he did not have time to make out the many others in minuscule before Galen closed the book again. The last service rendered by the ghost of "Father Galen" before he disappeared was to recommend as a publisher Bernardinus Benalius of Bergamo, a friend of both Surianus himself and of his own recently deceased publisher, Octavianus Scotus.[2]

This fantastic *Preface* is not only a splendid advertisement for the superiority of the new edition and in particular, and rightly, for its text of *De motibus*, but it also represents Galen, although dressed in Greek garb, as a Latin author in a Latin university context. His "*archetypus*" corresponds in size and script to a typical late-medieval Latin manuscript of Galen's *Opera omnia*, he corrects it as a learned scholar, and he writes in Latin or, at the very least, knows that language well enough to remove the errors of Latin translators and copyists. Surianus' dream neatly shows Galen and Galenism at a crucial moment of transition, at a time when Greek manuscripts of Galen were already beginning to circulate and be discussed in Northern Italy. What were then regarded as Galen's complete works were first printed in 1490, comprising 79 treatises in medieval Latin translation, a quarter of them later shown to be spurious and all usually relying on a word-for-word translation from the Greek or on an Arabic or Hebrew intermediary. The 1490 printing, although, as Surianus was well aware, far from accurate and at times unintelligible, fixed the Galenic Corpus for almost forty years for doctors all over Europe, and was not replaced by a more modern collection in Latin until the 1540s.[3] Even after the appearance in print of the Greek Galen in 1525 had added many previously unknown or neglected treatises to the Corpus, Latin translations, more accurate and more elegant than their medieval predecessors, continued to exercise a greater influence on European medicine than the Greek original right down to the late nineteenth century.

By that stage Galen had been handed over almost entirely to classical philologists interested solely in the text rather than in his medical ideas. It was a dramatic fall for one whose ideas on medicine had dominated medicine for so long.[4]

Crafting a reputation

Such a long-lasting reputation would have gratified the philosopher-doctor from Pergamum, who had sedulously striven throughout his life to ensure that his merits were widely known and properly appreciated. Not only did he send copies of his writings to his friends around the Eastern Mediterranean in the expectation that they would pass them on in turn or deposit them in public libraries (something closely paralleled in the activities of another doctor-philosopher, Heraclitus of Rhodiapolis) but he also provided summaries and shorter versions for those unable to afford the larger books or fully comprehend all their subtleties.[5] Above all, he was concerned to avoid being misrepresented.[6] He wrote *My own Books* having reportedly overheard a dispute over whether a book available under the name of Galen was really his, and the preface to *My own Opinions* draws a parallel with a similar incident from the distant past involving the celebrated poet Parthenius.[7] In *The Order of my own Books* he also set out the most appropriate way of reading his huge oeuvre, and the final section of his *Art of Medicine* acts as a further guide to his writings.[8] Such concern for his own reputation goes for beyond what is known of any other author and helped to fix the image of Galen as supreme. In one of the opening illustrations in the celebrated Vienna Dioscorides, a codex copied around 512. for a Byzantine princess, Galen sits at the head of a group of distinguished pharmacologists, in the same pose and clothing as Chiron the centaur, the mythical inventor of pharmacology, on the previous page and as Jesus among his disciples in liturgical manuscripts.[9] Galen was right to worry about forgeries and misattributions for over the centuries many treatises that were not his circulated under his name and it was not until the 1540s that attempts were made to sort the wheat from the chaff. Some tracts, like the two theriac treatises, *The Properties of the Centaury*, and the (now lost) commentary on the Hippocratic *Nature of the Child* that was later ascribed to his teacher Pelops, seem to be contemporary writings from his library swept up along with his own at his death. Others are later summaries or compilations from scattered texts, and still others, particularly from the sixteenth century, are Greek pastiches incorporating some genuine material, often retranslated from Oriental sources. Their very existence is further testimony to the authority the mere name of Galen could confer.[10]

Reactions to his writings from his contemporaries focus as much on his philosophy as on his medicine.[11] Alexander of Aphrodisias, above, p. 124 considered some of his ideas on time, motion and cosmology important enough to be worth detailed refutation, while a group of Christians led by Theodotus the shoemaker repaid his interest in their beliefs by attempting to combat his strictures about their defective logic.[12] Their adoration for him quickly led to their being stigmatised as heretics, but some more significant theologians seem to have profited from his writings. Clement of Alexandria (c. 150–c. 215), the leading Christian teacher at Alexandria, drew heavily on Galen for his theory of demonstration as well as for other sections relating to medicine in his *Miscellanies* and *The Tutor*, while his successor there, Origen (c. 184–c. 253), may well have been referring to Galen when he explained that physicians who practise dissection can explain how Providence has designed each part of the body, even the smallest, for a specific purpose.[13] Further evidence for his reputation in Egypt comes from several sources. Their contemporary Athenaeus of Naucratis included him as a famous writer on medicine and philosophy among the interlocutors at his imaginary learned banquet, describing two of his interventions, and a papyrus fragment of his *The Opinions of Hippocrates and Plato* written around 230, has been discovered at Oxyrhynchus. Even more remarkable for a Greek writer is his mention by a Latin writer on foodstuffs, Gargilius Martialis, who lived in North Africa around 250, although, like those in Athenaeus, none of his quotations can be identified for certain among Galen's extant books.[14]

His reputation and authority continued to grow, especially at the expense of Hippocrates, who became known more and more at one remove only through texts Galen had commented upon or through ideas that he had espoused. Indeed, some Arabic translations of Hippocratic texts were not made from the originals, but from passages excerpted and discussed by Galen.[15] This was a process that continued into the late sixteenth century. The first printing of our Hippocratic Corpus in Latin translation did not appear until 1525, thirty five years after the first similar printing of the complete works of Galen, and it was not until the following year, 1526, that the first edition in Greek was published, a year after the similar Aldine printing of Galen in Greek. A widespread medieval legend neatly illustrates their relationship. Galen, the apprentice of his uncle, Hippocrates, became so successful that he took over many of his uncle's patients. Envious and angry at being supplanted, Hippocrates murdered Galen while he was inspecting plants in his herb garden. He did not go unmourned, however, and on his deathbed, the penitent Hippocrates was forced to acknowledge that he had indeed been surpassed by his brilliant nephew.[16] In a Latin epigram put into the mouth of Galen a renaissance poet and medical professor Eobanus Hessus (1488–1540) explained why:

> Remove Hippocrates, first then shall I be.
> My debts to him are many, but so are his to me.
> Things left undone, obscure, I leave complete,
> A thousand volumes, crystal clear and neat.
> A tiny island bore him, me the mighty land
> Of Asia. He a few things, I a myriad penned.
> He gave us building blocks from which a citadel
> I built for medicine. Apollo guards it still.[17]

Cutting Galen down to size

But for all Galen's achievements, the sheer bulk of his writings posed a major problem. Sometimes it was a question of style. An Arabic commentator on the neo-Platonist philosopher Porphyry contrasted Galen's verbosity with the brevity of Hippocrates: both extremes made for very difficult reading.[18] But more often it was Galen's desire for completeness that was to blame. A Byzantine satirist explained Galen's absence from a court hearing by saying that he had been delayed adding yet more information to an already immense work in progress, while an exasperated medieval reader was more succinct. "You would have made a mattress out of a few threads", was his comment in the margin of his copy.[19]

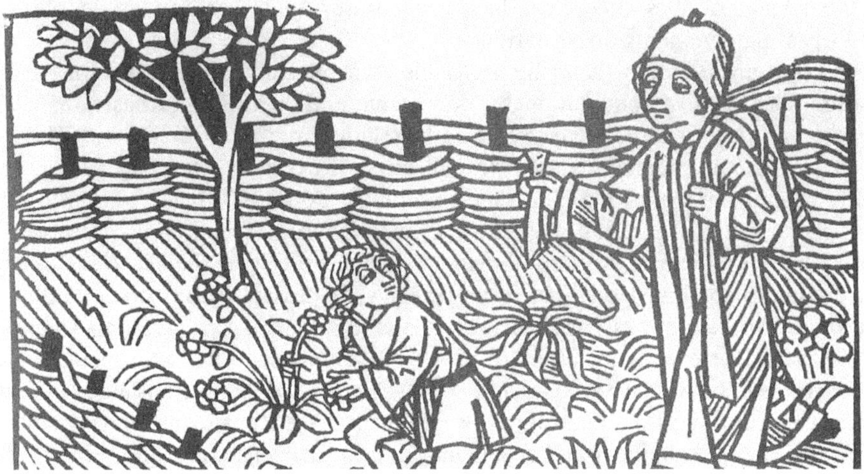

Figure 6.1 A widespread medieval legend. Hippocrates murders his nephew Galen out of envy at his success. Woodcut from *Die cyben weisen meister*, Augsburg, 1497, n.p.

Three different processes combined to make Galen's oeuvre more accessible. Many treatises, especially the non-medical, were simply never copied or recopied, and even where they were, like the *Introduction to Logic*, they seem to have been little read. Bigger books and those only tangentially related to therapy were particularly at risk. Only occasional fragments of his most important contribution to logic, *Demonstration*, survive today in Greek, although it was widely cited and discussed by Arabic and Hebrew scholars, and the full Arabic version may well be awaiting discovery in an Eastern library.[20] Another survivor in Arabic, the second part of *Anatomical Procedures*, seems to have disappeared in Greek by 1300, probably because its detailed advice on dissection was difficult, if not impossible, to follow when dissection was nigh unknown.[21] When some of these treatises were lost can be determined only vaguely. Late medieval Byzantine manuscripts contain fewer tracts than the 129 recorded by Hunayn Ibn Isḥāq around 860 as being already available in Arabic, and some shorter texts, like the two little treatises on causation or *Problematical Movements* that were translated from the Greek into Latin by Niccolò da Reggio in Naples around 1330, had disappeared by 1500. This was a process of attrition, halted only by the advent of printing.[22]

The second response to Galen's prolixity involved some form of abbreviation. Galen himself had provided summaries of his larger works on pulses and the *Method of Healing*, but later authors devised other methods of presenting his ideas as well.[23] By 380, his medical works were being excerpted and included in massive encyclopedias of medicine. The three most important, compiled by Oribasius (about 320–400), doctor to the emperor Julian, by Aetius of Amida in the first half of the sixth century, and by Paul of Aegina, around 630, included excerpts from many of his writings, some, like his commentary on *Airs, Waters and Places*, now lost to us in Greek.[24] Over the years, the percentage of Galenic extracts in these compilations continued to increase at the expense of lesser figures such as Rufus: sometimes they swallowed up other authors, while still bearing the name of Galen. Alternatives to Galen were being pushed aside, and the format of these encyclopedias also ensured that there was little place for Galen's passing comments or hesitations.

Sometimes an author or a scribe made his own selection of passages for his own purposes. The massive compilation by the Arabic author al-Rāzī, Rhases (850–932), the *Kitab al-Hāwī*, or in its medieval Latin translation, the *Liber Continens* (*The Book that has Everything*), represents his own collection of extracts, often pages long, occasionally taken from works, like *The Voice*, no longer extant in Greek.[25] The Byzantine scribe of Paris, BNF gr. 2332, copied in Constantinople around 1450 short sections from a variety of treatises, keeping Galen's wording, order and the shape of his argument.[26] Others combined sections from Galen with passages from other authors to make their own handbooks. Two teachers in medieval Paris, Jean de Saint-Amand (fl. 1261–98) and Pierre de Saint-Flour (fl. 1349–80), composed their own medical Latin dictionaries out of a cento of Galenic passages that had been translated.[27] Similar summaries of Galenic works and ideas proliferated in the Renaissance, giving students a guide to Galen's main ideas and arguments, even if they left much out. None of them was short. Luigi Mondella's massive *Theatrum Galeni* (*The Theatre of Galen*) covered 685 folios, while one of the shortest, Juan Carlos Amat's *Fructus medicinae ex Galeni variis locis decerpti* (*The Fruits of Medicine plucked from various places in Galen*), of 1623, still ran to 284 duodecimo pages. Even Andrea Laguna's popular *Epitome Galeni* (*An Epitome of Galen*), took up five volumes in its Venice edition of 1548 or almost 655 folio pages in its final printing at Strasbourg in 1604.[28] The last such selection for medical students was the nearly seven hundred pages of John Redman Coxe's *The Writings of Hippocrates and Galen* of 1846, although his assertion that "our teachers refer to them *ex cathedra*; our books continually quote them" should be taken with a pinch of salt. After all, Coxe had been made to retire from his chair of materia medica and pharmacy at the University of Philadelphia in 1835 because his teaching was too conservative and focused exclusively on an exposition of "the doctrines and opinions of the earlier fathers of Physic".[29]

The third method of dealing with Galen, probably initiated in Alexandria in the fourth or fifth century, long remained influential, even in today's Muslim world.[30] It reduced his essential writings to a syllabus of sixteen (or, in a modern numbering, twenty) books, that in turn were studied and commented on in a lecture, in the same way as Galen had treated Hippocrates. It was a carefully chosen and organised syllabus, beginning with *Sects* and *The Art of Medicine*, two works that provided an overall introduction to the theory (and vocabulary) of medicine and to its practice, before going on to short texts on pulses, general therapy and anatomy. Then followed what might be termed physiology (*Elements, Mixtures, Natural Faculties*) and pathology, before ending with diagnosis, therapeutics and, sometimes, guidance on general health. The early books were all short, and none equalled in length the drug books, *Anatomical Procedures* or *The Method of Healing*. All presumed a previous acquaintance with (especially Aristotelian) philosophy and logic – indeed, some lecturers, like Stephanus of Athens, around 600, also wrote commentaries on Aristotle, and most would have required a good teacher in order to explain the meaning of Galen's concise statements. Notes from several such lectures survive from teachers active in the sixth century in Alexandria and in Ravenna, an outpost of Byzantium in Northern Italy, the latter in Latin. Whether the sixteen books were in fact always studied is not at all clear – the first introductory texts appear to have been

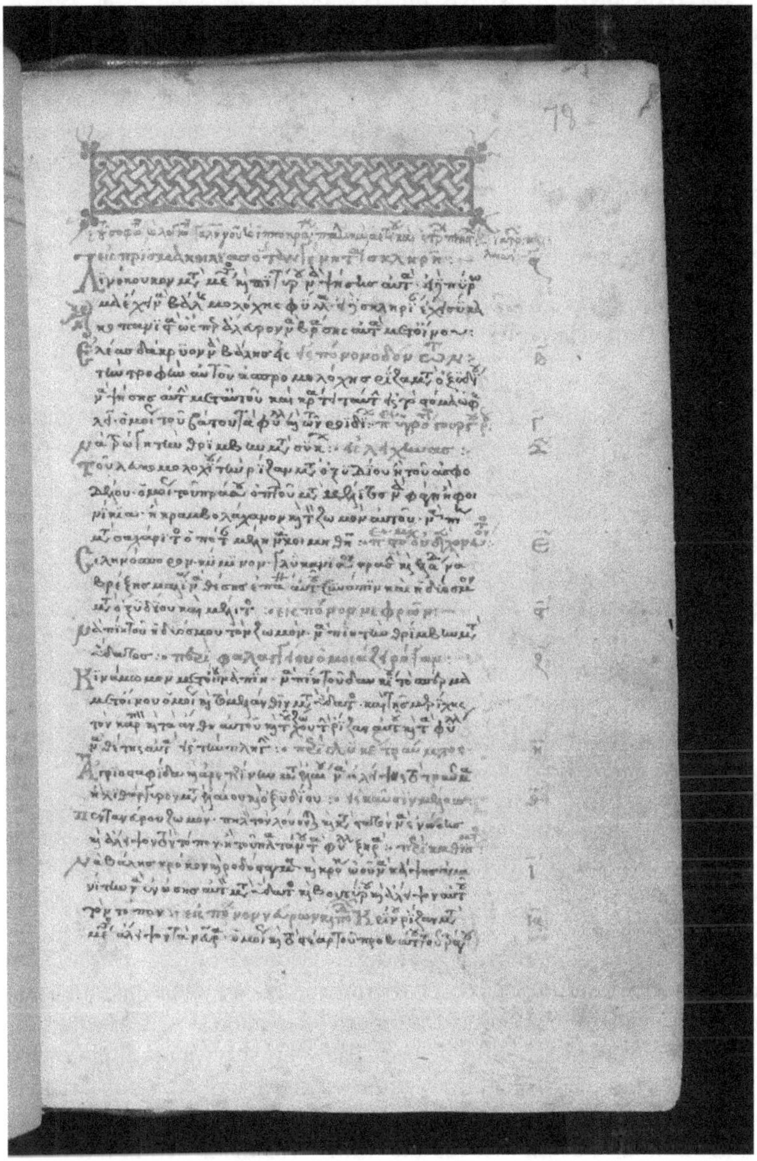

Figure 6.2 Greek extracts taken from "the most wise and learned Galen, Hippocrates, Paulus, Aetius, and many other ancient physicians". Wellcome Library, MSMSL60, fol. 78r. A fifteenth-century manuscript from Constantinople.

most popular – but summaries of most of them intended for students circulated widely and were later translated into Arabic and Hebrew.[31] Alongside them were used short texts by teachers such as Magnus (c. 400?) that brought together scattered passages in Galen on urine and pulses. The result was Galenism rather than Galen, as these abridgements of Galen's treatises became more influential than the originals. So, for example, what later became the cornerstone of Galenist therapeutics, attention to the so-called six non-naturals – food and drink; sleep; rest and exercise; excretions; the environment; and the emotions – had its origin in the work of a summariser who extended a specific observation by Galen on pulses to form a statement of a general principle by which the doctor could organise any therapy.[32]

The triumphs of Galenism

Galenism fared less well in the Latin-speaking world, where Methodist medicine continued to flourish in North Africa. The little handbook of Cassius Felix (active in 447), an attempt to combine Methodist and Galenic medicine, and the Ravenna lectures are exceptions in their inclusion of Galenic theory.[33] This is not surprising, for the Latin world was far poorer than the Greek and lacked the institutional traditions in both philosophy and medicine found in the major cities of the East. To Latin doctors before 1000, Galen was little more than a name, the last in a line of great doctors that began with Hippocrates, the author of recipes and of a (pseudonymous) alphabetical guide to medicinal plants.[34]

Far more significant was the spread of Galenism among the non-Greek speakers of the Near East. At least twenty-six of his texts were translated in the early sixth century into Syriac, the language of Christians there, by a Syrian doctor and cleric, Sergius of Resaena, who had studied at Alexandria and who also translated some works on philosophy. His successors were unfairly critical of the accuracy of his versions in order to puff their own translations and downplayed his significance in establishing Galenism as the supreme medical theory of the region.[35] Doctors began to write their own Galenist handbooks in the vernacular – one by an otherwise unknown Aaron seems to have been particularly popular – and towns like Edessa and Nisibis became centres of medical education, a development not always welcomed by those who saw potential clerics seduced away from the church by the prospects of a more lucrative career.[36]

But, in general, Galen's high ethical standards, his interest in Christians and, above all, his belief in a purposeful Creator helped ensure his survival as a 'philosopher of the cosmos', as one Byzantine hagiographer approvingly described him.[37] In some Byzantine monastic frescoes he was depicted alongside other worthies of Antiquity who allegedly had foretold or acknowledged the truths of Christianity. In late medieval Italy he found a place in a stained-glass window in Milan Cathedral, while, further South, at Anagni, he is portrayed discussing with Hippocrates the divine basis of the cosmos.[38] Writers as different as the fourth-century bishop Nemesius of Emesa, the Byzantine polymath Michael Psellos (1018–78) or the fourteenth-century Jewish moralist Ibn Falaquera quoted from recherché Galenic treatises to back up their philosophical or theological arguments.[39] Others, like the Muslim al-Razi (d. 925/935) and the Jew Maimonides (1138–1204), while accepting much of his teleology, took pains to refute what seemed to them Galen's objectionably agnostic views on the eternity of creation or the nature of the soul.[40]

The initial expansion of Galenism took place within a Syriac-speaking world that stretched from Egypt in a crescent round to modern Iran, and even to Eastern China. Long after the Muslim conquests of the sixth century, Christians remained in a majority in the Middle East, and medicine was for many centuries dominated by Syriac Christians even in the new capital of Baghdad. In the ninth century, the Caliphs supported a programme that sought to introduce into the Arabo-Islamic world many aspects of Greek philosophy and science, principally Aristotle and Galen. With the support of many members of the court elite, a remarkable physician, Ḥunayn Ibn Isḥāq (d. 873), assisted by his son and nephew, embarked on a massive project to translate the surviving works of Galen into Syriac and subsequently Arabic.[41] In a letter composed while he was in prison, Hunayn listed his own and earlier versions of 129 works, adding his own comments on their authenticity and their translators, as well as on his difficulties in tracking down Greek codices in Alexandria, Damascus and possibly even in the Byzantine Empire. Some treatises were common and had been often translated, particularly those that formed the standard syllabus of learned medicine, but others survived only in fragmentary copies or defective translations. Later, in a second tract, he listed those books that were omitted from Galen's autobibliography, some because they had been thought lost, others through inadvertence, and at least one, *My own Opinions*, because it had not yet been written. His translations were based on collating Greek manuscripts, where possible, and on abandoning a word-for-word equivalence in favour of a more stylish presentation of the sense. It was a remarkable achievement that not only provided Arabic-speakers with a sophisticated new vocabulary of medicine, but also secured Galenism as the basis of medicine for centuries in the Muslim world and even further afield.[42] Many of its leading practitioners, such Ibn Sina (Avicenna, d. 1037), Ibn Rushd (Averroes, d. 1198) or Maimonides, continued the Galenic tradition of the philosopher-doctor, and his agnosticism and his logical inconsistencies were discussed well beyond the medical school.[43] Doctors, like Hunayn himself in his treatise *On the Eye*, added new material to a basic summary of Galen, while others incorporated relevant information from lands scarcely mentioned by classical authors.[44] Al-Bīrūnī (973–1051), for example, investigated herbs from modern Afghanistan and India, and compared aspects of Indian religion and culture to Asclepius cult.[45] Some Galenic texts might be adapted for new purposes. Ubaidallah Ibn Buhtishu'a (d. after 1058), the scion of a famous family of court physicians in Baghdad, wrote a commentary on a pseudonymous Galenic treatise, *Apparent Death*, a topic particularly relevant in a society where burial was expected to occur within a very short period of time after death, and where failure to notice signs of life might lead to an accusation of murder.[46] New and larger compendia were produced to bring together thematic material scattered across the Galenic Corpus, as well as to reconcile discrepancies within it. The most famous of them, Avicenna's *al-Qānūn* (*The Canon*), constituted a huge, logical synthesis of Galenic medicine that remains today the basis of an officially supported medicine, Yūnānī (Ionian/Greek), medicine in India as well as in Pakistan and several other Muslim countries.[47] Despite both Byzantine and Arabic expertise in surgery and the substantial development of Galenic ideas on pharmacology little attempt was made to go beyond Galen's own anatomy.[48] This is probably because Muslim and Jewish religious requirements made investigating dead bodies almost impossible. The observation of Abd-al-Latīf (1162–1231) that neither the sacrum nor the lower jaw of skeletons who died in an Egyptian famine of 1200 were composed of several parts as Galen had stated is a rare exception, Debate still rages over the extent to which the 'discovery' of the circulation of the blood by Ibn an-Nafī s (d. 1288) was the result of his own dissections or of a combination of what he had observed during surgery with meditation upon information already to be found in Galen.[49] Whatever one decides, it cannot be denied that his conclusions, proposed in a commentary on *The Canon* and subsequently repeated by other later Arabic commentators, never excited debate or stimulated further research in the same way as did those of William Harvey in the West three and a half centuries later.

With the consolidation of Galenic medicine came also an interest in Galen's life. The literate public wanted to know more about this great doctor, and in response scholars combed the Galenic Corpus for fascinating incidents or simply hints of what might have been.[50] Some of what they found may be genuine: the medical biographer Ibn abī Usaibi'a (1203–1270) is particularly scrupulous in indicating his sources in books now lost to us.[51] Others are plausible: Galen is cited for the belief that true love occurs between two rational beings as a result of their similarity of intellect, for the stupid cannot follow an ordered course or agree on how to compose their differences.[52] Others are unjustified interpretations of genuinely Galenic material: the story of his friendship with Cleopatra derives from his quotation at second-hand of recipes from a book on cosmetics that passed under her name. In a biography later widely circulated in many languages, Al-Mubashshir ibn Fatik (fl. 1048) modelled his image of Galen on the recommendations for the ideal doctor's dress and behaviour that he had read in the commentary on *Epidemics* VI. One can also see how he came to the conclusion that Galen never stopped talking or that his wonderful library had once contained the writings of the early Greek philosopher Anaxagoras along with expensive books written on silk.[53] Readers of Galen were also eager to know where and when he died. Travellers to Sicily were told where they might see the tomb of Galen, just outside Palermo, "on the left going from Qasr al-Amīrī towards the capital".[54] An alternative (and equally flawed) tradition placed his death at Perama at the mouth of the Nile while on a pilgrimage to the Holy Land, an exaggerated expansion of his interest in Jews and Christians.[55] Even more fanciful are stories that link him with Mary Magdalene and St Peter, whose wife he is reported to have cured.[56] A desire to make Galen into a sexologist may lie behind the production and circulation of the equally pseudonymous *The Secrets of Women* and *The Secrets of Men.*[57] Even if modern scholars dismiss them as legendary, the very survival of these stories would have only added to his reputation as a miraculous and authoritative healer.

Although it had its critics, whether in Greek, Arabic or Latin, scholastic Galenism, was far from being rejected. Indeed, the centuries-long survival of medical practices and a humoral theory that went back to Hippocrates only appeared to confirm their essential validity: patients did often recover through these measures, even if others died. Besides, reliance on something that had worked in the past was better than doing nothing or trusting to some novelty.[58] Rather, the debate in both Byzantium and the Islamic world centred upon the extent to which all worthwhile medical ideas could be found within the Galenic Corpus or required to be supplemented from elsewhere. In Byzantium, around 550, the widely travelled Alexander of Tralles, brother of an imperial lawyer as well as of the architect of Hagia Sophia in Constantinople, contrasted his own willingness to employ a variety of therapies, some, *more galenico*, obtained from peasants in Italy, Spain and even Armenia, with the reluctance of book-bound and nigh-on murderous Galenists to depart from the words of the master.[59] A similar argument took place around 1060 in the East between the Egyptian Ibn Ridwan, who argued that failings in Galenism were due to the misunderstandings and ignorance of the Galenists themselves, and the Syrian Ibn Butlan, who took a more inclusive view of other therapies.[60] At around the same time in Byzantium, a doctor and court official, Simeon Seth, openly boasted of his introduction of therapies from India and further East in the face of resistance from hide-bound Galenists.[61]

Medieval and Renaissance Galenism

Such debates could not have taken place in the contemporary early medieval West, whose exposure to the riches of Galenism began only in the late eleventh century, when Constantine, an African monk at the monastery of Monte Cassino, began a series of translations from Arabic into Latin, mainly of the standard set texts.[62] These were soon being studied at Salerno, a South Italian city with a long medical tradition and strong links with his monastery. Other Latin translations from Arabic followed in Sicily and Spain, beginning with the major Arabic compendia, and only later including individual Galenic treatises, principally translated by Gerard of Cremona (d. c. 1187) and the slightly younger Mark of Toledo.[63] Others were made directly from the Greek at Constantinople by Burgundio of Pisa (d. 1193): several of the Greek manuscripts that he owned and used survive today and bear his comments in their margins.[64] By 1220 the first great wave of Galenic translations ended, but it may not have been for another fifty years that they became at all commonly available or found a place in the medical curriculum at the new Western universities. Medicine arrived late here but from 1270 or so, the 'new Galenism' became established as the foundation of learned medicine. Its basis in Aristotelian philosophy and logic fitted well with the wider Aristotelianism of the medieval schools, and its elitism (for few could afford, or had the necessary skills to profit from, a university course) and its pretensions to both intellectual and professional superiority were further reasons for its success.[65] Its leading proponents, such as Pietro d'Abano (1250–1316) in Padua or Jacques Despars (d. 1465) in Paris, were remarkable connoisseurs of Galen, although few of their students appear to have been interested in more than the basic texts. The extremely accurate word-for-word translations made in the first half of the fourteenth century at Naples by Niccolò da Reggio are found in only a handful of manuscripts, in part because they dealt with specific points or themes largely irrelevant to general medical practice.[66] Hartmann Schedel's report that around 1450 a volume of Niccolò's translations lay rotting on top of a Bavarian sacristy cupboard warns against the assumption that medieval doctors were always eager to read everything their great predecessor had written.[67] As late as 1524, Wolfgang Reichart, a graduate of Padua, was advising his student son that all he needed for his studies there was a copy of the so-called *Articella*, a short collection of Byzantine and Classical Greek texts, including Galen's *Art of Medicine*, that had been first assembled in Salerno at least three centuries earlier.[68] Modern medicine, he argued, was merely an extension of these fundamental (and largely Galenic) principles.

University medicine was at first little affected by the rise of so-called humanism, the renaissance of interest in, and the privileging of, Classical Antiquity. The rediscovery of Celsus' *Medicine* at Siena in 1426 provided a new stylistic model for writing about medicine, and information on pre-Galenic medicine could be found in the voluminous pages of Pliny's *Natural History*, but both were avowedly dependent on Greek sources that were unavailable even to the handful of scholars who knew Greek. The situation began to change in 1453 with the Ottoman conquest of Constantinople which drove many Greeks westward, particularly to Venice and Florence, bringing with them Greek medical manuscripts.[69] Wealthy collectors, most notably the Medici in Florence and the exiled Greek Cardinal Bessarion (1403–72), now endeavoured to obtain a complete library of Greek medical and scientific manuscripts. Greek was also being taught more widely in Northern Italy, and by 1490 humanists such as Politian (1454–94) in Florence or Urceus Codrus (1446–1500) in Bologna, as well as members of the Greek community in Venice and doctors like Alessandro Benedetti (1452–1512) who had served in some of the Venetian colonies in the Eastern Mediterranean, were reading Galen in Greek and exchanging ideas and textual emendations.[70]

The central figure in this Galenic revival was Niccolò Leoniceno (1428–1524), who taught medicine, mathematics and philosophy at Ferrara and Bologna. He had strong links with the Greek community in Venice as well as with the famous publisher Aldus Manutius (1447–1515) and his circle and was employed by the Dukes of Ferrara as both a doctor and a translator of Greek writings, especially on history and ethics. He had also personally amassed a remarkable library of Greek manuscripts on medicine and science, although his reluctance to share them led at least one of his contemporaries to call him a "book burier".[71] In 1492, two years after the first printing of the collected medieval Latin versions of Galen, he published with Aldus a short book, *The Errors of Pliny and Many Others in Medicine*, in which he showed conclusively that Latin medical writings, as far back as Pliny, were filled with mistakes caused by misunderstanding or mistranslating Greek. Herbs were misrepresented and misidentified, and phantom diseases were created through copying errors or the co-existence of two different Latin versions, one derived from the Arabic, the other direct from Galen's Greek. He argued that acquaintance with Greek and the abundance of previously unknown Greek medical texts would convey an instant benefit to the teaching and practice of medicine in a variety of ways. So, for example, in a short essay that accompanied some of his first Galenic translations, he explained that in the compressed opening sentence of *The Art of Medicine*, almost the first thing a medical student would read, Galen had been talking simply about how medicine might be taught, and not, as medieval commentators had debated at length, about different methods of logical analysis.[72] He was less convincing in his further claim that even apparently new diseases, such as syphilis, that were now ravaging Europe could be identified in classical Greek texts, along with their cures.

Other North Italians quickly followed his example. His pupil and successor at Ferrara, Giovanni Manardi (1461–1536), applied Leoniceno's methodology to the identification of ancient diseases, while Giorgio Valla (1447–1500) and Alessandro Benedetti did the same for anatomical terms. Benedetti's book, which bore the provocative Greek title *Anatomice or an Enquiry into the Human Body* and was printed in elegant italic script, aroused the anger of the Paduan anatomist Gabriele Zerbi (d. 1505), who denounced Benedetti's less extensive experience of actual anatomical dissection in many double columns of old-fashioned gothic type.[73] Zerbi's murder at the hand of Greek brigands seemed to some of his opponents appropriate revenge.[74]

But, as the German physician Leonhard Schmaus complained in 1519, these claims for Greek were worthless to those who knew only Latin and who had perforce to rely on medieval Latin versions such as those edited by Surianus in 1502.[75] True, Leoniceno and others had produced more accurate versions of the texts contained in the *Articella*, but scarcely any previously unknown tract was published in translation before 1525. Leoniceno's plan for a complete translation of Galen ended with his death, and all that was published by Aldus from among the Galenic codices he had amassed for a collected edition was the short and pseudo-Galenic *History of Philosophy* that appeared in the first edition of the Greek Aristotle in 1497. A rival project, by the Venetian printers Callierges and Vlastos, produced a splendid printing of the two treatises on the *Method of Healing* in 1500 (*Fig. 5.1*), but its high costs seem also to have deterred them from publishing anything further for almost a decade.[76] The sheer size of Galen once again proved a major handicap. Symphorien Champier's 1516 vision of a *Symphony of Hippocrates, Plato, Aristotle and Galen* remained no more than that, and his prefatory illustration depicting Galen as the leader of a classical string quartet was no more than an elegant metaphor.[77]

The situation changed dramatically in 1525–6 with the publication by the Aldine Press in Venice of a complete Galen in Greek.[78] There was now a market for Greek that extended beyond Northern Italy, and, indeed, Professor Opizzoni's team included a German, Georg Agricola, and three Englishmen, Thomas Lupset, Edward Rose and John Clement, all associates of Thomas Linacre (1460–1524), who had himself studied at Padua and produced some of the first humanist translations of Galen on the basis of Greek manuscripts in his own collection (*Fig. 2.1*). An opportune period of peace meant that there was a large supply of metal in Venice that might otherwise have been used for cannon but could now be bought and turned into type. Even if they could make use of only some of Bessarion's manuscripts in the Marciana Library, Leoniceno's death gave the Aldine editors at least limited access to his collection, and there were other manuscripts in the city and in Northern Italy, as well as those that had been copied earlier for Aldus.[79]

Reactions to the publication of the Aldine Galen were lukewarm. It was a hasty and at times careless production: one passage was printed with a large gap after a printer had allowed a candle to fall on the manuscript while it was being copied for the press. Agricola was later said to have filled several volumes with his corrections, while visitors to the Leiden University Library today can still see the many changes that Clement made in the margins of his own copy.[80] Several were passed on to the editors of the next edition of Galen's complete works in Greek, published at Basle in 1538, and most were also copied by the Englishman John Caius (1510–73), who filled his copy of the Basle edition with emendations as well as readings taken down from manuscripts and books in Italy and England. A handful of newly recovered texts were added and many small corrections made in the later editions by René Chartier in the seventeenth century and by Carl Gottlob Kühn in the nineteenth, but, for all its faults, the Aldine edition remains even today the basis of scholarly understanding of several of Galen's works, particularly his pharmacological treatises.[81] Furthermore, compared with the steady attrition of the Galenic writings available during the age of manuscripts, no work once printed has since been lost.

Nonetheless, the contemporary significance of the Aldine Galen lay less in the text itself than in the opportunity it now gave to translators around Europe to translate into Latin works previously unknown or neglected.[82] The leading humanist of the day, Desiderius Erasmus, one of the stiffest critics of the Aldine's Greek, was also alert to the main chance, publishing within a matter of months Latin versions of tracts of wider cultural interest, the *Exhortation to the Arts, The Best Method of Teaching* and *The Best Doctor is also a Philosopher.* He was followed by a whole phalanx of translators, from Spain to Poland, turning out Latin versions in large numbers.[83] The figures are impressive. Between 1500 and 1525 there were, on average, two or three printings a year, rising to a maximum of seven in 1523. Between 1526 and 1556, the number jumps to an annual average of just over twelve, before sinking back to three for the rest of the century. Seventeen editions were published in 1528, twenty-one in both 1538 and 1547, and thirty-one in 1549, many containing more than one Galenic treatise. From the late 1530s onwards printers in Venice, Basle, and Lyons competed to produce multi-volume editions of the complete works of Galen in modern Latin translation, frequently improved by having the translations checked against the readings of Greek manuscripts.[84] Those put out by the Juntine Press in Venice from 1551 onwards included in a separate volume (*Fig.1.2*) a huge index compiled by Antonio Musa Brasavola (1500–55), Manardi's successor at Ferrara, that still remains useful as a quick guide to Galen's ideas. These new versions allowed doctors with Latin but little or no Greek to participate in this new learning: knowledge of Greek, however, retained a social cachet as well as allowing those who had it to claim a superiority over all other purveyors of healing. This newly Latinised Galen was introduced wholesale into Renaissance universities such as Jena, as well as into older ones such as Ingolstadt and Freiburg when they modernised their curricula.[85] The Statutes of the London College of Physicians, founded by Thomas Linacre in 1518, either in its original Statutes or, more likely, in revisions under Edward Wotton in 1542 or under John Caius around 1562, imposed a stiff entrance examination in Galen and Hippocrates on aspiring members. The date of this innovation is less important than the strongly Galenist tone of the College – Wotton was one of the Aldine editors and Caius edited and translated many Galenic texts – which was shared with similar medical Colleges across Europe.[86]

The Aldine edition and the subsequent translations, some also into vernacular languages, reintroduced works of Galen that had been unknown or neglected for centuries. For the first time it was possible, with the aid of treatises such as *The Opinions of Plato and Hippocrates*, to see clearly how Galen's medicine and philosophy interacted. Galen's dietetics, his pharmacology and his ideas on venesection or fevers were given a new precision. His commentaries on Hippocrates not only established anew the authority of the Father of Medicine but also helped to create a new model for the Renaissance physician seeking to understand his ancient Greek texts. Uroscopic diagnosis and medical astrology, which had been the badge of the learned doctor in the fifteenth century, were by 1600 firmly associated with quackery, replaced among elite doctors by full physical diagnosis and new ideas about the importance of climate. The personal stories scattered throughout the Galenic Corpus, and the outlines of his life sketched in *Prognosis, for Epigenes* and *My own Books*, the former only rarely accessed in Niccolò da Reggio's medieval version, the latter newly published for the first time, became the basis for new and more accurate biographies of Galen and for new histories of medicine.[87] Catholic and Protestant disputed the extent and nature of Galen's Christian beliefs, classifying the events of his life according to the way they displayed the cardinal virtues, to the surprise of today's scholars unaccustomed to viewing Galen as an exemplum of charity and self-restraint.[88] The techniques used by Galen in investigating the authenticity of Hippocratic writings were adopted by editors of Galen working to distinguish, usually correctly, the genuine from the spurious among the treatises that passed under his name. Their conclusions formed, until very recently, the basis for all later studies of Galen's life and works. Illustrations on printed frontispieces (*Figs 1.2; 2.1; 3.2; 5.1*) helped further to fix a visual image of Galen that continues to be reproduced today, to the confusion of the unwary.

Supporters of the new Galen, like the young men who in the 1540s founded a "New Academy" in Florence, emphasised two major advances over later medieval medicine: Galenic anatomy and Galenic methodology.[89] The availability of Greek and of more accurate (or simply more stylish) versions had given greater precision to the details of many medical doctrines, e.g. on venesection. They had also highlighted Galen's constant repetition of the need to employ both logic and experience, both book-learning and practical skills, in a therapeutic *method* that was more sophisticated and wider-ranging than anything the Middle Ages had known. To Galenists like John Caius, the Frenchman Jean Fernel (1497–1558), the German Johann Crato von Crafftheim (1522–97), the Dutchman Pieter van Foreest (1522–1597) and the Spaniard Luis Mercado (1520–1606), Galen had not only laid down the guidelines for proper medical practice but had given in his voluminous writings innumerable indications of the proper method to be followed in specific cases, which they in turn transmitted to students and colleagues in handbooks. Caius, Crato and van Foreest had all studied at Padua with Giambattista da Monte (1498–1551), the most influential champion of this new method of healing, which demanded an enormous spread of learning in order to carry out a differential diagnosis that paid attention to all aspects of the individual patient.[90] Da Monte linked the theoretical and the practical by going directly from the lecture room to visit the sick, when topics just discussed in a lecture would then be further expounded at the bedside and colleagues and students asked to comment on the specific features of the case.[91] Other distinguished physicians, like Girolamo Fracastoro (1483–1553) or Girolamo Mercuriale (1530–1606), applied evidence in large part derived from Galen to produce novel syntheses of matters as diverse as physical exercise and contagious diseases like plague and syphilis, both of which were striking with greater virulence in this period.[92]

But the defects of Galenic method were also clear. It was far from easy to reach a conclusive judgment swiftly when, as Galen had insisted, so many factors had to be taken into account, and when relevant passages from across the Galenic Corpus had to be recalled, often from memory. Da Monte's lectures neatly, if inadvertently, demonstrate the problem. He had so much material at his disposal that in commenting on the Galenic text he rarely managed to say all that he wanted. Printed transcripts of his individual lectures and his courses as a whole often end with apologies for running over time or for failing to deal with everything in the set text.

But it was 'anatomy' even more than 'method' that became the shibboleth of Renaissance Galenism. The Latin Middle Ages had known relatively little about Galen's major anatomical writings, except for a far from accurate abridgement of *The Use of Parts, De juvamentis membrorum*, and doctors were in no position to appreciate the wider role of anatomy in Galen's thought.[93] Descriptions of the human body in post-Galenic Greek and Arabic sources merely repeated Galen's conclusions briefly as a preliminary to more extensive discussions of therapeutics. The first university anatomy, by Mondino de' Liuzzi in Bologna around 1315, inspired by his acquaintance with the 'new Galen', introduced the visual evidence of a dissected corpse into medical education.[94] But the highly ritualised nature of the event, performed once a year, ensured that it was far more a visual reinforcement of truths already described in writing and in lectures than an encouragement to young physicians to dissect for themselves. The actual cutting of the body was done by a surgeon, a junior professor read out Galenic passages, and a third teacher pointed out and explained to students what might be visible and required to be put into context. Such university dissections, however, were far from common. Very few universities outside Italy had an annual anatomy before 1520, and where one was demanded by the Statutes, local pressures and problems might prevent a dissection taking place for years on end. Even at the end of the sixteenth century, a prison governor at Wittenberg refused to hand over the body of an executed criminal for dissection for fear of reprisals, despite the agreement and authorisation of all civic and religious authorities.[95] As the death records from Rome show, even in Italy it was deemed preferable to dissect criminals who had no known relatives and came from a long way away.[96]

Although as we have seen, above p. 142, Benedetti and Giorgio Valla had already produced their own syntheses of Galenic anatomy, and medical teachers such as Matteo Corti (1475–1542), the best paid medical professor in Italy, were demanding a return to the new Greek Galenic anatomy, it was the publication of the Aldine edition in 1525 and of subsequent translations that marked the crucial turning point. In Paris, for example, an interest in anatomy does not feature in a series of *éloges* of students in the mid-1520s: half a dozen years later anatomy was all the rage, as students of all faculties struggled to get into an overcrowded anatomy lecture room.[97] It is easy to see why the new Galenists were so enthusiastic about anatomy. For the first time for centuries, physicians could read the first half of *Anatomical Procedures* (as well as Galen's introductory anatomical books). From *The Use of Parts* and *The Opinions of Hippocrates and Plato*, they could gain not only new information about the body but also a deeper understanding of the contribution of dissection to wider philosophical and medical problems. Above all, they saw a new side to Galen – no longer the dogmatist but the experimentalist, the dissector, encouraging others to see for themselves and dissect as regularly as he had done. To young physicians, whose guild had previously taken care to distinguish itself from 'manual operators', this new material was exciting, if not revolutionary. Anatomy now stood at the very centre of the up-to-date medical curriculum.

Universities like Oxford and Cambridge, where dissections had been unknown, now instituted anatomical teaching; where it had been sporadic, it was now carried out on a regular basis. John Caius in the statutes for his re-founded Cambridge College demanded a regular dissection for the medical students of the College, in addition to those provided by the University.[98] At Louvain, student pressure for the introduction of the new anatomy into the curriculum led to the dismissal of two professors who held firmly to the older Galenism.[99] At Protestant Wittenberg, the Lutheran reformer Philip Melanchthon (1497–1560) required all students, whatever their Faculty, to become acquainted with anatomy through attending lectures on Aristotle's *The Soul*, where they would learn about the majestic handiwork of the Creator and the constraints of the earthly body that, temporarily, housed the immortal soul. The same message was promoted just as much in a Catholic university like Ingolstadt as in a Protestant one like Jena.[100]

Anatomy became the new renaissance science. In Paris in the late 1530s Jacobus Sylvius (1478–1555) illustrated his lectures on *The Use of Parts* to a packed audience at the Collège de Tréguier with specimens of animals he had recently dissected.[101] The blood and the smell did not deter his audience, who came from all over Europe and was not confined to medical students. Old projects were revived. A Latin version of

Anatomical Procedures, prepared around 1500 by the Greek exile Demetrius Chalcondylas (c. 1424–1511), was revised and published in 1529 by the professor of surgery at Bologna, Berengario da Carpi, although it was never to achieve the same impact as the version by Johann Guinter von Andernach (1505–74) that appeared at Paris only two years later. Emblematic is the frontispiece to the 1530 Paris reprint of Linacre's translation of the *Method of Healing* (*Fig. 2.1*) which depicts Galen cutting up a human figure in front of an eager audience – even though the work itself contains almost nothing relating to dissection.[102]

Galenic anatomy had apparently triumphed. The leading exponents of anatomy around Europe in the 1530s, like Sylvius or Corti at Bologna, were fervent Galenists. Sylvius, Guinter and another young Parisian teacher, Andrés Laguna (1499–1559), and, in Italy, Berengario and the Venetian Niccolò Massa (1485–1569), all expounded Galenic methods in handbooks of anatomy for students. In London, John Caius gave lectures on anatomy to the Barber-Surgeons at the express request of King Henry VIII.[103] Even if some of these teachers did not carry out the actual cutting up of the corpse themselves, either because their manual dexterity was weak or because they believed that the duty of the teacher was to place what could be seen into a proper medical context, they all stressed the need for everyone to have a detailed understanding of the human body based on at least witnessing a dissection.

Replacing Galen

Yet obeying Galen's injunction to dissect personally swiftly revealed an unexpected problem. Not everything he had said appeared to be confirmed by the evidence of observation. Initially, these anomalies could be explained away as isolated or pardonable errors. It was well known, for instance, that Galen had carried out many of his dissections on animals, and thus the reason for the anomaly might lie with the corpse, not with the dissector. It was the achievement of Andreas Vesalius (1514–64) to have seen that these anomalies were neither isolated nor accidental, but the result of Galen's systematic reliance on animal rather than human bodies.

Vesalius had received a humanist education at Louvain before studying medicine in Paris, where his talent with the knife had been quickly recognised with an invitation to act as the dissector at Guinter's anatomical lectures.[104] In 1538 he was appointed to the chair of surgery in Padua, the rival of Bologna as the greatest medical school in Europe. He was immediately called upon to perform the annual dissection, supplementing his lectures with references to Guinter's *Principles of Anatomy according to Galen*, in his view the best available student textbook. He was also quickly called upon by Da Monte to revise the Latin versions of Galen's anatomical works for the 1541–2 Juntine edition of the *Opera Omnia*. In this his methodology was entirely Galenic: along with his flatmate John Caius, he collated Greek manuscripts and notes loaned to him by another distinguished Galenist, Antonio Gadaldino (1478–1568), in order to create a sounder text on which to base his revisions of the Latin. For his lectures in 1539 he made two innovations: he not only lectured but performed the actual dissection personally, and he provided the students with visual illustrations in the form of printed sheets. He also published an unauthorised revision of his master's textbook, still with the same title, but including many changes of wording as well as some of his recent discoveries. Notes in his own copy show that he was in the middle of preparing yet a further edition when he changed his mind and began instead on a different and larger book, *De humani corporis fabrica, The Make-up of the Human Body.*[105] In it, as he had already asserted in a bitter argument with Corti at Bologna in 1540, the evidence of human dissection was to take precedence over whatever Galen had said.[106] Galen, he insisted, had got it wrong because he had never dissected a human corpse, and in a neat appeal to ancient authority, he claimed in his preface to be reverting to a (lost) Alexandrian anatomy, that of Herophilus and Erasistratus, both famous for dissecting condemned criminals.[107]

The appearance of the *Fabrica* in 1543 provoked sharply contrasting reactions among Galenists. Some, like Hieronymus Gemusaeus (1505–44), one of the editors of the 1538 Basle Galen in Greek, immediately acknowledged it as a masterpiece in every way.[108] Melanchthon, who swiftly read his own copy from cover to cover, eagerly adopted its conclusions for the second edition of his treatise *On the Soul.* Like many other readers at Wittenberg, he accepted that Vesalius was working in the Galenic tradition, following in practice a methodology that Galen himself had been able only to advocate but not realise.[109] Guinter himself had left university teaching, but his wholesale adoption in his own revision of his textbook of the changes made by Vesalius to his earlier *Anatomical Principles*, and, indeed, the improvements he introduced into it himself, do not indicate strong opposition.[110]

But other Galenists were scandalised at what they saw as impiety towards their master, not least when large parts of the *Fabrica* were taken over directly from Galen – and without acknowledgment. Besides, ‘everyone knew’, that Galen had dissected animals, and had warned against excessive trust in his descriptions. To accuse Galen of never seeing a human body was simple misrepresentation, for Vesalius had carefully hidden all the passages where Galen had referred to examining a human body – Caius was not the only person to draw up a list of the relevant sentences and write them in the front of his copy of the Greek Galen. Others accused Vesalius of ignorance and mistranslation, a charge accepted in very small part by Vesalius in his second edition of 1555. The German translator and professor of medicine Janus Cornarius (1500–58) removed with ferocious strokes of the pen all reference to Vesalius’ involvement from his own copy of Vesalius’ Latin translations of Galen’s anatomical writings that he was revising for the Basle printers Froben and Episcopius. Others argued that the fault lay further back, with ignorant copyists, and that a better Greek text, produced after a careful search for manuscripts, would eliminate many of the mistakes signalled by Vesalius.[111] John Caius filled the margins of his own books with variant readings and comments directed at the shortcomings of ‘Wesalius’.[112] In his much later *Autobibliography* he cunningly mentioned his friendship with Vesalius, the great dissector, citing only passages where Vesalius had accepted his corrections in order to give an impression of their widespread agreement.[113] Others wondered whether it was not the human body which had changed since Galen’s time. After all, dog breeders were well aware that the characteristics of a hound could be changed over time through breeding choices, so why could not the same be true of human development?

While some of these objections to Vesalius were valid, witness the changes he made in his second edition of 1555 and in the annotations he made in preparation for a never-published third edition, most were irrelevant: Galenic anatomy was indeed largely animal anatomy.[114] Conservative Galenist anatomists continued to call down anathemas on Vesalius, but they were a fast diminishing minority, and by 1600 Galenic anatomy in its pre-Vesalian form was confined to the fringes of academia or to Spain. Here the brief flourishing of Vesalian anatomy in the 1550s was ended by the fiat of the

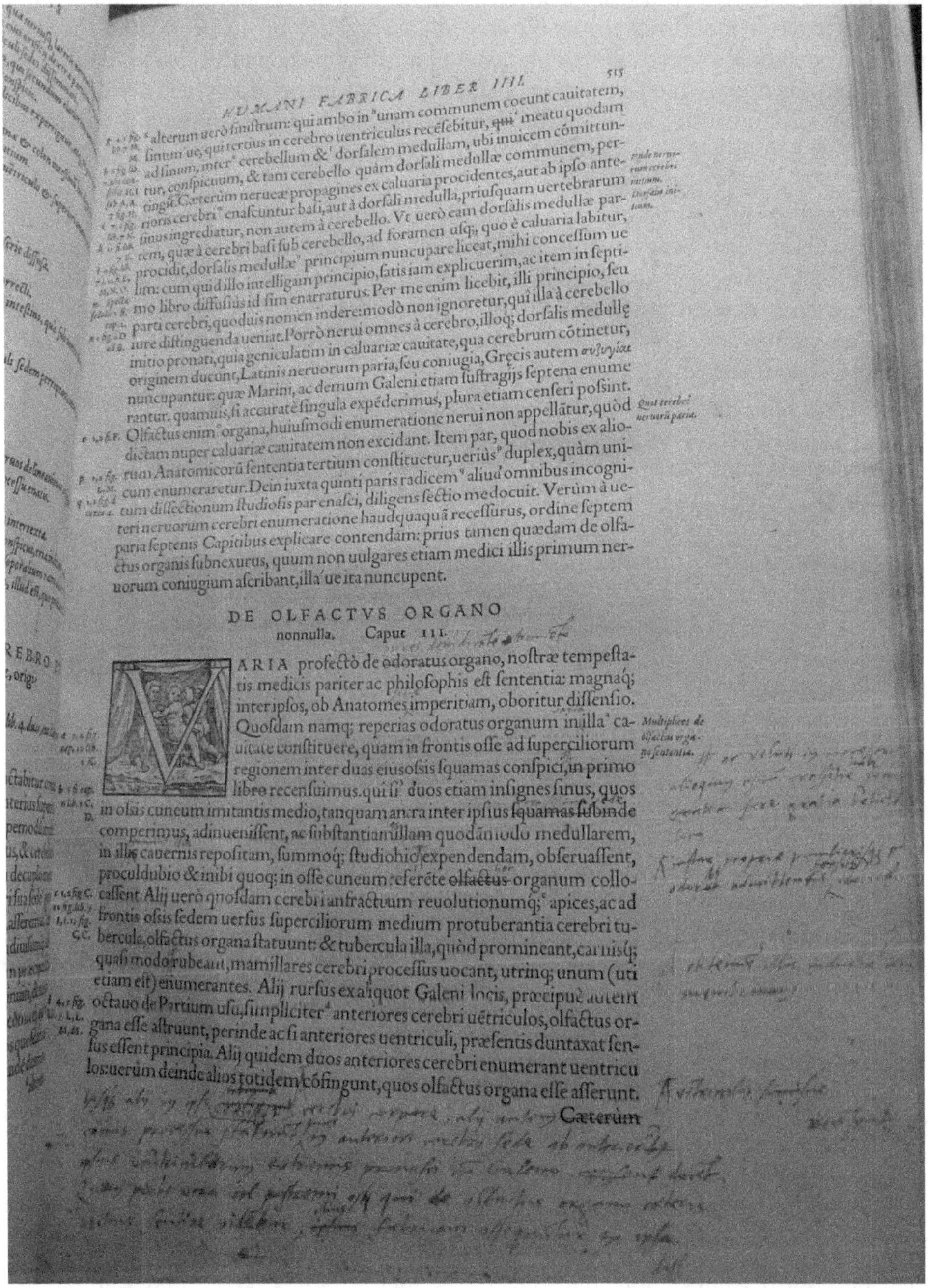

Figure 6.3 Vesalius revises his own revision of the *Fabrica* by reverting to some of Galen's original description of the organ of smell. Andreas Vesalius, De *humani corpris fabrica*, ed. 2, Basle: J. Oporinus, 1556, p. 515. Toronto, Thomas Fisher Rare Book Library. Copyright: G. Vogringic.

Galenist Luis Mercado, whose position as royal protomedico, chief physician, gave him oversight of all types of healing within the realm. Like other Spanish colleagues, he preferred to consult *The Use of Parts*, on the grounds that its emphasis on function and purpose made it more relevant to the day-to-day practice of medicine than the mere study of bones and organs.[115] A similar conservatism prevailed in Bologna well into the seventeenth century. One lecturer, Paolo Mini, ended his anatomy course in 1679 by exhorting his students to abandon dissection as useless, "performed only by persons of little talent and little brains", since the study of Galen's *The Use of Parts* was sufficient in itself.[116]

A second assault on Galen represented the culmination of a centuries-long debate between Aristotelian believers in a unified soul, who predominated in the faculties of Arts and Theology, and the Galenist physicians who favoured tripartition. Strategies had long been devised on both sides to accommodate both views within an overall Christian framework. It was argued, for example, that the three systems of the body did not indicate a tripartite soul, but merely three instruments by which the faculties of the unitary soul controlled the body.[117] The publication in 1628 of William Harvey's anatomical demonstration of the circulation of the blood resolved the argument by combining Aristotelian notions of circularity and unity with Galenic experimentalism.[118] Following his Paduan teacher, Fabrizio of Aquapendente (1533–1610), Harvey showed by careful experiments on humans and animals that Galen's venous and arterial systems formed a continuum (although visual proof of the existence of the linking capillaries had to wait until 1661). His arguments drew on both Galen and Aristotle to establish a conclusion that, within a generation or so, effectively ended any appeal to Galen's anatomy and physiology. Even if they were not entirely wrong, they were outmoded.

What Harvey's discovery did not do was to put an end to Galenic medicine, even if direct citation and use of Galenic texts lessened.[119] After all, one of Harvey's arguments for the circulation of the blood was that it provided a better explanation for Galenic therapeutics. He himself was a ferocious examiner at the London College of Physicians, and he saw no reason to change his methods of practice, even if his reluctance to adopt new drugs and treatments was, according to his friend John Aubrey, at least as likely to harm his patients as to benefit them.[120] But the advent of new drugs from America and the Indies, the chemical remedies of the Paracelsians and, later, from the 1650s onwards, a variety of mechanistic explanations of the body all combined to reduce Galen's direct influence still further. Molière was not the only playwright or satirist to depict Galenism as useless conservatism, as expensive as it was ineffective.[121]

But Galen did not entirely disappear from medical schools. Lively debates among practitioners over the interpretation of Galen lasted well into the eighteenth century, and the flexibility of Galenism allowed adoption of therapies, such as Paracelsian mineral drugs, that had once been regarded as incompatible. Conrad Gessner (1516–65), one of the editors of the 1542 Basle edition of the collected works of Galen in Latin, incorporated many new chemical remedies into his *Treasury of Euonymus*, a pharmaceutical compendium that quickly became a best-seller around Europe and was translated into many vernacular languages.[122] Johann Guinter, Vesalius's old teacher, produced at the end of his life a substantial volume, 867 pages long, devoted to reconciling Paracelsian and Galenic medicine. He eschewed Paracelsian cosmological speculation, while emphasising their shared belief in the notion of health as a balance.[123] Within therapeutics the medical vocabulary of 'temperament', 'constitution' and 'faculty' remained central, and medical semiotics rarely deviated from the advice of Galen. The general appeal to Hippocrates as the founder of true medicine also hid the extent to which this father-figure was still largely Galen in disguise. Indeed, at the end of the eighteenth century, there may even have been a return to Galen among the so-called eclectics, who were dissatisfied with all the proposed medical systems, and who turned to Galen in search of therapies with a proven record of efficacy.[124] This was one of the reasons why Carl Gottlob Kühn (1754–1840), professor of medicine at Leipzig, the most flourishing medical school in Germany, brought out between 1821 and 1833 an edition of Galen in twenty-two stubby volumes containing over 20,000 pages. Its purpose was medical, not philological; to provide a repository of potentially useful therapies, accessible via a modified version of Brasavola's index.[125]

The victory of the philologists

Within little more than a decade, even Kühn's limited aim was abandoned as new developments in medicine combined to remove Galen and Galenic medicine entirely from the purview of Western medical practitioners.[126] Galen was now a classical text to be interpreted by philologists or antiquarian doctors. The thirty years between 1884, when a Galenic text was first published in the Teubner series, and 1914, saw a massive renewal of interest in editing Galen, at least in Germany. From Bonn to Erlangen, from Greifswald to Ansbach, in *Festreden, Schulprogramme* and dissertations, doctorands, schoolmasters, and even the occasional professor set their hand to editing a Galenic *opusculum*. The first volume of Galen in the *Corpus Medicorum Graecorum*, an international project, but one firmly under the control of Berlin professors, appeared in 1914. It was devoted to three Hippocratic commentaries, for Galen was not then seen as worth editing for himself – the verdict of Professor Wilamowitz-Moellendorf, "that great windbag", was damning – but only as a first stage in the recovery of the infinitely more valuable words of the great Hippocrates. Others elsewhere also made major contributions to Galenic studies – Charles Daremberg's exposition of Galen's physiology and Johann Ilberg's pioneering essays on the chronology of his writings, for instance – but aroused little interest among doctors.[127] The publication by Max Simon in 1906 of the previously lost books of *Anatomical Procedures* in Arabic, along with a German translation and a detailed commentary, was no more than a nine days' wonder.[128] In any case, the First World War effectively ended this Galenic revival. Volumes in the *Corpus Medicorum* continued to appear sporadically afterwards, and German exiles, principally Ludwig Edelstein (1902–65) and Owsei Temkin (1902–2002), transplanted a little knowledge of Galen into the U.S.A.[129] The recognition that there were yet more texts preserved in Arabic could proceed only slowly because of the rarity of scholars, usually German, with a sound knowledge of both Greek and the relevant Oriental languages. Galen's ghost in the 1950s was very pallid indeed.

The situation began to change in the mid-1960s. Particularly in Britain and Italy students of ancient philosophy began to take seriously post-Aristotelian philosophy for its own sake, and not merely as a repository of earlier material.[130] Galen's merits as a logician and an independent thinker were recognised for almost the first time since his death. Ancient historians also became aware that Roman history did not end chronologically with the death of the Emperor Domitian in 96 or geographically at the

Ionian Sea, and, aided by the increasing accessibility of lands in the Eastern Mediterranean, began to investigate the culture of cities once familiar to Galen.[131] Feminism played a smaller role in this Galenic revival than in other branches of classics, for Galen said relatively little about women, and the first substantial investigation into his ideas on gender had to wait until 2000.[132] Cynics might also argue that, given the relatively circumscribed range of topics available to Classicists, it was inevitable that, as in the 1890s, thesis-seekers would inevitably alight on Galen, *faute de mieux.*

The first International Galen Conference, held at Cambridge in 1979, can be taken to mark a change from the earlier purely philological interest in Galen.[133] It brought together many younger scholars from Europe and America who approached Galen and Galenism from a variety of standpoints and with varied linguistic expertise. Since then there has been a veritable explosion in Galenic studies.[134] The *Corpus Medicorum*, having survived communism and, so far, capitalism, now also includes vernacular translations and commentaries by scholars from around the world, and faces competition from the revived American Loeb library and the French Budé series of texts and commentaries. Recent volumes in the latter series have remarkably included two pseudo-Galenic texts, long neglected precisely because they were not by Galen.[135] Major treatises have been published for the first time, including *Examining the Physician* and *My Own Opinions*, the latter published first from medieval Latin versions but then rediscovered in the original Greek along with previously lost portions of *My own Books and The Order of my own Books*, and, most spectacular of all, the previously unknown *Avoiding Distress.*[136] There have been frequent conferences devoted to Galen and his influence, as well as an international journal that bears his name. The task of compiling a Galenic bibliography, relatively easy a generation ago, is now immense, even with the aid of the computer, which has also brought original Greek manuscripts to one's worktop. Even the most diligent of researchers is likely to miss important publications appearing around the world and in journals with very varied focuses. Doctors too have turned their attention to Galen again, appreciating what he was trying to do in circumstances different from their own: he may have been wrong, but he was rarely foolish.[137] A leading American child psychologist, Jerome Kagan (b. 1929), has even argued that Galen's theory of temperament is a more useful starting point in understanding child development than Freud.[138] Further blood has been returned to Galen's ghost by scholarly biographers as well as by the more imaginative reconstructions of novelists in English and Italian.[139]

Galen and Galenism, as this chapter has shown, cannot be entirely separated. Perceptions of Galen, whether in the second or the twenty-first century, have affected how his writings have come down to us, and how they have been studied, whether by doctors, philosophers, philologists, or historians. Long-lasting legends of his acquaintance with Cleopatra or his conversion to Christianity helped to establish his authority with a general public that had little access to his actual writings. Galen's own attempts to define his legacy by listing his genuine works and explaining how they should be read succeeded only in part, and modern historians have been able to do far more than simply repeat the incidents that he thought most noteworthy by placing his activities in context and by carefully scrutinising his arguments and observations. His reputation has risen and fallen, and arguably risen again over the last forty years, with a corresponding increase or decrease in scholarly and medical interest in what he said and wrote. Few doctors, of any period, can be credited with such an influence, whether as a living presence or as a ghost.

Notes

1 The most detailed biography of Surianus (d. 1522), who later became a Camaldolensian monk and head of his order, is given by Mittarelli and Costadoni 1764: 33–34.
2 Surianus 1502: pref; Fortuna 2005: 473–5; 2012; 2019a; Nutton and Bos 2011: 79–81.
3 Fortuna 2012, 2019a.
4 Temkin 1973 remains fundamental for its insights.
5 Galen, *Ind.*, 20–1: pp. 8.11–9.5 BJP; pp. 84–5 tr. Nutton; for Heraclitus, above, p. 11.
6 Raiola 2015; Petit 2018: 210–54.
7 Galen, *Lib.Prop.* 1,1–3: 19,50 K; pp. 134–5 BM; p. 3 tr. Singer PN; *Prop.Plac.*1,1; p. 172 BMP; pp. 56–9 Garofalo-Lami; p. 186 Vegetti.
8 *Ord.Lib.Prop.* 1: 19,49–61 K; pp. 88–103 BM; pp. 30–4 tr. Singer PN.
9 Lazaris 2019: 616, seeing a parallel also with the images of the Seven Sages; his list, pp. 611–2, shows that medieval images of Galen are found in a variety of contexts.
10 Savino 2019. For Hunayn's earlier bibliography, which comments on their authorship, see above, p. 139.
11 Pietrobelli 2019a: 20–22; Pietrobelli 2020 discusses critical reactions to Galen down to the Renaissance.
12 Gero 1990; Barnes 2002.
13 Grant RM 1983; Havrda 2011; Ramelli 2015: 139–44; Pietrobelli 2019a: 26–29.
14 Nutton 2008: 358–9; Pietrobelli 2019a: 16–19, 30–1.
15 Weisser 1989.
16 Regenbogen 1961: 125–7. A drawing of this incident, from around 1450, is found in a medieval English manuscript of surgery, British Library MS, Sloane 6, fol. 175v.
17 Hessus 1533: 21v; my translation.
18 Gyekye 1979: 30.
19 *Timarion*, p. 75 Romano, cf. Temkin 1973: 63–4; the annotator was Niccolò de Leonardis, fl. 1430, in his copy of Galen, Cesena, Biblioteca Malatestiana, S.V.4, fol. 132va.
20 For the use of Galen in medieval Jewish philosophy, Zonta 1995; Caballero-Navas 2019; Langermann 2019. The textual history of the Galenic Corpus is succinctly surveyed by Boudon-Millot 2007: xci–ccxxix. For *Demonstration*, see von Müller 1897: 410, citing a report of 1616 that a complete Greek text existed in a noble library in Wallachia. John Caius in the 1560s had also heard similar rumours of its existence in an Italian episcopal library, see Nutton 1987: 94, 98.
21 A complete copy was said by the lexicographer Calepinus to have been in the possession of one Antonio Visconti around 1500, Nutton, *ibid.*
22 Boudon-Millot 2007: clxix cxcviii; Nutton 2013d; Lamoreaux 2016; Degni 2019.
23 *Syn.Puls.*: 9,431–549 K; Garofalo 1999.
24 Bouras-Vallianatos 2019a: 38–44.
25 Fancy 2019.
26 Pietrobelli 2019b: ccxi–iii.
27 Jacquart 1998: 183–94.
28 Mondella 1568; Amat 1623; Laguna 1548, 1604.
29 Edelstein 1967: 465–6.
30 Duffy 1984; Palmieri 2002; Garofalo 2019: 62–5.
31 Garofalo 2019: 65–74, noting also the use of schematic visual aids to memory.
32 García Ballester 1993; Walbridge 2014: 18, 111–2.
33 Bouras-Vallianatos 2019a: 53–4, arguing also for a knowledge of Galen by another Latin (but possibly bilingual) author, Theodore Priscian, around 500.
34 Fischer 2003; Everett 2012.
35 Hugonnard-Roche 1989, 1997; Bhayro 2017, 2019: 163–8.
36 Kessel 2019.
37 Delehaye 1909: 219.
38 Lazaris 2019, who omits the Milan windows (Belloni 1984) and the remarkable illuminated MS, painted in Paris around 1460, Dresden, Db 92–93 (above, *Figs 4.1* and *5.2*); Nutton 2011; Pressouyre 1966.
39 Sharples and Van der Eijk 2008; Bouras-Vallianatos 2019b: 86–8; Volk 1990; Stathakopoulos 2019: 144–6; Zonta 1995.

40 Koetschet 2019c; Schacht and Meyerhof 1937b.
41 Cooper 2011b, 2019; Lamoreaux 2016.
42 In Armenia (Orengo 2019) and possibly Tibet and China (Yoeli-Tlalim 2019), although the extent and timing of the arrival of Galenism remains obscure.
43 Caballero-Navas 2019; Chandelier 2019; Langermann 2019; Strohmaier 2019. For al-Razi's *Doubts on Galen*, see Koetschet 2019a, b, c; and for Maimonides' criticisms, Schacht and Meyerhof 1937b.
44 Savage-Smith 2002.
45 Strohmaier 1988: 127–8.
46 Kahl and Bos 2018.
47 Strohmaier 2019.
48 Hamarneh 1997.
49 Fancy 2019.
50 The scribe of Paris, BNF, ms. grec 2425, attempted a synchronism of his life with that of Ptolemy, Boudreaux 1912: 95. See also Figs. *1.2; 2.1; 4.1*; and *5.2* for visual depictions of Galen's life.
51 Swain 2007a; Alessi 2019; Savage-Smith *et al.* 2020.
52 Meisami 1989: 275–6, perhaps a hint that the highly rational Galen never married: we hear of no relations with members of the opposite sex or of any close friends.
53 Rosenthal 1975: 35; Swain 2007a: 402–3. For Anaxagoras, see above, p. 93, note 19.
54 Amari 1897; Strohmaier 2007.
55 Al-Istakhrī, ed. De Goeje 1870: I: 53.
56 Swain 2007a: 401–2.
57 Levey and Souryal 1968.
58 For the ubiquity of Galen and Galenic remedies in Byzantium, see Bouras-Vallianatos 2019b; Zipser 2019.
59 Bouras-Vallianatos 2019a: 44–52.
60 Schacht and Meyerhof 1937a.
61 Bouras-Vallianatos and Xenophontos 2015; Cronier et al. 2015; Bouras-Vallianatos 2019b: 98–100. His criticisms of Galen seem not to have been widely read.
62 Green MH 2019.
63 Long B 2019.
64 Urso 2019: 364–9.
65 O'Boyle 1998; Green MH 2018; McVaugh 2019.
66 Nutton 2013d; Fortuna 2019b.
67 Stauber 1908: 58. He later acquired the manuscript, now Munich, Staatsbibliothek, CLM 2.
68 Ludwig 1999: 265–9. The title *Articella*, 'Little Art', is not attested before the age of printing, and may have been student slang.
69 Nutton 1987; Gundert 2006; Fortuna 2019a. Jackson DF 2012 suggests that very little interest was taken in specifically medical codices as such until the end of the fifteenth century: they were bought but not studied. It may be no coincidence that several Mss have links with a circle of doctors and teachers at the Kral Hospital in Constantinople between 1440 and 1470, see now Pietrobelli 2019b: ccxxxxix–ccxli.
70 Nutton 1987: 22–5.
71 Mugnai Carrara 1991 remains fundamental.
72 Leoniceno 1508.
73 Benedetti 1503; Ferrari 1996, 1998. The 1517 Pavia edition was printed in Gothic script and reverted to medieval ligatures and abbreviations.
74 French 1999: 81–91.
75 Arbenz 1891: 248.
76 Nutton 1979: 29; Fogelmark 2015: I,5–7.
77 Temkin 1973: pl.4. For the background, see Copenhaver 1978: 67–70; 116–7.
78 Nutton 1987; Fortuna 2019a. Potter 1998 shows that the final volume (containing the Hippocratic commentaries) must have appeared a year later than the others.
79 Perilli 2018: 68 suggests that Leoniceno had already lent some of his Mss to the Aldine Press for their long-delayed edition, and that it was his death, and the wish of his heirs to sell the Mss, that speeded up the editorial process.

80 Gundert 2006.
81 For Caius, Nutton 1987, 2018; for Chartier (1572–1654), see Boudon-Millot et al. 2012; for Kūhn (1754–1840), Nutton 2002b.
82 And even to produce forgeries of Galenic Greek texts, Savino 2019.
83 Details of printings are taken from Durling 1961 and Fortuna 2019a; vernacular translations are considerably fewer and mostly in French of treatises of interest to learned surgeons. For Erasmus, see Perilli 2012.
84 Fortuna 2019a.
85 Pielmeyer 1981.
86 Clark 1964.
87 Nutton 2009b.
88 Several versions of the so-called '*Conversion of Galen*' (*Fig. 3.2*) were printed in the eighteenth and nineteenth centuries.
89 *Nova Academia Florentina* 1533. For wider discussions of this new Galenism, see Siraisi 1990, 2001; Maclean 2002; Bigotti 2019; Nutton 2019.
90 Ferretto 2012.
91 Ongaro 1994, pointing out that Da Monte was by no means the first at Padua to do this.
92 Pastore and Peruzzi 2006; Arcangeli and Nutton 2008.
93 French 1979.
94 Some texts are translated in Lind 1975.
95 Nutton 1993b: 18. But one should not forget that there were also private dissection classes, either on animals or human osteology.
96 Carlino 1999.
97 Nutton 2003.
98 Nutton 2018: 34.
99 O'Malley 1964: 65–6.
100 Nutton 1983; Helm 2001.
101 Nutton 2017: 22.
102 Maddison et al. 1977: pl. VI.
103 Nutton 2018: 70.
104 O'Malley 1964; Nutton 2014a; Joffe 2014; Van Hee 2014; Vons 2016; Canalis and Ciavolella 2018.
105 Nutton 2017 publishes previous unknown notes by Vesalius.
106 Eriksson 1959.
107 Vesalius 1543: pref.
108 Nutton 1998.
109 Nutton 1993a.
110 Nutton 2017: 42–5. He had been assisted in his Paris dissections by Michael Servetus (1511–53), later a discoverer of the circulation of the blood.
111 Nutton 2019, forthcoming 1.
112 Nutton 1987.
113 Nutton 2018: 35–6.
114 Richardson and Carman 1998–2009; Nutton 2012c; Garrison and Hast 2014. For immediate reactions from readers, Margócsy *et al.* 2018. Baker 2016: 62 gives an example of Vesalius' unacknowledged reversion to Galen.
115 Skaarup 2015.
116 Adelmann 1966: 87; Gnudi and Webster, 1950: 148, 198, emphasise the significance of Galenic functional and teleological anatomy for medical practice over and against Vesalius. Similar arguments are used in modern debates about the place of anatomy and dissection in the UK medical curriculum.
117 Nutton 1990b; Bigotti 2019; Hirai forthcoming.
118 French 1994; for some wider considerations, O'Rourke Boyle 2018.
119 Donato 2019.
120 Keynes 1978 remains standard.
121 Dandrey 1998, 2006.
122 Gessner 1554.
123 Guinter 1571.

124 Broman 1996.
125 Nutton 2002b.
126 Nutton 2002b; Tassinari 2019
127 Daremberg 1854–56; Ilberg 1889–97.
128 Simon 1906.
129 Edelstein 1967; Temkin 1973.
130 Michael Frede, Geoffrey Lloyd, Paul Moraux and Mario Vegetti were also leading participants in the *Symposia Aristotelica.*
131 Bowersock 1969. One of my teachers, Joyce Reynolds, was just beginning her work on the inscriptions of Aphrodisias, South of Pergamum.
132 Flemming 2000.
133 Nutton 1981.
134 One can compare the Bibliography below with those in Hankinson 2008a; Boutras-Vallianatos and Zipser 2019 and Laskaris *et al.* forthcoming.
135 Petit 2009; Boudon-Millot 2016a.
136 Iskandar 1988; Nutton 1999; Boudon-Millot and Pietrobelli 2005; Boudon-Millot 2007; Boudon-Millot *et al.* 2010.
137 E.g. Siegel 1968, 1970; Brain 1986; Manzoni 2001; Rocca 2002; Powell 2003; Johnston 2006. See also the Appendix.
138 Kagan 1994.
139 Prantera 1991, Magri 2002, 2004.

7 Conclusion

Galen was his own worst enemy, and it is easy to list his many failings. Egotistic, verbose, dogmatic, unscrupulous in argument and pedantic in learning, he has been accused of holding back the development of medicine for centuries almost single-handedly.[1] Indeed, the history of medicine is often written in terms of a decline from the great days of Classical Greece and early Alexandria until its final emancipation from Galen in the sixteenth century. His belief in humours and his failure to recognise the circulation of the blood, coupled with his promotion of bloodletting as therapy, have earned him a place amongst the great sinners of medicine. His description of the body is condemned as a confused amalgam of animal and, all too rarely, human anatomy, while the thousands of pages of his recipes remain almost entirely unread and are dismissed as ineffective as well as being largely copied verbatim from earlier sources. Francis Clifton, a London doctor of the eighteenth century, blamed everything on his passion for theorising compared with Hippocrates: "the one's [practice] was founded chiefly upon experience and observation, the other's upon reasoning: so that Hippocrates has occasion'd very little dispute among physicians, while Galen had laid a foundation for eternal dispute".[2]

Classicists have until recently shared this medical disdain. The prestigious Loeb series contained until 2011 but a single work of Galen, published as long ago as 1916, while the equivalent French Budé series had none at all until 2007. Even the promoters of the *Corpus Medicorum Graecorum*, the home of the best modern editions for almost a century, began with Galen, not for himself, but for what he could reveal about the text of Hippocrates and about medicine five or six centuries before his time.[3] His philosophy was likewise seen as derivative, a falling away from the exciting innovations of the pre-Socratics or the challenging thoughts of Plato and Aristotle, and, along with most of the rest of Hellenistic and later Greek philosophy, it was left to the occasional intrepid or foolish investigator. Even after the first modern revival of interest in the editing of Galenic Greek texts in the late nineteenth century, largely the achievement of young German doctoral students, studies in Galenic medicine and Galenic ideas were few and far between.

His reputation until recently was damaged by two related factors. He was, if judged by modern medical criteria, frequently wrong, and the dogmatism of many of his presentations of his results was acknowledged by friend and foe alike. But the first is true of any medic, not least in today's world where the speed of change has become ever faster and where long-held certainties can be overturned almost overnight, and the second relates at least as much to Galenism as to Galen himself. His enormous oeuvre could only be made useful by a process of deletion and summary, which meant that the great majority of doctors, both in his own time and, still more, in later centuries, were familiar with only a handful of his writings. Those that they read preserved the main lines of his thought but omitted his nuances, his hesitations and uncertainties and, most significantly, his experimentalism. They were treatises that, on the whole, presented his conclusions succinctly and definitively rather than the methods by which they were reached, didactic textbooks rather than accounts of investigations. Their message was reinforced by the preliminary training leading doctors received down at least to the seventeenth century, which was heavily based on Aristotelian logic and natural philosophy, attuned to the demands of theoretical debate at least as much as to practical medicine. This is the Galenism satirised by writers like Molière, and while Galen himself cannot entirely escape censure for it, a rigid adherence to his every word was foolish when he himself was always prepared to add or to modify, as some leading proponents of Galenic medicine, from Alexander of Tralles in the sixth century onwards, pointed out. The eleventh-century debates between Ibn Butlan and the far more conservative Ibn Ridwan in the Middle East, and between Simeon Seth and more orthodox Galenists in Byzantium, demonstrate clearly the range of opinions that could exist within the framework of Galenism. The flexibility and adaptability of Renaissance Galenism was one of the reasons for its survival as a major system of therapeutics long after Galenic anatomy and physiology were superseded.

But, as this book has tried to show, there is another side to the story. It is not surprising that in a writing career that lasted perhaps more than seventy years Galen should have produced so many treatises or that his method of composition, frequently oral expositions taken down by his amanuenses and then further recopied by others, should have led to repetitions and inconcinnities, particularly if works written decades apart are placed side by side. A good teacher, like a good orator, has to repeat the main points of his or her presentation more than once for it to be fully grasped by the audience, and, particularly when speaking extempore, there are triggers that result in the reiteration of familiar phrases or even sentences. Given that Galen was a practising physician engaged in often heated argument in a combative environment, his mistakes in logic are relatively few, and his eye for the failings of others unerring. Indeed, the fact that thinkers of the calibre of Alexander of Aphrodisias or Clement of Alexandria regarded him as an authority or a worthwhile opponent is a strong indication of the respect in which he was held by contemporaries. Had we more of his *Demonstration*, the treatise he considered his most important contribution to logic, we would be in a better position to compare him with Aristotle and the early Stoics, and to make a more secure assessment of his abilities as a philosopher. But, even without this, there can be no doubt of his independence of mind, or of his conviction of the necessity for a doctor to exercise thought in his day-to-day practice.

But to provide an assessment of Galen, the thinking doctor at the bedside, is no easy task, since so much of our information comes from Galen himself, and his vigorous assertion of his own merits is bound to provoke a sceptical counter-reaction. One can see through many of the strategies he uses to demolish his opponents and admire, without being convinced by, the artful rhetoric by which he accepts the plaudits of those who consider his successful cases miraculous, while at the same time playing down any suggestion of magic and quackery. Yet there is much to support the notion that he was an excellent physician: his remarkable powers of observation whether of the world around him, the anatomy of the body or the patient before him, his prodigious learning in an age that valued learning as a mark of social as well as intellectual standing, his manual dexterity and his demands for high ethical standards, even if he may seem today to fall short of them on many occasions. That many of his therapies were, in modern eyes, ineffective (although today's practising herbalists would disagree) should not blind us to the fact that others were valuable. Even if he is inclined to exaggerate in his accounts, especially when referring to cases long past, and to misremember details of what he had once done, he is still far from deliberately inventing his successes, especially as many of his readers or audience would have been with him at the bedside and in a position to check his story. He would have been tactful at least in front of the sick, to judge both from his exposition of the merits of the true Hippocratic doctor and from his long service at court. No one could have been a royal physician, let alone survived for more than a decade the murderous uncertainties of a Commodus, without an acute understanding of the arts of the courtier. Besides, if his claims are in any way true, he was also accessible to anyone in need, from a slave and those injured in the gymnasium to members of the imperial family, and it was not only the followers of Theodotus the shoemaker who recognised his abilities. The long list of patients he claims to have cured as well as a reputation that brought letters seeking advice from far away and led to a position at court can hardly have been built on nothing. Surviving treatises by other ancient doctors show that his choice of therapies was more extensive, and scarcely more dangerous, than those of his competitors, and he was undoubtedly well placed to obtain the finest ingredients for his recipes. He was also constantly looking for new information or making further qualifications to his dogmatic utterances, as the Byzantine satirical author of the *Timarion* noted. Galen at the bedside would have appeared extremely knowledgeable, and his various tricks to disguise the source of his apparently amazing information about his patients, their history and their surroundings would only have added to the impression of a great authority who could not be gainsaid. His use of 'common Greek', as opposed to neologisms or the faux-Ionic of his contemporary Aretaeus of Cappadocia, would also have assisted what Laín Entralgo called the therapy of the word.[4] Galen was only too well aware of the importance of what he called the living word in presenting a case and in convincing the sick person in front of him.[5] But one would have had to exercise patience to listen to his diatribes, splendidly rhetorical though some were, and one wonders how many of his associates ever had the opportunity to express their own opinion, let alone convince the great man to change his mind or modify his therapy.

But the strongest argument for the importance of Galen's personal example rather than the derivative Galenism as a system rests on the impact that his writings made once they became accessible to physicians outside the Greek world. The great flowering of Arabic medicine between the ninth and the twelfth century cannot be understood without the Galenic translations made by Hunayn and his school, which not only gave to the Arabic language a new and broader vocabulary of medicine and made largely unknown works of Galen available to those who knew no Greek, but also established the Galenic philosopher-doctor as the *beau ideal*. Philosophy as well as medicine would be poorer without such distinguished exponents as Avicenna, Averroes and Maimonides, to give them their Latin names. A similar upsurge of intellectual excitement following the arrival of Galenic texts can be demonstrated for eleventh century Salerno and, even more, for the later Western Middle Ages where Latin translations of Arabic Galenist authors and then, from 1200 onwards, of Galen himself led to what Luis García Ballester called the New Galenism and its implantation into the burgeoning universities of Western Europe. Appeals to the authority of Galen not only acknowledged his importance but strengthened the position of his new followers at a time when they were seeking to establish themselves against other practitioners.

Yet more striking was the effect of Galen when Greek manuscripts of his writings first appeared in Northern Italy at the end of the fifteenth century. Not only did it stimulate new ideas on medical practice, leading to the general rejection of astrology and uroscopy as prime diagnostic methods, but it established anatomy as the new science that every doctor with pretensions to learning should know. The triumph of an exclusively Galenic anatomy and physiology was relatively brief, as the discovery of both his errors and new structures in the human body quickly made his anatomy outdated. But one should remember that the same fate also befell Vesalius and Colombo and many others as their own syntheses were in turn jettisoned in favour of others that were more modern and more accurate. But Galen's achievements in dissection were never entirely forgotten (*Fig. 7.1*). The professors of Vienna, whose Medical School in the late nineteenth century was one of most progressive in the whole of Europe, acknowledged their debt to Galen in 1888 by placing his statue, holding his *The Use of Parts*, at the head of the main staircase of their new Anatomical Institute.[6] The following year, he was commemorated, along with Hippocrates and Aretaeus, in a large stained-glass window on the equally grand staircase of the Medical School at Sydney.[7] His personality, visible throughout his writings, continues equally to fascinate or repel even today, a tribute to the forceful rhetoric of his self-presentation as well as to his wide-ranging curiosity and his unique insights. Even if his arguments are rejected, they cannot be ignored, and they rarely fail to provoke.

But any student of Galen is compelled to struggle not only against Galen's insistence on his own superiority, but, still more. against his determination to leave behind the portrait of Galen that he himself wished us to have. He was far from alone in this. The Emperor Augustus had copies of his own account of his achievements set up in stone in cities around the Roman Empire, and historians of the early church would be the poorer without the *Confessions* of St Augustine. The *Sacred Tales* of Galen's contemporary, Aelius Aristides, are a vivid and detailed account of his relationship with the healing god Asclepius, while the huge inscription set up at around the same time at Oenoanda in Lycia (Southwest Turkey) by the Epicurean Diogenes is only the most substantial exposition of a personal belief in a particular philosophical creed.[8]

But Galen goes beyond mere confession. No other ancient author has bequeathed so many detailed instructions as to how his books should be read and his ideas discussed, or used so many incidents from his own life to exemplify how medicine should be practised.[9] The Roman politician Cicero notoriously (and unsuccessfully) invited a historian to write an account of his achievements as consul, providing him with the appropriate guidelines to follow.[10] Galen has no need of a mediating author to influence how he should be viewed. He crafts his own *persona* with great care, portraying himself as an outsider who reached the summit of his profession despite the hostility and ignorance of his rivals. His views are not only correct, but also maintained against overwhelming odds. Belief in Hippocratism is a minority position, and his own interpretations require to be successfully defended even against other Hippocratics. He buttresses his claims not only by experiment and demonstration, but also by placing himself in a direct line of great physicians from Hippocrates onwards. His description of his discovery that the wife of Justus was in love with an actor is deliberately

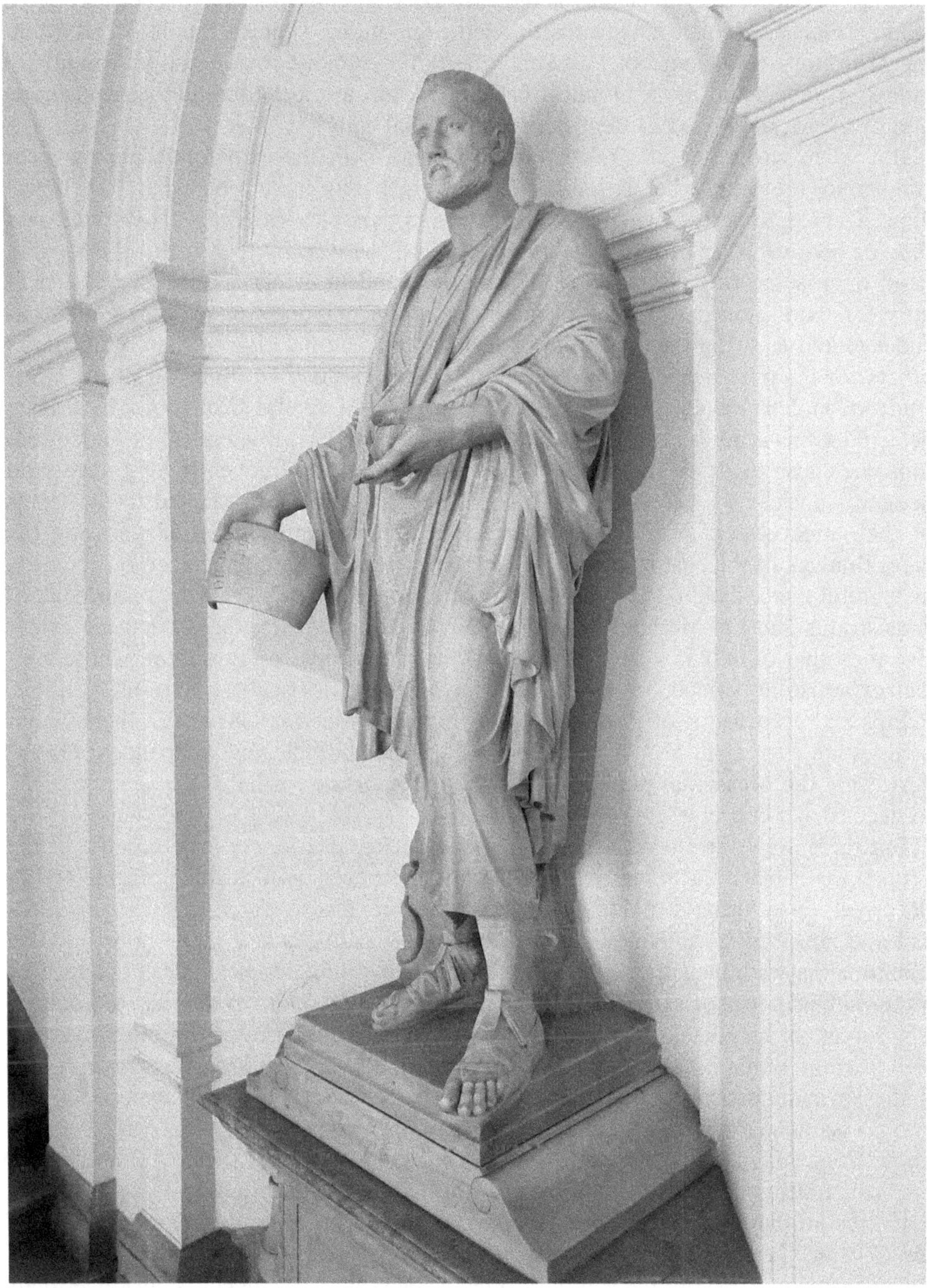

Figure 7.1 Galen holding a copy of *The Use of Parts.* Statue, 1888, by Hugo Haerdtl (1846–1918) at the head of the grand staircase of the new Anatomical Institute of the Vienna Medical School. Photo: Herwig Swoboda.

modelled on a series of famous stories of the medical diagnosis of lovesickness that have as their heroes Hippocrates and Erasistratus among others. No one hearing or reading Galen's account could miss this self-promotional subtext. Similarly, his often-repeated story of his cure of Pausanias the Syrian sophist is not just a demand for others to understand the anatomical basis of certain medical conditions, but also sets him in the social context of the Roman intellectual elite.

But when writing about Galen, far more than with the emperor Augustus or St Augustine, the biographer is limited by having to rely largely on what the subject himself chose to reveal, whether deliberately as part of a carefully constructed *persona* or because what he left out was, in his view, not directly relevant to the topic in hand or in some way discreditable. Where independent evidence does exist, particularly for the arguments of his philosophical opponents, one can see how Galen has endeavoured to swing the debate in his favour. His manipulation of the arguments of others for his own purposes has been amply demonstrated by Teun Tieleman in his study of Galen's relationship with earlier Stoics, and similar distortions have been detected in his attitudes to the Methodists.[11] But even here, it is typical of Galen that those he chose to attack by name in his writings were also frequently long dead, and he leaves unclear the extent to which contemporary sectarians adhered to the tenets of their predecessors, while at the same time representing himself as knowing the great thinkers of the past better than their followers. Far more difficult to overcome is his careful concealment of his debts to others, save for his father. Our knowledge of Erasistratus and the Methodists, with whom he argued at length, is far more extensive than that of individual Empiricists, such as Heraclides of Tarentum, whose clinical expertise he valued, let alone those of Hippocratics such as Satyrus, Quintus, Pelops and even Rufus of Ephesus, from whom he gained much, or of others whom he does not even mention.[12] The self-portrait of the infallible and independent Galen, bestowing the occasional plaudit on a fellow Hippocratic, is hard, if not impossible, to deconstruct entirely.

But there are several ways of resolving this Galenic puzzle, not least because of the abundance of material, of various kinds, that throws light on medicine in Rome and in the Greek East during his lifetime.[13] It provides a context in which to situate his medical and non-medical activities. His distribution of his books to and, he hoped, by his friends, along with his gifts to colleagues places him within a typical ancient context of mutual obligation that extended far beyond the morning *salutatio* that he so despised. The success of his enemies the Methodists can be easily confirmed from inscriptions as well as from within his own writings, even if it would be unwise to conclude with him that their many patients had all been taken in by their claims to simplicity and to swift and pleasant treatment. Parts of his career can also be paralleled elsewhere. We now know from epigraphy, as well as from his own reminiscences, that other well-to-do medical students travelled a long distance for a medical education: at least one other made the journey from Pergamum to Alexandria, and the author of *The Properties of the Centaury* had left behind a brother in the Greek world while he visited patients in Rome with a mentor. But the length of time Galen spent as a student is far longer than any other known to us, which is a measure of his family wealth at least as much as of his passion for knowledge. Nor was he the only prolific scribbler among doctors. Julian's exposition of the Hippocratic *Aphorisms* alone ran to 48 books and was but a fraction of the 156 books written a century earlier by Tiberius Claudius Menecrates, the founder of his own "logical" sect.[14] He was not alone in his claim to be both doctor and philosopher. Heraclitus of Rhodiapolis made similar boasts about his own literary and medical prowess, and, to prove it, this "Homer of medical poetry" could show the honours he had received from distinguished groups around the Eastern Mediterranean. These examples show that Galen was not always as unique as his rhetoric tries to suggest.

But contextualisation, however useful, can take us only so far in evaluating Galen the scholar-doctor and his achievements. He was not a typical doctor in the age of the Antonines, and to extrapolate from him to the ancient medical profession in general is foolhardy. He was an elite physician, whose career would have been impossible for all but a tiny handful of medical practitioners in ancient Greece and Rome. His family wealth and his long education, not only in medicine, played a considerable part in his success, and the help he claims to have given in the form of books, instruments and the like to other doctors less fortunate than he reveals the gulf between him and some of his fellow practitioners, even if it is not always easy to be precise about its extent.

But the sheer scale and variety of his surviving writings offers an opportunity to penetrate the Galenic carapace, even if, as Caroline Petit wittily puts, it is also a school for patience.[15] One can admit that there was much that he got wrong – and that later Galenists made worse by disregarding his careful qualifications and by failing to share his passion for experiment. But, given the technological and social constraints on his medicine, it is also remarkable how much he discovered and how much he observed that escaped the notice of others or is not otherwise recorded. Although he made regular changes to his writings, usually in the form of cross-references, the fact that many of books originated as oral presentations, dictated to or copied down by a scribe, provides a greater opportunity to see into his mind than when dealing with more careful or more private authors. Some of his works are less firmly structured than others, and one can follow his hesitations and qualifications, and sometimes his meandering train of thought, that were edited out from his shorter didactic works or in later Galenism. Much of his writing deserves to be criticised for its repetitiveness – a common feature of teachers now as then – but some is extremely elegant, clear and varied, all qualities highly regarded in a period when style was also an indication of status. His anecdotes also offer a rare glimpse into the court world around the emperors, where doctors and their supporters jockeyed for position and where, in the reign of Commodus, a wrong decision might lead to banishment or even death. No other author, not even Cicero in his letters, allows such access to his private thoughts.

Two things stand out above all. His capacity for observation and his demand that the doctor should be a thinking doctor. Like his critic Andreas Vesalius, fourteen hundred years later, he has a remarkable eye, whether for the smallest structures in the human body, the individuality of his patients or the wider world around him. He is acutely aware of the complexities of medicine and medical practice. While the doctor can hope for, and occasionally achieve, certainty, the vagaries of human nature and life itself rarely allow more than a choice between different degrees of plausibility. One must work often by approximation, not secure knowledge.[16] But his hesitations and qualifications, visible in his longer or more narrowly focussed works, are minimised in the shorter writings intended for students that were most often copied and read. In them he instructed others how to profit from his own experiences by following the intellectual guidelines he had constructed for himself, preferring, like a good teacher, clarity and succinctness to overwhelming detail. Later Galenism only added to his reputation for dogmatism by concentrating on a mere handful of didactic texts.

Leaving aside his biting, and often unfair, criticism of others, one cannot fail to be impressed by the extent of his learning and, still more, by his commitment to the medical art and the sheer energy that he must have displayed in travelling, writing and attending to thousands of patients from morning to night over a career of fifty, if not nigh on seventy years. He may not always be right in his conclusions, and comparison with other ancient medical texts from roughly the same period and milieu, whether by Rufus of Ephesus, Aretaeus of Cappadocia or the anonymous author of the pseudo-Galenic *Introduction to Medicine*, reveals some of his weaknesses.[17] But his prescription for the thinking doctor and his own example are still as valuable today as they were when he penned his *Method of Healing*. Even in today's medicine modern technology still requires human thought in order to be used properly, and some of Galen's dilemmas when faced with a patient are still with us.

To attempt within a short compass to describe the achievements of Galen is no easy task. The sheer abundance of his surviving writings, the great variety of his interests, the authority he wielded over some aspects of medicine for more than a millennium and a half and, not least, the careful investigations of scholars particularly over the last half century, all present different obstacles to a brief synthesis. Much must perforce be left out, or else overwhelm the reader. Yet one major obstacle remains, whatever the length of the exposition. Whether by his language, his argumentative strategies as a whole or his manifold examples of his own success, Galen is constantly pushing the reader towards an acceptance of his point of view. There is always the danger of taking him at his own valuation, and of being induced by his powerful rhetoric and his destructive criticisms of the views of others either to agree with him uncritically or to feel driven to an equally vigorous rejection of all he stood for. He is not an author who invites a dispassionate analysis. Yet this ability to provoke, whether positively or negatively, allows a way towards understanding Galen that is unusual in an ancient author. It is a rare chapter that does not contain something to make one sit up and take note, and his asides are at times more interesting than the point he is trying to make. One can agree with his detractors that he was frequently overbearing and longwinded, not always careful to distinguish the merely plausible from the certain, and all the time convinced of his own rightness – and not afraid to declare it. But that has been a small price to pay for acquaintance with a physician of undoubted genius.

Notes

1 Wootton 2007; for his egotism compared with that of other medical writers, see Nutton 2009c.
2 Clifton 1732: 86–7, a reference I owe to Sam Taylor.
3 Kollesch 2019: 242, a valid judgment if applied only to the actual text of the Hippocratic writings; Nutton 2008: 380.
4 Deichgräber 1971; Lain Entralgo 1970.
5 *Comp.Med.Loc.* VI,1: 12,894 K; cf. *Alim.Fac.* I,1,47: p. 39 tr. Powell; *SMT* VI, pr.: 11.791 K.
6 I am grateful to Herwig Swoboda, who first showed me the statue, and Kerstin Kohl for details of its inauguration.
7 "'Galen, Hippocrates, and Aretaeus of Cappadocia', Window, The University of Sydney," *Medievalism in Australian Cultural Memory*, accessed October 19, 2019, http://ausmed.arts.uwa.edu.au/items/show/723. The image appears on the cover of Rocca 2003 as a tribute to the author's *alma mater*.
8 Petsalis-Diomidis 2010; Hammerstaedt and Smith 2014, 2018 give the latest news of Diogenes' inscription.

9 Raiola 2015; Petit 2018.
10 Cicero, *Letters to Friends* V,12.
11 Tieleman 2009; Tecusan 2004. Tieleman 1996: xxii, on Galen's "backward-looking" independence.
12 Guardasole 1997.
13 Nutton 2010, 2013b.
14 Nutton 2013a: 4.
15 Petit 2018, a fascinating study of Galen's language and rhetorical strategies in their cultural context.
16 *MM* IX,16: 10,653 K; II, p. 653 tr. Johnston-Horsley.
17 For these authors, see respectively Pormann 2008; Oberhelman 1994; and Petit 2009.

Appendix

Titles and abbreviations of Galen's books

Abbreviation	*Latin title*	*English title*	*Editions and translations*
AA	*De anatomicis administrationibus* (2,215–731 K)	*Anatomical Procedures*	Singer C (1956 E); Duckworth, Lyons and Towers (1962 E); Garofalo (1991 I)
Adv.Jul.	*Adversus Julianum* (18A,246–99 K)	*Against Julian*	Wenkebach (*CMG* 1951 Edn); Tecusan (2004 E)
Adv.Lyc.	*Adversus Lycum* (18A,196–245 K)	*Against Lycus*	Wenkebach (*CMG* 1951 Edn)
Adv.Typ.Scr.	*Adversus eos qui de typsis scripserunt* (7,475–512 K)	*Against Those Who Have Written on Disease Types*	
Aff.Dig.	*De propriorum animi cuiusque affectuum dignotione et curatione; De animi cuislibet peccatorum dignotione et curatione* (5,1–103 K)	*The Diagnosis and Treatment of the Affections and Errors Peculiar (Affections and Errors)*	De Boer (*CMG* Edn); Singer PN (2013 E)
Alim.Fac.	*De alimentorum facultatibus* (6,453–748 K)	*The Properties of Foodstuffs*	Helmreich (*CMG* 1923 Edn); Powell (2003 E); Wilkins (2013 Edn F)
Ant.	*De antidotis* (14,1–209 K)	*Antidotes*	
[*An Ut.*]	*An animal sit quod in utero geritur* (19,151–81 K)	*Whether What is in the Womb is an Animal*	
Ars Med.	*Ars medica* (1,305–412 K)	The *Art of Medicine*	Singer *PN* (1997 E); Boudon-Millot (2000 Edn F); Johnston (2016 E)
Art.Sang.	*An in arteriis natura sanguis contineatur* (4,703–36 K)	*Whether Blood is Naturally Contained in the Arteries*	Furley and Wilkie (1984 Edn E)
At.Bil.	*De atra bile* (5,104–48 K)	*Black Bile*	De Boer (CMG 1937 Edn); Grant M (2000 E)

Abbreviation	*Latin title*	*English title*	*Editions and translations*
Bon.Hab.	*De bono habitu* (4,750–56 K)	*Good Condition*	Helmreich (1901 Edn); Singer PN (1997 E)
Bon.Mal. Suc.	*De bonis malisque succis* (6,749–815 K)	*Good and Bad Juices*	Helmreich (*CMG* 1923 Edn)
CAM	*De constitutione artis medicae* (1,224–304 K)	*The Composition of the Art of Medicine*	Fortuna (*CMG* 1997 Edn I); Johnston (2016 E)
[*Cath.Med. Purg.*]	*Quos, quibus catharticis medicamentis et quando purgare oporteat* (11,343–56 K)	*Whom to Purge, with What Cleansing Drugs and When*	
Caus.Cont.	*De causis contentivis* (not surviving in Greek)	*Containing Causes*	Lyons (*CMG* 1969 Edn Arabic E)
Caus.*Morb.*	*De causis morborum* (7,1–41 K)	*Causes of Diseases*	Grant M (2000 E); Johnston (2016 E)
Caus.Proc.	*De causis procatarcticis* (not surviving in Greek)	*Antecedent Causes*	Bardong (*CMG* 1937 Edn); Hankinson (1998 Edn L E)
Caus.Puls.	*De causis pulsuum* (9,1–204 K)	*Causes of the Pulse*	
Caus.Resp.	*De causis respirationis* (4,465–9)	*Causes of Breathing*	Furley and Wilkie (1984 Edn E)
Caus.Symp.	*De causis symptomatum* (7,85–272 K)	*Causes of Symptoms*	Johnston (2006 E)
Comp.Med. Gen.	*De compositione medicamentorum per genera* (13,362–1058 K)	The *Composition of Drugs According to Kind*	
Comp.Med. Loc.	*De compositione medicamentorum secundum locos* (12,378–1007, 13,1–361 K)	*The Composition of Drugs According to Places*	
Cons.	*De consuetudinibus* (not in K)	*Habits*	Von Müller (1891 Edn); Schmutte and Pfaff (*CMG* Edn L and Arabic)
Cris.	*De crisibus* (9,550–768 K)	*Crises*	Alexanderson (1967 Edn)
Cur.Rat.Ven. Sect.	*De curandi ratione per venae sectionem* (11,250–316 K)	*Treatment by Bleeding*	Brain (1986 E)
[*Def.Med.*]	*Definitiones medicae* (19,346–462 K)	*Medical Definitions*	
Dem.	*De demonstratione* (not in K)	*Demonstration*	Von Müller (1895 Edn fragments)
Di.Dec.	*De diebus decretoriis* (9,769–941 K)	*Critical Days*	Cooper (2011 Edn Arabic E)
Di.Hipp. Morb.Ac.	*De diaeta Hippocratis in morbis acutis* (not in K)	*Hippocrates' Regimen*	Lyons (CMG 1969 Edn Arabic E)

(Continued)

(Cont.)

Abbreviation	*Latin title*	*English title*	*Editions and translations*
Diff.Feb.	*De differentiis febrium* (7,273–405 K)	*The Distinct Types of Fever*	
Diff. Morb.	*De differentiis morborum* (6,836–80 K)	*The Distinct Types of Disease*	Johnston (2006 E)
Diff.Puls.	*De differentiis pulsuum* (8,493–765 K)	*The Distinct Types of Pulse*	
Diff.Resp.	*De difficultate respirationis* (7,753–960 K)	*Difficulty in Breathing*	Minor (2011 Edn)
Dig.Insomn.	*De dignotione ex insomniis* (6,832–5 K)	*Diagnosis by Dreams*	Oberhelman (1983 E)
Dig.Puls.	*De dignoscendis pulsibus* (8,766–961 K)	*Pulses Diagnosis*	
Elem.	*De elementis ex Hippocrate* (1,413–508 K)	*Elements according to Hippocrates*	De Lacy (CMG 1996 Edn E)
Fasc.	*De fasciis* (18A,768–827 K)	*Bandages*	
Foet.Form.	*De foetuum formatione* (4,652–702 K)	*The Formation of the Foetus*	Singer PN (1997 E); Nickel (CMG 2001 Edn G)
Gal.Fasc.	*Ex Galeni* (18A,828–38 K)	*From Galen's Notes*	
Gloss.	*Glossarium* (19,62–157 K)	*Hippocratic Glossary*	Perilli (*CMG* 2017 Edn I)
[*Hipp.Alim.*]	*In Hippocratis* (15,224–417 K; inauthentic)	*Commentary on Hippocrates' Nutrition*	
Hipp.Aph.	*In Hippocratis Aphorimos* (17B,345–887; 18A,1–195 K)	*Commentary on Hippocrates' Aphorisms*	
Hipp.Art.	*In Hippocratis* (18A,300–767 K)	*Commentary on Hippocrates' Joints*	
Hipp.AWP	*In Hippocratis* (not surviving in Greek)	*Commentary on Hippocrates' Airs, Waters, and Places*	Wasserstein (1982 Edn Hebrew)
Hipp.Com.	*De comate secundum Hippocratem* (7,643–65 K)	*Coma according to Hippocrates*	Mewaldt (*CMG* 1915 Edn)
Hipp.Epid.I	*In Hippocratis Epidemiarum* (17A,1–302 K)	*Commentary on Hippocrates' Epidemics I*	Wenkebach (*CMG* 1934 Edn); Vagelpohl (*CMG* 2014 Edn Arabic: E)
Hipp.Epid.II	*In Hippocratis Epidemiarum* (inauthentic Greek text in 17A,303–479 K)	*Commentary on Hippocrates' Epidemics II*	Pfaff (*CMG* 1934 G from Arabic); Vagelpohl and Swain (*CMG* 2016 Edn Arabic: E)

Abbreviation	Latin title	English title	Editions and translations
Hipp.Epid.III	*In Hippocratis* Epidemiarum (17A,480–792 K)	*Commentary on Hippocrates' Epidemics III*	Wenkebach (*CMG* 1936 Edn)
Hipp.Epid.VI	*In Hippocratis Epidemiarum* (18A, 793–1009; 17B,1–344 K)	*Commentary on Hippocrates' Epidemics VI*	Wenkebach and Pfaff (*CMG* 1956 I–VI Edn; VI–VIII G from Arabic)
Hipp.Fract.	*In Hippocratis* (18B,318–628 K)	*Commentary on Hippocrates' Fractures*	
[*Hipp.Hum.*]	*In Hippocratis* (15,1–488 K; largely inauthentic)	*Commentary on Hippocrates' Humours*	
[*Hipp.Jus*]	*In Hippocratis Jus* (not surviving in Greek)	*Commentary on Hippocrates' Oath*	Rosenthal (1956 fragments E)
Hipp.Off. Med.	*In Hippocratis* (18B,629–925 K)	*Commentary on Hippocrates' Surgery*	Lyons (*CMG* 1963 Edn Arabic E)
Hipp.Prog.	*In Hippocratis Prognosticum* (18B,1–317 K)	*Commentary on Hippocrates' Prognostic*	Heeg (*CMG* 1915 Edn)
Hipp.Prorrh.	*In Hippocratis* (16,489–840 K)	*Commentary on Hippocrates' Prorrhetic*	Diels (*CMG* 1915 Edn)
[*Hipp.Sept.*]	*In Hippocratis* (not surviving in Greek)	*Commentary on Hippocrates' Sevens*	Bergsträsser (*CMG* 1914 Edn Arabic G)
Hipp.Vict.	*In Hippocratis* (15,174–223 K)	*Commentary on Hippocrates' Regimen for Health (Commentary on Hippocrates' Human Nature, Book III)*	Mewaldt (*CMG* 1914 Edn)
[*Hipp.Vict. Morb.*]	*De victus ratione in morbis acutis ex Hippocratis sententia* (inauthentic Greek text at 19,182–221 K)	*Regimen in Acute Diseases according to Hippocrates*	Westenberger (*CMG* 1914 Edn)
[*Hist.phil.*]	*Historia philosophica* (19,222–345 K)	*History of Philosophy*	Diels (1879 Edn)
HNH	*In Hippocratis* (15,1–223 K)	*Commentary on Hippocrates' Human Nature*	Mewaldt (*CMG* 1914 Edn)
HRCIS	*De hirundinibus, revulsione, cucurbitula, incisione et scarificatione* (11,317–22 K)	*Leeches, Revulsion, Cupping, Incision, Scarification*	
[*Hum.*]	*De humoribus* (19,485–96 K)	*Humours*	Grant M (2000 E)
HVA	*In Hippocratis* (15,418–919 K)	*Commentary on Hippocrates' Regimen in Acute Diseases*	Helmreich (*CMG* 1914 Edn); Pietrobelli (2019, Book I *Edn)*
Inaeq.Int.	*De inaequali intemperie* (7,733–52 K)	*Uneven Bad Mixture*	Grant M (2000 E)

(Continued)

(Cont.)

Abbreviation	*Latin title*	*English title*	*Editions and translations*
Ind.	*De indolentia* (not in K)	Avoiding *Distress*	Boudon-Millot, Jouanna and Pietrobelli (Edn F); Garofalo and Lami (2012 Edn I); Vegetti (2013 Edn I)
Inst.Log.	*Institutio logica* (not in K)	*Introduction to Logic*	Kalbfleisch (1896 Edn); Kieffer (1964 E)
Inst.Od.	*De instrumento odoratus* (1I,857–86 K)	*The Organ of Smell*	Kollesch (*CMG* 1964 Edn G)
[*Int.*]	*Introductio seu medicus* (14,674–797 K)	*Introduction*	Petit (2009 Edn F)
Lib.Prop.	*De libris propriis* (19,8–48 K)	*My Own Books*	Singer PN (1997 E); Boudon-Millot (2007 Edn F).
Loc.Aff.	*De locis affectis* (8,1–452 K)	*Affected Places*	Siegel (1976 E); Gärtner (*CMG* 2015 Books I and II Edn G)
Marc.	*De marcore* (7,666–704 K)	*Marasmus*	Theoharides (1971 E)
Med.Exp.	*De experientia medica* (Greek fragments)	*Medical Experience*	Walzer and Frede (1985)
[*Mel.*]	*De melancholia* (19,699–720 K)	*Melancholy* according to Galen, Rufus etc.	
MM	*De methodo medendi* (10,1–1021 K)	*The Method of Healing*	Hankinson (1991 E, Books I and II); Johnston and Horsley (2011 E)
MMG	*De methodo medendi ad Glauconem* (11,1–146 K)	*The Method of Healing, for Glaucon*	Johnston (2016 E)
Mor.	*De moribus* (not surviving in Greek)	*Character Traits*	Kraus (1939); Mattock (1972 E); Davies (2013 E)
Morb.Temp.	*De morborum temporibus* (7,406–39 K)	*Opportune Moments in Disease*	Wille (1960 Edn G)
Mot.Dub.	*De motibus dubiis* (not surviving in Greek)	*Problematical Movements*	Nutton and Bos (2011 Edn Lat., Arabic, E)
Mot.Musc.	*De motu musculorum* (4,367–464)	*The Movement of Muscles*	Goss (1968 E); Rosa (2009 Edn I)
Musc.Diss.	*De musculorum dissectione* (18B,926–1026)	*The Anatomy of the Muscles*	Goss (1963); Garofalo and Debru (2005 Edn F)
Nat.Fac.	*De facultatibus naturalibus* (2,1–214 K)	*Natural Faculties*	Helmreich (1893 Edn); Brock (1916 E)
Nerv.Diss.	*De nervorum dissectione* (2,831–56 K)	*The Anatomy of the Nerves*	Goss (1966 E); Garofalo and Debru (2008 Edn F)

Abbreviation	*Latin title*	*English title*	*Editions and translations*
Nom.Med.	*De nominibus medicis* (not surviving in Greek)	*Medical Terminology*	Meyerhof and Schacht (1931 Edn Arabic G)
Opt.Const. Corp.	*De optima corporis constitutione* (4,737–49 K)	*The Best Constitution of our Bodies*	Helmreich (1901 Edn); Singer PN (1997)
Opt.Doct.	*De optima doctrina* (1,40–52 K)	*The Best Method of Teaching*	Barigazzi (*CMG* 1991 Edn I)
Opt.Med.	Quod *optimus medicus sit quoque philosophus* (1,53–63 K)	*The Best Doctor is also a Philosopher*	Brain (1977 E); Singer PN (1997 E); Boudon-Millot (2007 Edn F)
Opt.Med. Cogn.	*De optimo medico cognoscendo* (not surviving in Greek)	*Discovering the Best Physician*	Iskandar (*CMG* 1988 Edn Arabic E)
[*Opt.Sect.*]	*De optima secta* (1,106–223 K)	*The Best Sect*	
Ord.Lib. Prop.	*De ordine librorum propriorum* (19,49–61 K)	*The Order of My Own Books*	Singer PN (1997 E); Boudon-Millot (2007 Edn F)
Oss.	*De ossibus ad tirones* (2,732–78 K)	*Bones for Beginners*	Singer C (1952); Garofalo and Debru (2005 Edn F)
Part.Art. Med.	*De partibus artis medicae* (not surviving in Greek)	*The Parts of the Art of Medicine*	Kollesch, Nickel and Strohmaier (1969 Edn Lat); Lyons (1969 Arabic E)
Part.Hom. Diff.	*De partium homoeomerium differentia* (not surviving in Greek)	*The Difference Between Uniform Parts*	Strohmaier (*CMG* 1970 Arabic G)
Parv.Pil.	*De parvae pilae exercitio* (5,899–910 K)	Exercise with the Small Ball	Wenkebach (1938 Edn G); Singer PN (1997 E); Johnston (2018 E)
PHP	*De placitis Hippocratis et Platonis* (5,181–805 K)	*The Opinions of Hippocrates and Plato*	De Lacy (*CMG* 1978–84 Edn E)
Plat.Tim.	*In Platonis Timaeum* (not in Kühn: Greek fragments surviving)	*Commentary on the Medical Statements in the Timaeus*	Schröder (*CMG* 1934 Edn); Larrain (1992 Edn Frags G)
Plat.Tim. Comp.	*Timaei Platonis Compendium* (not in Greek)	*Compendium of Plato's Timaeus*	Kraus and Walzer (1951 Arabic and L.)
Plen.	*De plenitudine* (7,513–83 K)	*Fulness*	Otte (2001 Edn G)
[*Pond.Mens.*]	*De ponderibus et mensuris* (19,748–81 K)	*Weights and Measures*	Hutsch (1864 Edn)
Praec.	*De praecognitione ad Epigenem* (14,599–673 K)	*Prognosis, for Epigenes*	Nutton (*CMG* 1979 Edn E)
Praes.	*De praenotione* (19,497–511 K, part of *CAM*)	*Prognosis*	Fortuna (*CMG* 1988 Edn)

(Continued)

(Cont.)

Abbreviation	*Latin title*	*English title*	*Editions and translations*
Praes.Puls.	*De praaesagitione ex pulsibus* (9,205–430 K)	*Prognosis from the Pulse*	
[*Praes.Ver. Exp.*]	*De praesagitione vera et experta* (19,512–8 K)	*True and Expert Prognosis*	
[*Prog.Dec.*]	*Prognostica de decubitu ex mathematica scientia* (19,529–73 K)	*Prognosis Based on the Hour when a Patient goes to Bed Based on the Science of Astrology*	
Prolaps.	*De humero iis modis prolapso quos Hippocrates non vidit* (18A,346–422 K)	*Dislocations Unseen by Hippocrates*	
Prop.Plac.	*De propriis placitis* (not in K)	*My Own Opinions*	Nutton (*CMG* 1999 Edn Lat, E); Boudon-Millot and Pietrobelli (2005 Edn F); Garofalo and Lami (2012 Edn I); Vegetti (2013 Edn I)
Protr.	*Protrepticus* (1, 1–39 K)	*An Exhortation to Study the Arts*	Barigazzi (*CMG* 1991 Edn I); Singer PN (1997 E); Boudon-Millot (2000 Edn F)
Ptis.	*De ptisana* (6,816–31 K)	*Barley Gruel*	Hartlich (*CMG* 1923 Edn); Grant M (2000 E)
Puer.Epil.	*Puero epileptico consilium* (11,357–78 K)	*Advice for an Epileptic Boy*	Temkin (1934 E)
Puls.	*De pulsibus ad tirones* (8,453–92 K)	*Pulses for Beginners*	Singer PN (1997 E)
[*Puls.Ant.*]	*De pulsibus ad Antonium* (19,629–42 K)	*Pulses, for Antonius*	
Purg.Med. Fac.	*De purgantium medicamentorum facultatibus* (11,323–42 K)	*The Property of Purgatives*	Ehlert (1960 Edn)
QAM	*Quod animi mores corporis temperamenta sequantur* (4,767–822 K)	*The Soul's Behaviour Depends on Bodily Mixtures*	Bazou (2011 Edn); Singer (PN 2013 E)
[*Qual.Incorp.*]	*De qualitatibus incorporeis* (19,463–84 K)	*Qualities are Non-corporeal*	Giusta (1976 Edn I)
[*Rem.*]	*De remediis parabilibus* (14,311–581 K)	*Readily Available Remedies*	
[*Ren.Aff.*]	*De renum affectibus*	*Affections of the Kidneys*	
San.Tu.	*De sanitate tuenda* (6,1–452 K)	*Hygiene*	Koch (*CMG* 1923 Edn); Johnston (2018 E)
Sect.	*De sectis ad eos qui introducuntur* (1,64–105 K)	*Sects*	Helmreich (1893 Edn); Walzer and Frede (1985 E)

Abbreviation	*Latin title*	*English title*	*Editions and translations*
Sem.	*De semine* (4,512–651 K)	*Semen*	De Lacy (*CMG* 1992 Edn)
Sept.Part.	*De septimestri partu* (not in Kühn)	*The Seven-month Child*	Schöne (1933 Edn G); Walzer (1935 Edn Arabic G)
Sim.Morb.	*Quomodo simulantes morbum deprehendendi* (19,1–17 K)	*How to Detect Malingerers*	Deichgräber and Kudlien (*CMG* 1960 Edn)
SMT	*De simplicium medicamentorum facultatibus* (11,379–892; 12,1–377 K)	*The Properties of Simple Drugs*	
Soph.	*De sophismatibus penes dictionem* (14,582–98 K)	*Linguistic Sophisms*	Edlow (1977 E); Ebbesen (1981 E)
Sub.Nat.Fac.	*De substantia facultatum naturalium* (4,757–66 K, part of *Prop.Plac.*)	*The Substance of the Natural Faculties*	[See *Prop.Plac.*]
Subf.Emp.	*Subfiguratio empirica* (not surviving in Greek)	*A Sketch of Empiricism*	Deichgräber (1965 Edn); Walzer and Frede (1985 E)
[*Suc.*]	*De succedaneis* (19,721–47 K)	*Substitute Drugs*	
Symp.Diff.	*De symptomatum differentiis* (7,721–47 K)	*The Distinct Types of Symptom*	Johnston (2006 E); Gundert (2009 Edn G)
Syn.Puls.	*Synopsis de pulsibus* (9,431–549 K)	*A Synopsis of the Pulse*	Gossen (1907 Edn)
Temp.	*De temperamentis* (1,509–694 K)	*Mixtures*	Helmreich (1904 Edn); Singer PN and van der Eijk (2018 E)
[*Ther. Pamph.*]	*De theriaca ad Pamphilanum* (14,295–310 K)	*Theriac, for Pamphilianus*	
[*Ther.Pis.*]	*De theriaca ad Pisonem* (14,211–294 K)	*Theriac, for Piso*	Leigh (2015 Edn E); Boudon-Millot (2016 Edn F)
Thras.	*Thrasybulus sive Utrum medicinae sit aut gymnasticae hygiene* (5,806–98 K)	*Thrasybulus, whether Hygiene Belongs to Medicine or Physical Training*	Helmreich (1893 Edn); Singer PN (1997 E); Johnston (2018 E)
Tot.Morb. Temp.	*De totius morbi temporibus* (7,440–62 K)	*Opportune Moments in Diseases as a Whole*	Wille (1960 Edn G)
Trem.Palp.	*De tremore, palpitatione, convulsione et rigore* (7,584–642 K)	*Tremor, Spasm, Convulsion, and Shivering*	Sider and McVaugh (1979 E)
Tum.Pr.Nat.	*De tumoribus praeter naturam* (7,705–32 K)	*Unnatural Swellings*	Reedy (1968 Edn E); Lytton and Resuhr (1978 E)
Typ.	*De typis* (7,463–74 K)	*Types of Disease*	

(Continued)

(Cont.)

Abbreviation	*Latin title*	*English title*	*Editions and translations*
UP	*De usu partium* (3,1–939; 4,1–366 K)	*The Use of Parts of the Body*	Helmreich (1907–9 Edn); May (1968 E)
[*Ur.*]	*De urinis* (19,574–601 K)	*Urines*	
[*Ur.Comp.*]	*De urinis compendium* (19,602–8 K)	*A Synopsis of Urines*	
[*Ur.Comp. Gal.*]	*De urinis ex Hippocrate, Galeno* (19,609–28 K)	*A Synopsis of Urines, according to Hippocrates, Galen*	
Us.Puls.	*De usu pulsuum* (5,149–80 K)	*The Use of the Pulse*	Furley and Wilkie (1984 Edn E)
Us.Resp.	*De usu respirationis* (4,470–511 K)	*The Use of Breathing*	Furley and Wilkie (1984 Edn E)
Ut.Diss.	*De uteri dissectione* (2,887–908 K)	*The Anatomy of the Womb*	Goss (1962 E): Nickel (*CMG* 1971 Edn G)
[*Ven.*]	*De venereis* (19,911–4 K)	*Sexual Activity*	
Ven.Art.Diss.	*De venarum arteriarumque dissectione* (2,779–830 K)	*The Anatomy of Veins and Arteries*	Goss (1961 E); Garofalo and Debru (2008 Edn F)
[*Ven.Sect.*]	*De venae sectione* (19,519–28 K)	*Bloodletting*	
Ven.Sect.Er.	*De venae sectione adversus Erasistratum* (11,147–86 K)	*Bloodletting, against Erasistratus*	Brain (1986 E)
Ven.Sect.Er. Rom.	*De venae sectione adversus Erasistrateos Romae degentes* (11,187–249 K)	*Bloodletting, against the Erasistrateans in Rome*	Kotrc (1970 Edn E); Brain (1986 E)
Vict.Att.	*De victu attenuante* (not in Kühn)	*The Thinning Diet*	Kalbfleisch (*CMG* 1923 Edn); Marinone (1973 Edn); Singer PN (1997 E)
[*Virt. Cent.*]	*De virtutibus centaureae* (not surviving in Greek)	*The Properties of the Centaury*	Nutton (2015 Edn L E)
Voc.	*De voce* (fragments)	*The Voice*	Baumgarten (1962 Edn L G); Nutton (forthcoming Edn L E)

Bibliography

1 CMG editions of Galen

CMG V 1,1. Barigazzi, A. (1991) *Galeni de optimo docendi genere; Exhortatio ad medicinam (Protrepticus)*. Berlin: Akademie Verlag.

CMG V 1,2. DeLacy, P.H. (1994) *Galeni De elementis ex Hippocratis sententia*. Berlin: Akademie Verlag.

CMG V 1,5. Fortuna, S. (1997) *Galeni De constitutione artis medicae ad Patrophilum*. Berlin: Akademie Verlag.

CMG V 2,1. Nickel, D. (1971) *Galeni De uteri dissectione*. Berlin: Akademie Verlag.

CMG V 3,1. DeLacy, P.H. (1992) *Galeni De semine*. Berlin: Akademie Verlag.

CMG V 3,2. Nutton, V. (1999) *Galeni De propriis placitis*. Berlin: Akademie Verlag.

CMG V 3,3. Nickel, D. (2001) *Galeni De foetuum formatione*. Berlin: Akademie Verlag.

CMG V 4,1,1. De Boer, W. (1937) *Galeni De propriorum animi cuiuslibet affectuum dignotione et curatione; De propriorum animi cuiuslibet peccatorum dignotione et curatione; De atra bile*. Leipzig and Berlin: Teubner.

CMG V 4,1,2. DeLacy, P.H. (1978–84) *Galeni De placitis Hippocratis et Platonis*. Berlin: Akademie Verlag.

CMG V 4,2. Koch, K. (1923) *Galeni de sanitate tuenda*; Helmreich, G. *Galeni De alimentorum facultatibus libri III. De bonis malisque succis*; Kalbfleisch, K. *De victu attenuante*; Hartlich, O. *Galeni de ptisana*. Leipzig and Berlin: Teubner.

CMG V 5,1. Gundert, B. (2009) *Galeni De symptomatum differentiis*. Berlin: Akademie Verlag.

CMG V 6,1,1. Gärtner, F. (2015) *Galeni De locis affectis* I–II. Berlin: De Gruyter Akademie Forschung.

CMG V 8,1. Nutton, V. (1979) *Gale De praecognitione*. Berlin: Akademie Verlag.

CMG V 9,2. Diels, H. (1915) *Galeni in Hippocratis Prorrheticum I commentaria* III; Mewaldt, J. *Galeni De comate secundum Hippocratem*; Heeg, J *Galeni In Hippocratis Prognosticum commentaria* III. Leipzig and Berlin: Teubner.

CMG V 10,1. Wenkebach, E. (1934) *Galeni in Hippocratis Epidemiarum librum I commentaria* III; Pfaff, F. *Galeni in Hippocratis Epidemiarum librum II commentaria V*. Leipzig and Berlin: Teubner.

CMG V 10 2,1. Wenkebach, E. (1936) *Galeni in Hippocratis Epidemiarum librum III commentaria III*. Leipzig and Berlin: Teubner.

CMG V 10 2,2. Wenkebach, E. and Pfaff, F. (1956) *Galeni in Hippocratis Epidemiarum librum VI commentaria* I–VIII. Berlin: Akademie Verlag.

CMG V 10 2,3. Wenkebach, E. (1951) *Galeni adversus Lycum et adversus Iulianum*. Berlin: Akademie Verlag.

CMG V 10 2,4. Deichgräber, K. and Kudlien, F. (1960) *Die als sogenannte Simulantenschrift überlieferten Stücken des 2. Kommentars zu Epidemien II*. Berlin and Leipzig: Teubner.

CMG XI 2,1 Bergsträsser, G. (1914) *Pseudogaleni in Hippocratis de septimanis commentarium*.

CMG V 13,1. Perilli, L. (2017) *Galeni vocum Hippocratis glossarium*. Berlin: De Gruyter Akademie Forschung.

CMG Suppl. I. Schröder, H.O. (1934) *Galeni In Platonis Timaeum commentarii fragmenta*. Leipzig and Berlin: Teubner.

CMG Suppl. II. Bardong, K. (1937) *Galeni De causis procatarcticis*. Leipzig and Berlin: Teubner.

CMG Suppl. III. Schmutte, J.M. and Pfaff, E. (1941) *Galeni De consuetudinibus*. Berlin and Leipzig: Teubner.

CMG Suppl. V. Kollesch, J. (1964) *Galeni de instrumento odoratus*. Berlin: Akademie Verlag.

CMG Suppl. Or. I. Lyons, M.C. (1963) *Galeni in Hippocratis De officina medici commentariorum versio arabica.*. Berlin: Akademie Verlag.

CMG Suppl. Or. II. Kollesch, J., Nickel, D., and Strohmaier, G. (1969) *Galeni De partibus artis medicativae; De causis contentivis; libellorum versiones latinae*; Lyons, M.C. *Galeni De partibus artis medicativae; De causis contentivis.De diaeta in morbis acutis secundum Hippocratem libellorum versiones arabica*. Berlin: Akademie Verlag.

CMG Suppl. Or. III. Strohmaier, G. (1970) *Galeni De partium homoeomerium differentia*. Berlin: Akademie-Verlag.

CMG Suppl Or. IV. Iskandar, A.Z. (1988) *Galeni de optimo medico cognoscendo*. Berlin: Akademie Verlag.

CMG Suppl. Or. V 1. Vagelpohl, U. (2014) *Galeni In Hippocratis Epidemiarum librum I commentaria I-III*. Berlin: De Gruyter Akademie Forschung.

CMG Suppl. Or. V 2. Vagelpohl, U. and Swain, S. (2016) *Galeni In Hippocratis Epidemiarum librum II commentaria I–VI*. Berlin: De Gruyter Akademie Forschung.

II Secondary literature, including non-CMG editions and translations

Adamson, P., Hansberger, R., and Wilberding, J. (eds) (2014) *Philosophical Themes in Galen. Bulletin of the Institute of Classical Studies, Supplement* 114. London: Institute of Classical Studies.

Adelmann, H. (1966) *Marcello Malpighi and the Evolution of Embryology*. Ithaca, NY: Cornell University Press.

Afif, N., Bhayro, S., Pormann, P., Sellers, W., and Smelova, N. (2018) On Digamma and the Armenian Earth. *Le Muséon* 131(3–4): 391–414.

Albrecht, F. (1911) *Galeni Libellus An in arteriis natura sanguis contineatur*. Dissertation, University of Marburg.

Alessandrino, G. (1548) *Galeni enantiomaton aliquot liber*. Venice: Apud Iuntas.

Alessi, R. (2019) The Reception of Galen in Ibn Abī Uṣaybi'ah. In Bouras-Vallianatos and Zipser (eds): 279–303.

Alexanderson, B. (1967) *Galenos ΠΕΡΙ ΚΡΙΣΕΩΝ.Überlieferung und Text. Studia Graeca et Latina Gothoburgensia* 13. Gothenburg: Acta Universitatis.

Alexandru, S. (2011) Newly Discovered Witnesses Asserting Galen's Affiliation to the *gens Claudia*. *Annali della Scuola Normale Superiore di Pisa, ser*. 5, 3/2: 385–433.

Amari, M. (1897) Sul supposto sepolcro di Galeno alla Cannita. *Archivio storico Siciliano*, n.s. 11: 427–439.

Amat, J.C. (1623) *Fructus medicinae ex variis Galeni locis decerpti*. Lyons: L. Prost.

Andorlini, I. (2017) *πολλὰ ατρῶν ἐστι συγγράμματα. Scritti sui papiri e la medicina antica*. Milan: Mondadori.

André, J.M. (1985) *Les noms de plantes dans la Rome antique*. Paris: Les Belles Lettres.

Andrei, O. (1984) *A. Claudius Charax di Pergamo: interessi antiquari e antichità cittadine nell'età degli Antonini*. Bologna: Patron.

Arbenz, E. (ed.) (1891) *Die Vadianische Briefsammlung der Stadtbibliothek St. Gallen, II, Mitteilungen zur vaterländische Geschichte* 25.2. St. Gallen: Huber & Cie.

Arcangeli, A. and Nutton, V. (eds) (2008) *Girolamo Mercuriale. Medicina e cultura nell'Europa del Cinquecento*. Florence: Leo S. Olschki.

Arnott, W.G. (2007) *Birds in the Ancient World from A to Z*. London and New York, NY: Routledge.

Asper, M. (2005) Un personaggio in cerca di lettore: Galens *Grosser Puls* und die "Erfindung" des Lesers. In Fögen, T. (ed.) *Ancient Technical Texts*. Berlin and New York, NY: W. de Gruyter: 21–39.

Bailey, A. (2002) *Sextus Empiricus and Pyrrhonean Scepticism*. Oxford: Clarendon Press.

Baker, T. (2016) Why All This Jelly? Jacopo Zabarella and Hieronymus Fabricius ab Aquapendente on the Usefulness of the Vitreous Humour. In Goldberg, B., Ragland, E.R., and Distelzweig, P. (eds) *Early Modern Medicine and Natural Philosophy*. Dordrecht, Heidelberg, New York, and London: Springer: 59–88.

Baldwin, B. (1973) *Studies in Lucian*. Toronto: Hakkert.

Baldwin, B. (1975) The Career of Oribasius. *Acta Classica* 18: 85–97.

Barbier de Meynard, C. (1861–77) *Al-Mas'ūdī, Les prairies d'or*. Paris: Imprimerie Nationale.

Barnes, J. (1991) Galen on Logic and Therapy. In Kudlien and Durling (eds): 50–102.

Barnes, J. (1997) Logique et pharmacologie. À propos de quelques remarques d'ordre linguistique dans le *De simplicium medicamentorum temperamentis ac facultatibus* de Galien. In Debru (ed.): 3–34.

Barnes, J. (2002) Galen, Christians, Logic. In Wiseman, T.P. (ed.) *Classics in Progress: Essays in Ancient Greece and Rome*. Oxford: Oxford University Press: 399–419.

Barnes, J. (2003) Proofs and Syllogisms in Galen. In Barnes *et al.* (eds): 1–24.

Barnes, J., Jouanna, J., and Barras, V. (eds) (2003) *Galien et la philosophie*. Vandoeuvres: Fondation Hardt.

Bartels, E.M., Swaddling, J., and Harrison A.P. (2006) An Ancient Greek Pain Remedy for Athletes. *Pain Practice* 6(3): 212–218.

Barton, T.S. (1994) *Power and Knowledge. Astrology, Medicine and Physiognomics under the Roman Empire*. Ann Arbor, MI: University of Michigan Press.

Baumgarten, H. (1962) *Über die Stimme*. Göttingen: University of Göttingen.

Baykan, D. (2012) *Allianoi Tip Aletler*. Istanbul: Institutum Turcicum.

Bazou, A. (2011) *Ὅτι ταῖς τοῦ σώματος κράσεσιν αἱ τῆς ψυχῆς δυνάμεις ἕπονται,*. Athens: University of Athens.

Beccaria, A. (1971) Sulle tracce di un antico canone latino di Ippocrate e Galeno. *Italia medioevale e umanistica* 14: 1–24.

Belloni, L. (1984) Die Zunft der Mailänder Apotheker und das Glasfenster vom heiligen Johannes dem Damazener im Dom von Mailand. In Baur, O. and Glandien, O. (eds) *Zusammenhang. Festschrift für Marielene Putscher*. Cologne: Wienand Verlag: 177–188.

Benedetti, A. (1503) *Historia corporis sive Anatomice*. Venice: B. Guerraldo.

Benedetti, A. (ed. Ferrari, G.) (1998) *Alessandro Benedetti, Historia corporis sive Anatomice*. Florence: Giunti.

Benedum, J. (1971) Statilios Attalos. *Medizinhistorisches Journal* 6: 264–277.

Berengario da Carpi, J. (1521) *Commentaria…super Anatomia Mundini*. Bologna: H. de Benedictis.

Berengario da Carpi, J. (1522) *Isagogae breves…in anatomiam humani corporis*. Bologna: H. de Benedictis,

Berengario da Carpi, J. (tr. Lind, L.R.) (1959) *A Short Introduction to Anatomy*. Chicago, IL: Chicago University Press.

Bergsträsser, G. (1925) *Hunain ibn Ishaq, über die syrischen und arabischen Galen-Übersetzungen, Abhandlungen für die Kunde des Morgenlandes* 17, 2.

Bergsträsser, G. (1932) *Neue Materialien zu Hunain Ibn Ishaq's Galen-bibliographie, Abhandlungen für die Kunde des Morgenlandes* 19, 2.

Bhayro, S. (2017) Galen in Syriac: Rethinking Old Assumptions. *Aramaic Studies* 15: 132–154.

Bhayro, S. (2019) The Reception of Galen in the Syriac Tradition. In Bouras-Vallianatos and Zipser (eds): 163–178.

Bigotti, F. (2019) *Physiology of the Soul. Mind, Body and Matter in the Galenic Tradition of the Late Renaissance (1550–1630). The Age of Descartes/Descartes et son temps* 3. Turnhout: Brepols.

Boatwright, M.T. (2000) *Hadrian and the Cities of the Roman Empire.* Princeton, NJ: Princeton University Press.

Bobzien, S. (2002) Pre-Stoic Hypothetical Syllogistic in Galen's *Institutio Logica.* In Nutton (ed.): 57–72.

Bos, G., McVaugh, M., and Shatzmiller, J. (2014) Transmitting a Text through Three Languages; the Future History of Galen's *Peri Anomalou Dyskrasias. Transactions of the American Philosophical Society* 104, part 5.

Boudon, V. (1994) Les oeuvres de Galien pour les débutants. In *ANRW* II,37,2: 1421–1467.

Boudon, V. (2000) *Galien*, Tome II, *Exhortation à l'étude de la médecine.* Paris: Les Belles Lettres.

Boudon-Millot, V. (2007), *Galien*, Tome I, *Introduction générale. Sur l'ordre de ses propres livres. Sur ses propres livres. Que l'excellent médecin est aussi philosophe.* Paris: Les Belles Lettres.

Boudon-Millot, V. (2012) *Galien de Pergame, un médecin grec à Rome.* Paris: Les Belles Lettres.

Boudon-Millot, V. (2013) What is a Mental Illness and How can it be Treated? Galen's Reply as a Doctor and Philosopher. In Harris, W.V. (ed.): 129–146.

Boudon-Millot, V. (2015) Mystère autour d'une petite balle: à quel jeu jouaient Galien et Marc Aurèle? *Galenos* 9: 37–56.

Boudon-Millot, V. (2016a) *Galien, Tome VI. Thériaque à Pison.* Paris: Les Belles Lettres.

Boudon-Millot, V. (2016b) Vésale lecteur de Galien et d'Hippocrate. In Vons, J. (ed.), *La Fabrique de Vésale.* Paris: Bibliothèque universitaire de Santé: 11–26.

Boudon-Millot, V. (2016c) Aelius Aristide et Galien: regards croisés de l'orateur et du médecin sur la maladie. In Pernot, L., Abbamonte, G., and Lamagna, M. (eds). *Aelius Aristide écrivain.* Tournai: Brepols: 393–414.

Boudon-Millot, V. (2018) Galen's Hippocrates. In Pormann, P.E. (ed.) *The Cambridge Companion to Hippocrates.* Cambridge: Cambridge University Press: 292–314.

Boudon-Millot, V. (2019) Galien de Pergame ou le médecin qui voulait se faire philosophe. In Crignon and Lefebvre (eds): 109–128.

Boudon-Millot, V., Cobolet, G., and Jouanna, J. (eds) (2012) *René Chartier (1572–1654), éditeur et traducteur d'Hippocrate et de Galien. Actes du colloque de Paris (7–8 octobre 2011).* Paris: De Boccard.

Boudon-Millot, V., Jouanna, J., and Pietrobelli, A. (2010) *Galien*, Tome IV, *Ne pas se chagriner.* Paris: Les Belles Lettres.

Boudon-Millot, V. and Pietrobelli, A. (2005) Galien ressuscité: édition princeps du texte grec du *De propriis placitis. Revue des Études grecques* 118: 168–213.

Boudreaux, P. (1912) *Catalogus codicum astrologorum graecorum, pars tertia*, Tome VIII,3. Brussels: H. Lamertin.

Boulogne, J. and Drizenko, A. (eds) (2006) *L'enseignement de la médecine chez Galien. Collections UL3; Travaux et Recherches.* Lille: Éditions du Conseil Scientifique de l'Université Charles de Gaulle – Lille 3.

Bouras-Vallianatos, P. (2019a) Galen in Late-Antique Medical Handbooks. In Bouras-Vallianatos and Zipser (eds): 38–62.

Bouras-Vallianatos, P. (2019b) Galen in Byzantine Medical Literature. In Bouras-Vallaniatos and Zipser (eds): 86–110.

Bouras-Vallianatos, P. and Xenofontos, S. (2015) Galen's Reception in Byzantium: Symeon Seth and his Refutation of Galenic Theories on Human Physiology. *Greek, Roman, and Byzantine Studies* 55: 431–469.

Bouras-Vallianatos, P. and Zipser, B. (eds) (2019) *Brill's Companion to the Reception of Galen.* Leiden and Boston, MA: Brill.

Bouyges, M. (1927) *Al-Ghazzālī, Tahāfut al-Falāsifat*. Beirut: Imprimerie catholique.
Bowersock, G.W. (1969) *Greek Sophists in the Roman Empire*. Oxford: Clarendon Press.
Brain, P. (1986) *Galen on Bloodletting*. Cambridge: Cambridge University Press.
Broadbent, W.H. (1890) *The Pulse*. London: Cassell.
Brock, A.J. (1929) *Greek Medicine*. London and Toronto: J.M. Dent and Sons.
Brockman, C., Brunschön, C.E.W., and Overwien, O. (eds) (2009) *Antike Medizin im Schnittpunkt von Geistes- und Naturwissenschaften. Internationale Fachtagung aus Anlass des 100-Jährigen Bestehens des Akademievorhabens "Corpus Medicorum Graecorum/Latinorum"*. Berlin: W. de Gruyter.
Broman, T.W. (1996) *The Transformation of German Academic Medicine, 1750–1820*. Cambridge: Cambridge University Press.
Burnyeat, M.W. (1997) Postscript on Silent Reading. *Classical Quarterly* 47: 74–76.
Caballero Navas, C. (2019) The Reception of Galen in Hebrew Medieval Scientific Writing. In Bouras-Vallianatos and Zipser (eds): 537–558.
Canalis, F.R. and Ciavolella, M. (eds) *Andreas Vesalius and the Fabrica in the Age of Printing. Art, Anatomy, and Printing in the Italian Renaissance*. Turnhout: Brepols.
Caplan, J.J., McCartney, J., and Sisti, D.A. (eds) (2004) *Health, Disease and Illness. Concepts in Medicine*. Ashington, DC: Georgetown University Press.
Carlino, A. (1999) *Books of the Body: Anatomical Ritual and Renaissance Learning*. Chicago, IL: Chicago University Press.
Carroll, M. (2018) *Infancy and Earliest Childhood in the Roman World*. Oxford: Oxford University Press.
Carter, K.C. (2017) *The Decline of Therapeutic Bloodletting and the Collapse of Traditional Medicine*. London: Routledge.
Cassia, M. (2012) *Andromaco di Creta. Medicina e potere nella Roma neroniana*. Acireale and Rome: Bonanno editore.
Chandelier, J. (2019) Médecine et philosophie selon Averroès. In Crignon and Lefebvre (eds): 171–196.
Chaniotis, A. (1999) Milking the Mountains. Economic Activities and the Cretan Uplands in the Classical and Hellenistic Period. In Chaniotis, A. (ed.) *From Minoan Farmers to Roman Traders. Sidelights on the Economy of Ancient Crete*. Stuttgart: Steiner: 181–220
Chaniotis, A. (2004) Epigraphic Evidence for the Philosopher Alexander of Aphrodisias. *Bulletin of the Institute of Classical Studies* 47: 79–81.
Chiaradonna, R. (2009a) Le traité de Galien Sur la démonstration et sa postérité tardo-antique. *Philosophia Antiqua* 1: 43–77.
Chiaradonna, R. (2009b) Galen and Middle Platonism. In Gill *et al.* (eds):243–268.
Chiaradonna, R. (2014) Galen on What is Persuasive (pithanon) and What Approximates to Truth. In Adamson *et al.* (eds): 61–88.
Chiaradonna, R. (2019) Langage ordinaire et connaissance médicale selon Galien. In Crignon and Lefebvre (eds): 129–168.
Christol, M. and Drew-Bear, T. (2004) Caracalla et son médecin L. Gellius Maximus à Antioche de Pisidie. In Colvin, S. (ed.) *The Greco-Roman East: Politics, Culture, Society*. New Haven, CT: Yale University Press: 85–118.
Clark, Sir G. (1964) *A History of the Royal College of Physicians*. Oxford: Clarendon Press, for the Royal College of Physicians.
Clifton, F. (1732) *The State of Physick, Ancient and Modern, Briefly Consider'd: with a Plan for the Improvement of it*. London: J. Nourse.
Coarelli, F. (2016) *Pergamo e il Re: Forma e funzioni di una capitale ellenistica*. Pisa and Rome: F. Serra.
Coker, A. (2019) Galen and the Language of Old Comedy: Glimpses of a Lost Treatise at *Ind. 23b-68*. In Petit (ed.): 63–90.
Cooper, G.M. (2011a) Galen and Astrology: A Mésalliance. *Early Science and Medicine* 16: 120–146.

Cooper, G.M. (2011b) *Galen, De diebus decretoriis, from Greek into Arabic.* Farnham and Burlington, VT: Ashgate.

Cooper, G.M. (2019) Ḥunayn Ibn Isḥāq and the Creation of an Arabic Galen. In Bouras-Vallianatos and Zipser (eds): 179–195.

Copenhaver, B.P. (1978) *Symphorien Champier and the Reception of the Occultist Tradition in France.* The Hague and New York, NY: Mouton.

Coqueugniot, G. (2013) Where was the Royal Library of Pergamum? An Institution Found and Lost Again. In König *et al.*(eds): 109–123.

Cosans, C.E. (1998) The Experimental Foundations of Galen's Teleology. *Studies in the History and Philosophy of Science* 29(1): 63–80.

Craik, E.M. (2015) *The 'Hippocratic' Corpus. Content and Context.* London and New York, NY: Routledge.

Crignon, C. and Lefebvre, D. (eds) (2019) *Médecins et philosophes. Une histoire.* Paris: CNRS Éditions.

Cronier, M., Guardasole, A., Magdelaine, C., and Pietrobelli, A. (2015) Galien en procès à Byzance. L'Antirrhétique de Syméon Seth. *Galenos* 9: 71–121.

Curry, A. (2008) The Gladiator Diet. *Archaeology* 61(6): 28–30.

Dandrey, P. (1998) *La médecine et la maladie dans le théâtre de Molière.* Paris: Klingsieck.

Dandrey, P. (2006) *Monsieur de Pourceaugnac ou le carnaval des fourbes.* Paris: Klingsieck.

Daremberg, C.D. (1854–56) *Œuvres anatomiques, physiologiques et médicales de Galien*, 2 vols. Paris: Baillière.

Das, A.R. (2014) Re-evaluating the Authenticity of the Fragments from Galen's On the Medical Statements in Plato's Timaeus (Scorialensis Graec. Φ-III-11, ff. 123r–126v). *Zeitschrift für Papyrologie und Epigraphik* 192: 93–103.

Das, A.R. (2018) New Materials from Galen's On the Authentic and Spurious Works of Hippocrates. *Classical Philology* 113: 305–329.

Das, A.R. (2019) Probable New Fragments and a Testimonium from Galen's Commentary on Plato's Timaeus. *Classical Quarterly* 69: 384–401.

Davies, D. (2013) Character Traits. In Singer, P.N. (ed.): 107–201.

Debru, A. (1994) L'Expérimentation chez Galien. *ANRW*, II, 37, 2: 1718–1756.

Debru, A. (1995a) Les démonstrations médicales à Rome au temps de Galien. In van der Eijk *et al.* (eds): 69–82.

Debru, A. (1995b) L'ordre de formation des organes embryonnaires: la retractio de Galien. *Bulletin d'Histoire et d'Epistémologie des Sciences de la Vie* 2: 156–163.

Debru, A. (ed.) (1997) *Galen on Pharmacology. Philosophy, History and Medicine.* Leiden: Brill.

Debru, A. (1999) Doctrine et tactique doxographique dans *l'*Anonyme de Bruxelles: une comparaison avec *l'*Anonyme de Londres. In van der Eijk (ed.): 453–472.

Debru, A. (2008a) Physiology. In Hankinson (ed.): 263–282.

Debru, A. (2008b) Les enseignements de la torpille dans la médecine antique. In Boehm, I. and Luccioni, P. (eds) *Le Médecin initié par l'animal. Animaux et médecine dans l'Antiquité grecque et latine.* Lyon: Maison de l'Orient et de la Méditerranée: 39–47.

De Carolis, S. (ed.) (2009) *Ars medica. I ferri del mestiere. La domus 'del Chirurgo' di Rimini e la chirurgia nell'antica Roma.* Rimini: Guaraldi.

Degni, P. (2019) Textual Transmission of Galen in Byzantium. In Bouras-Vallianatos and Zipser (eds): 124–139.

De Goeje, M.J. (1870) *Al-Istakhri, Viae regnorum: descriptio ditionis Moslemicae*, Bibliotheca geographicorum arabicorum I. Leiden: E. J. Brill.

Deichgräber, K. (1950) Professio medici. Zum Vorwort des Scribonius Largus. *Abhandlungen der Akademie der Wissenschaften in Mainz.* Mainz: Steiner.

Deichgräber, K. (1956) Parabasenverse aus Thesmophoriazusen II des Aristophanes bei Galen. *Sitzungsberichte der deutschen Akademie der Wissenschaften zu Berlin.*

Deichgräber, K. (1957) Galen als Erforscher des menschlichen Pulses: ein Beitrag zur Selbstdarstellung des Wissenschaftlers (De dignotione pulsuum I 1). *Sitzungsberichte der Deutschen Akadademie der Wissenschaften zu Berlin.*

Deichgräber, K. (1965) *Die griechische Empirikerschule*, ed. 2. Berlin and Zurich: Weidmann.

Deichgräber, K. (1970) Medicus gratiosus. *Abhandlungen der Akademie der Wissenschaften in Mainz*. Mainz: Steiner.

Deichgräber, K. (1971) Aretaeus von Kappadokien als medizinischer Schriftsteller. *Abhandlungen der sächsichen Akademie der Wissenschaften* 63(3).

Deichgräber, K. (1976) Ausgewähltes aus der medizinischen Literatur der Antike, I. *Philologus* 101: 135–147.

DeLacy, P.H. (1988) The Third Part of the Soul. In Manuli and Vegetti (eds): 43–63.

Delehaye, H. (1909) *Les légendes grecques des saints militaires.* Paris: Alphonse Picard et Fils.

Desideri, P. (2000) Galeno come intellettuale. In Manetti, D. (ed.) *Studi su Galeno. Scienza, filosofia, retorica e filologia. Atti del seminario, Firenze, 13 novembre 1998*. Florence: Università degli studi, Dipartimento di scienze dell'antichità 'Giorgio Pasquale'.

Diels, H. (1879) *Doxographici Graeci.* Berlin: Weidmann.

Dillon, J. (1993) *Alcinous. The Handbook of Platonism.* Oxford: Clarendon Press.

Dillon, J. and Long, A.A. (eds) (1985) *The Question of 'Eclecticism'. Studies in Later Greek Philosophy.* Berkeley, CA: University of California Press.

Dols, M. (1992) *Majnun: The Madman in Medieval Islamic Society.* Oxford: Clarendon Press.

Donato, M.P. (2019) Galen in an Age of Change (1650–1820). In Bouras-Vallianatos and Zipser (eds): 487–507.

Donini, P.L. (1985) The History of the Concept of Eclecticism. In Dillon and Long (eds): 15–33.

Donini, P.L. (1992) Galeno e la filosofia. *ANRW* II,36,5: 3484–3504.

Donini, P.L. (2008) Psychology. In Hankinson (ed.): 184–209.

Duckworth, W.L.H., Lyons, M.C., and Towers, B. (1962) *Galen on Anatomical Procedures. The Later Books.* Cambridge: Cambridge University Press.

Duffy, J.M. (1984) Byzantine Medicine in the Sixth and Seventh Centuries: Aspects of Teaching and Practice. *Dumbarton Oaks Papers* 38: 21–27.

Duncan-Jones, R.P. (2018) The Antonine Plague Revisited. *Arctos* 52: 41–72.

Dunkle, R. (2013) *Gladiators: Violence and Spectacle in Ancient Rome.* London: Routledge.

Durling R J (1961) A Chronological Census of Renaissance Editions and Translations of Galen. *Journal of the Warburg and Courtauld Institutes* 24: 230–305.

Ebbesen, S. (1981) *Commentators and Commentators on Aristotle's Sophistici Elenchi.* Leiden: Brill.

Edelstein, E.J. and Edelstein, L. (1945) *Asclepius. Collection and Interpretation of the Testimonies.* Baltimore, MD: Johns Hopkins University Press.

Edelstein, L. (1967) *Ancient Medicine. Select Papers of Ludwig Edelstein.* Baltimore, MD: Johns Hopkins University Press.

Edlow, R.B. (1977) *Galen on Language and Ambiguity.* Leiden: Brill.

Edwards, C. and Woolf, G. (eds) (2003) *Rome the Cosmopolis.* Cambridge: Cambridge University Press.

Ehlert, J. (1960) *Galeni De purgantium medicamentorum facultate.* Göttingen: University of Göttingen.

El-Abbadi, M. (1992) *Life and Fate of the Ancient Library of Alexandria*, ed. 2. Alexandria: UNESCO.

Eriksson, R. (1959) *Andreas Vesalius' first Public Anatomy at Bologna 1540*. Uppsala and Stockholm: Almqvist and Wiksell.

Everett, A. (2012) The *Alphabet of Galen. Pharmacy from Antiquity to the Middle Ages.* Toronto, Buffalo, NY and London: University of Toronto Press.

Evershed, R. (2004) Roman Face Cream Reproduced. On-line at https://www.bristol.ac.uk/news/2004/590.html. Accessed on 11 July 2019.

Fabricius, C. (1972) *Galens Exzerpte aus älteren Pharmakologen*. Berlin: W. De Gruyter.

Fagan, G.G. (1999) *Bathing in Public in the Roman World.* Ann Arbor, MI: University of Michigan Press.

Fancy, N. (2019) Galen and Ibn al-Nafīs. In Bouras-Vallianatos and Zipser (eds): 263–278.

Fausti, D. (2017) Farmacologia e medicina popolare: un rapporto complesso. *Medicina nei Secoli* 29(3): 799–824.

Fazzo, S. (2002) Alexandre l'Aphrodise contre Galien: la naissance d'une légende. *Philosophie antique. Problèmes, renaissances, usages* 2: 109–144.

Feissel, D. (1999) Le Roufinion de Pergame au 6e siècle d'après un sceau nouvellement publié. *Revue des Études byzantines* 57: 263–270.

Ferrari, G. (1996) *L'esperienza del passato. Alessandro Benedetti filologo e medico umanista.* Florence: Leo S. Olschki.

Ferrari, G. (ed.) (1998) *Alessandro Benedetti, Historia corporis humani sive Anatomice.* Florence: Giunti.

Ferretto, S. (2012) *Maestri per il metodo di trattare le cose. Bassiano Landi, Giovan Battista da Monte e la scienza della medicina nel xvi secolo.* Padua: CLEUP.

Fischer, K.D. (2003) Galeni qui fertur ad Glauconem Liber tertius. In Garofalo and Roselli (eds): 101–132, 283–346.

Fischer, K.D. (2009) Galen, Pardalas and Sundry Delights for the Student of Ancient Greek Medicine. *Galenos* 3: 161–176.

Fischer, K.D., Nickel, D., and Potter, P. (eds) (1998) *Text and Tradition: Studies in Ancient Medicine and its Transmission Presented to Jutta Kollesch.* Leiden: Brill.

Flashar, H. (1966) *Melancholie und Melancholiker in den medizinischen Theorien der Antike.* Berlin: De Gruyter.

Flashar, H. and Jouanna, J. (eds) (1997) *Médecine et Morale dans l'Antiquité.* Vandoeuvres, Switzerland: Fondation Hardt.

Flemming, R. (2000) *Medicine and the Making of Roman Women.* Oxford: Oxford University Press.

Flemming, R. (2002) The Pathology of Pregnancy in Galen's Commentaries on the Epidemics. In Nutton (ed.): 101–112.

Flemming, R. (2007) Galen's Imperial Order of Knowledge. In König and Whitmarsh (eds): 241–277.

Flemming, R. (2008) Commentary. In Hankinson (ed.): 323–354.

Flemming, R. (2009) Demiurge and Emperor in Galen's World of Knowledge. In Gill *et al.* (eds): 59–84.

Flemming, R. (2017) Galen and the Christians. Texts and Authority in the Second Century AD. In Carleton Paget, J. and Lieu, J. (eds) *Christianity in the Second Century: Themes and Developments.* Cambridge: Cambridge University Press: 172–186.

Flemming, R. (2018) Galen's Generation of Seeds. In Hopwood, N., Flemming, R., and Kassell, L. (eds) *Reproduction. Antiquity to the Present Day.* Cambridge: Cambridge University Press: 95–108.

Flemming, R. (2019) Galen and the Plague. In Petit (ed.): 220–244.

Fogelmark, S. (2015) *The Kallierges Printer a Study in Renaissance Greek Scholarship and Printing.* Cologne: Jūrgen Dinter.

Forcada, M. (2019) The Reception of Galen after Avicenna (Eleventh-Twelfth Centuries). In Bouras-Vallianatos and Zipser (eds): 227–243.

Fortuna, S. (2005) Galeno latino, 1490–1533. *Medicina nei Secoli* 17: 469–505.

Fortuna, S. (2012) The Latin Editions of Galen's Opera omnia (1490–1625) and their Prefaces. *Early Science and Medicine* 17/4: 391–412.

Fortuna, S. (2019a) Editions and Translations of Galen from 1490–1540. In Bouras-Vallianatos and Zipser (eds): 432–452.

Fortuna, S. (2019b) Il Corpus delle traduzioni di Niccolò da Reggio (fl. 1308–1345). In *La medicina nel,basso medioevo. Tradizioni e conflitti. Atti del LV Convegno storico internazionale Todi, 14–16 ottobre 2018.* Spoleto: Centro italiano di studi sul alto medioevo: 285–312.

Fraser, P.M. (1969) The Career of Erasistratus of Ceos. *Rendiconti dell Istituto Lombardo, Classe di Lettere e Scienze Morali e Storiche* 103: 518–537.

Fraser, P.M. (1972) *Ptolemaic Alexandria*. Oxford: Clarendon Press.

Frede, M. (1981) On Galen's Epistemology. In Nutton 1981a (ed.): 65–86.

Frede, M. (1982) The Method of the so-called Methodical School of Medicine. In Barnes, J., Brunschwig, J., Burnyeat, M., and Schofield, M. (eds) *Science and Speculation*. Cambridge: Cambridge University Press: 1–23.

Frede, M. (1987) *Essays in Ancient Philosophy*. Oxford: Clarendon Press.

Frede, M. (2003) Galen's Theology. In Barnes *et al.* (eds): 73–126.

Frede, M. and Walzer, R. (1985) *Galen. Three Treatises on the Nature of Science*. Indianapolis, IN: Hackett.

French, R.K. (1979) De Juvamentis Membrorum and the Reception of Galenic Physiological Anatomy. *Isis* 70: 96–109.

French, R.K. (1994) *William Harvey's Natural Philosophy*. Cambridge: Cambridge University Press.

French, R.K. (1999) *Dissection and Vivisection in the European Renaissance*. Aldershot and Brookfield, VT: Ashgate.

Friedländer, L. (1862–71) *Darstellungen aus der Sittengeschichte Roms in der Zeit von August bis zum Ausgang der Antonine*. Leipzig: S. Hirzel.

Furley, D.J. and Wilkie, J.S. (1984) *Galen On Respiration and the Arteries*. Princeton, NJ: Princeton University Press.

García Ballester, L. (1972) *Galeno en la sociedad e la ciencia de su tiempo*. Madrid: Ediciones Guadarrama.

García Ballester, L. (1993) On the Origin of the "Six Non-natural Things" in Galen. In Kollesch and Nickel (eds): 105–115.

García Ballester, L. (1994) Galen as a Clinician: his Methods in Diagnosis. *ANRW* II,37,2: 1636–1672.

Garnsey, P.D.A. (1988) *Famine and Food Supply in the Graeco-Roman World: Responses to Risk and Crisis*. Cambridge: Cambridge University Press.

Garofalo, I. (1988) *Erasistrati Fragmenta*. Pisa: Giardini.

Garofalo, I. (1991) *Galeno, Procedimenti anatomici*. Milan: BUR.

Garofalo, I. (1994) La traduzione araba dei compendi alessandrini delle opere del canone di Galeno. Il compendio dell'Ad Glauconem. *Medicina nei Secoli* 6: 329–348.

Garofalo, I. (1999) Una nuova opera di Galeno in traduzione araba. *Studi classici e orientali* 47: 9–19.

Garofalo, I. (2019) Galen's Legacy in Alexandrian Texts written in Greek, Latin, and Arabic. In Bouras-Vallianatos and Zipser (eds): 62–85.

Garofalo, I. and Debru, A. (2005) *Galien, Tome VII. Les os pour les débutants. L'anatomie des muscles*. Paris: Les Belles Lettres.

Garofalo, I. and Debru, A. (2008) *Galien, Tome VIII. L'anatomie des nerfs. L'anatomie des artères*. Paris: Les Belles Lettres.

Garofalo, I. and Lami, I. (2012) *Galeno. L'anima e il dolore. De indolentia. De propriis placitis*. Milan: BUR.

Garofalo, I. and Roselli, A. (eds) (2003) *Galenismo e medicina tardoantica. Fonti greche, latine e arabe. Seminario internazionale di Siena, Certosa di Pontignano, 9 e 10 settembre, 2002*. Naples: Istituto universitario orientale.

Garrison, D. and Hast, M.H. (trans.) (2014) *Vesalius, the Fabric of the Human Body*. Basle: Karger.

Garzya, A. (ed.) (1996) *Storia e ecdotica dei testi medici greci*. Naples: M. D'Auria.

Garzya, A. and Jouanna, J. (eds) (1999) *I testi medici greci. Tradizione e ecdotica*. Naples: M. D'Auria.

Gavrilov, A.K. (1997) Techniques of Reading in Classical Antiquity. *Classical Quarterly* 47: 56–73.

Georges, T. (ed.) (2017) *Ephesos. Die antike Metropol im Spannungsfeld von Religion und Bildung*. Tübingen: Mohr Siebeck.

Gero, S. (1990) Galen on Jews and Christians. A Reappraisal of the Arabic Evidence. *Orientalia Christiana et Patristica* 56: 371–411.

Gessner, C. (1554) *Thesaurus Euonymi philiatri*. Zurich: A. Gesner.

Gill, C. (2010) *Naturalistic Psychology in Galen and Stoicism*. Oxford: Oxford University Press.

Gill, C. (2013) Philosophical Theory as Preventive Psychological Medicine. In Harris, W.V. (ed.): 339–360.

Gill, C., Whitmarsh, T., and Wilkins, J. (eds) (2009) *Galen and the World of Knowledge*. Cambridge: Cambridge University Press.

Giusta, M. (1976) *L'opusculo pseudogalenico ὅτι α ποιότητες ἀσώματοι*. Turin: Paravia.

Gleason, M.W. (2005) Greek Cities under Roman Rule. In Potter, D.S. (ed.) *Blackwell's Companion to the Roman Empire*. Oxford: Blackwell: 228–249.

Gleason, M.W. (2009) Shock and Awe: The Performance Dimension of Galen's Anatomical Demonstrations. In Gill *et al.* (eds): 85–114.

Gnudi, M.T. and Webster, J.P. (1950). *The Life and Times of Gaspare Tagliacozzi, Surgeon of Bologna 1545–1599*. New York, NY: Herbert Reichner.

Goltz, D. (1976) *Mittelalterliche Pharmazie und Medizin*. Stuttgart: Enke.

Goss, C.M. (1961) On the Anatomy of Veins and Arteries by Galen of Pergamos. *The Anatomical Record* 141: 355–366.

Goss, C.M. (1962) On the Anatomy of the Uterus. *The Anatomical Record* 144: 77–83.

Goss, C.M. (1963) On the Anatomy of Muscles for Beginners by Galen of Pergamon. *The Anatomical Record* 145: 477–501.

Goss, C.M. (1966) On the Anatomy of the Nerves by Galen of Pergamon. *American Journal of Anatomy* 118: 327.

Gossen, J. (1907) *De Galeni libro, qui Σύνοψις περ σφυγμῶν inscribitur*. Dissertation, University of Berlin.

Gourevitch, D. (2001) *I giovani pazienti di Galeno: per una patocenosi dell'impero romano*. Rome: Laterza.

Gourevitch, D. (2013) *Limos kai Loimos: A Study of the Galenic Plague*. Paris: De Boccard.

Gourevitch, D. (2016) Popular Medicines and Practices in Galen. In Harris, W.V. (ed.): 251–271.

Grant, M. (2000) *Galen on Food and Diet*. London: Routledge.

Grant, R.M. (1983) Paul, Galen and Origen. *Journal of Theological Studies* 34: 533–536.

Green, M.H. (2018) Richard de Fournival and the Reconfiguration of Learning in the mid-13th Century. In Ducos, J. and Lucken, C. (eds) *Richard de Fournival et les sciences au XIIIe siècle*. Florence: SISMEL: 179–206.

Green, M.H. (2019) Gloriosissimus Galienus: Galen and Galenic Writings in the Eleventh- and Twelfth-Century Latin West. In Bouras-Vallianatos and Zipser (eds): 319–342.

Green, R.M. (1951) *A Translation of Galen's Hygiene (De Sanitate tuenda)*. Springfield, IL: C. C. Thomas.

Grimaudo, S. (2004) La medicina ellenistica in Plutarco. In Gallo, I. (ed.) *La Biblioteca di Plutarco. Atti del IX. Convegno plutarcheo, Pavia, 13–15 giugno 2002*. Naples: M. D'Auria: 417–442.

Grimaudo, S. (2008) *Difendere la salute. Igiene e disciplina del soggetto nel De sanitate tuenda di Galeno*. Naples: Bibliopolis.

Grmek, M.D. and Gourevitch, D. (1988) L'École médicale de Quintus et de Numisianus. *Mémoires du Centre Jean Palerne* 8: 43–60.

Grmek, M.D. and Gourevitch, D. (1994) Aux Sources de la doctrine médicale de Galien: l'enseignement de Marinus, Quintus et Numisianus. *ANRW* II,37,2: 1491–1528.

Guardasole, A. (1997) *Eraclide di Taranto. Frammenti*. Naples: M. D'Auria.

Guardasole, A. (2014) Galen of Pergamum: A Witness of Scribonius Largus' Œuvre. In Maire, B. (ed.) *'Greek' and 'Roman' in Latin Medical Texts: Studies in Cultural Change and Exchange in Ancient Medicine*. Leiden and Boston, MA: Brill: 316–329.

Guardasole, A. (2015) Les extraits de Scribonius Largus transmis dans les traités de pharmacologie de Galien. *Semitica et Classica* 8: 73–88.

Guinter, J. (1571) *De medicina veteri et nova facienda*. Basle: ex off. Henricpetrina.

Gundert, B. (2006) Zu den Quellen der Basler Galen-Ausgabe (1538). In Müller, C.W., Brockmann, C., and Brunschön, W. (eds) *Ärzte und ihre Interpreten. Medizinische Fachtexte der Antike also Forschungsgegenstand der Klassischen Philologie. Fachconferenz zu Ehren von Diethard Nickel*. Munich and Leipzig: K.G. Saur: 81–100.

Gyekye, K. (1979) *Ibn al-Tayyib. Commentary on Porphyry's Eisagoge*. Albany, NY: S.U.N.Y. Press.

Habicht, C. (1969) *Die Inschriften des Asklepieions, Altertümer von Pergamon* VIII.3. Berlin: W. De Gruyter.

Hahn, J. (1989) *Der Philosoph und die Gesellschaft. Selbstverständnis, öffentliche und populäre Erwartungen in der hohen Kaiserzeit*. Stuttgart: Franz Steiner Verlag.

Hahn, J. (2011) Philosophy as Socio-political Upbringing. In Peachin, M. (ed.) *The Oxford Handbook of Social Relations in the Roman World*. Oxford: Oxford University Press: 119–143.

Hamarneh, S.K. (1997) *Yunani (unani), Arabic and Islamic Medicine and Pharmacy*. Karachi: Hamdard Foundation.

Hammerstaedt, J. and Smith, M.F. (2014) *The Epicurean Inscription of Diogenes of Oenoanda. Ten Years of New Discoveries and Research*. Bonn: Habelt Verlag.

Hammerstaedt, J. and Smith, M.F. (2018) Diogenes of Oinoanda: The New and Unexpected Discoveries of 2017 (NF 21–219), with a re-edition of fr. 70–72. *Epigraphica Anatolica* 51: 43–79.

Hands, M.W. (2013) Myth and History. Galen and the Alexandrian Library. In König *et al.* (eds): 364–376.

Hankinson, R.J. (1988) Galen Explains the Elephant. In Matthen, M. and Linsky, B. (eds) *Philosophy and Biology, Canadian Journal of Philosophy, Suppl.* 14: 135–157.

Hankinson, R.J. (1989) Galen and the Best of all Possible Worlds. *Classical Quarterly* 39: 206–227.

Hankinson, R.J. (1990) Saving the Phenomena. *Phronesis* 35: 195–215.

Hankinson, R.J. (1991a) *Galen On the Therapeutic Method, Books I and II*. Oxford: Clarendon Press.

Hankinson, R.J. (1991b) Galen's Anatomy of the Soul. *Phronesis* 36: 197–233.

Hankinson, R.J. (1992) Galen's Philosophical Eclecticism. *ANRW* II,36,5: 3505–3522.

Hankinson, R.J. (1998a) *Galen: On Antecedent Causes*. Cambridge: Cambridge University Press.

Hankinson, R.J. (1998b) *Cause and Explanation in Ancient Greek Thought*. Oxford: Clarendon Press.

Hankinson, R.J. (2003) Causation in Galen. In Barnes *et al.* (eds): 31–66.

Hankinson, R.J. (ed.) (2008a) *The Cambridge Companion to Galen*. Cambridge: Cambridge University Press.

Hankinson, R.J. (2008b) The Man and his Work. In Hankinson (ed.) 1–33.

Hankinson, R.J. (2008c) Epistemology. In Hankinson (ed.): 157–183.

Hankinson, R.J. (2008d) Philosophy of Nature. In Hankinson (ed.): 219 241.

Harig, G. (1974) *Bestimmung der Intensität im medizinischen System Galens*. Berlin: Akademie Verlag.

Harig, G. (1987–8) Zur Datierung der Reisen Galens. Ein Nachtrag. *Beiträge zur Hochschul- und Wissenschaftsgeschichte Erfurts* 21: 13–20.

Harris, C.R.S. (1973) *The Heart and the Vascular System in Ancient Greek Medicine*. Oxford: Clarendon Press.

Harris, W.V. (ed.) (2013) *Mental Disorders in the Classical World*. Leiden and New York, NY: Brill.

Harris, W.V. (ed.) (2016) *Popular Medicine in Graeco-Roman Antiquity: Explorations*. Leiden and Boston, MA: Brill.

Harris, W.V. (ed.) (2018) *Pain and Pleasure in Classical Times*. Leiden and Boston, MA: Brill.

Harris, W.V. and Ruffini, G. (eds) (2004) *Ancient Alexandria between Egypt and Greece*. Leiden and Boston, MA: Brill.

Hasluck, F.W. and Hasluck, M.M. (1929) *Christianity and Islam under the Sultans*. Oxford: Clarendon Press.

Havrda, M. (2011) Galenus Christianus ? The Doctrine of Demonstration in Stromata *VIII* and the Question of its Source. *Vigiliae Christianae* 65: 343–375.

Havrda, M. (2015) The Purpose of Galen's Treatise On Demonstration. *Early Science and Medicine* 20(3): 265–287.

Heilen, S. (2018) Galen's Computation of Medical Weeks: Textual Emendations, Interpretation, History, Rhetorical and Mathematical Examinations. *SCIAMUS* 19: 201–279.

Heitsch, E. (1964) Die griechischen Dichterfragmente der rőmischen Kaiserzeit. *Abhandlungen der Akademie der Wissenschaften zu Gőttingen, phil.-hist. Kl.* 58.

Helm, J. (2001) Religion and Medicine: Anatomical Education at Wittenberg and Ingolstadt. In Helm, J. and Winkelmann, A. (eds) *Confessions and the Sciences in the Sixteenth Century.* Leiden: Brill: 51–68.

Helmreich, G. (1893) *Claudii Galeni Pergameni Scripta Minora*, vol. III. Leipzig: Teubner.

Helmreich, G. (1901) *Galenus, De optima corporis constitutione. Idem de bono habitu.* Hof: kgl. Gymnasium.

Helmreich, G. (1904) *Galenus, De temperamentis.* Leipzig: Teubner.

Helmreich, G. (1907–9) *Galenus, De usu partium.* Leipzig: Teubner.

Hessus, E. (1533) *Bonae salutatis conservandae praecepta.* Paris: S. De Colines.

Hillert, A. (1990) *Antike Ārztedarstellungen.* Frankfurt: Peter Lang.

Hillgruber, M. (2010) Liebe, Weisheit und Verzicht. Zu Herkunft und Entwicklung der Geschichte von Antiochos und Stratonike. In Brüggemann, T., Meissner, B., Mileta, C., Pabst, A., and Schmitt, O. (eds) *Studia Hellenistica et Historiographica. Festschrift für Andreas Mehl.* Gutenberg: Computer Druck Satz und Verlag: 73–102.

Hirai, H. (forthcoming) Galen in Early Modern Debates. In Laskaris *et al.* (eds).

Hodge, A.T. (2002) *Roman Aqueducts and Water Supply*, ed. 2. (London: Duckworth).

Hoffmann, A. (1998) The Roman Remodelling of the Asklepieion. In Koester (ed.): 41–62.

Holmes, B. (2013) Disturbing Connections: Sympathetic Affections, Mental Disorders and the Elusive Soul in Galen. In Harris, W.V. (ed.): 147–176.

Hood, J. (2010) Galen's Aristotelian Definitions. In Charles, D. (ed.) *Definition in Greek Philosophy.* Oxford: Oxford University Press: 450–466.

Horstmanshoff, H.F.J. (1995) Galen and his Patients. In van der Eijk *et al.* (eds): 83–99.

Horstmanshoff, H.F.J. (ed.) (2010) *Hippocrates and Medical Education. Selected Papers presented at the XIIth International Hippocrates Colloquium, Universiteit Leiden, 24–26 August 2005.* Leiden and Boston, MA: Brill.

Hugonnard-Roche, H. (1989) Aux Origines de l'exégèse orientale de la logique d'Aristote: Sergius de Res'aina (+536), médecin et philosophe. *Journal Asiatique* 277: 1–17.

Hugonnard-Roche, H. (1997) Note sur Sergius de Res'aina, traducteur du grec en syriaque et commentateur d'Aristote. In Endress, G. and Kruk, R. (eds) *The Ancient Tradition in Christian and Islamic Hellenism: Studies on the Transmission of Greek Philosophy and Science Dedicated to H. J. Drossaert Lulofs.* Leiden: Brill: 121–143.

Hultsch, F. (1864) *Metrologicorum scriptorum reliquiae*, I. Leipzig: Teubner.

Ilberg, J. (1889–97) Über die Schriftstellerei des Klaudios Galenos. *Rheinisches Museum* 44: 207–239; 47: 489–514; 51: 165–196; 52: 591–562: repr. Darmstadt: Wissenschaftliche Buchgesellschaft (1974).

İplikçioğlu, B. (2014) Heraklit von Rhodiapolis, ein gefeierter Arzt der trajanischen Zeit. In Fischer, J. (ed.) *Der Beitrag Kleinasiens zur Kultur-und Geistesgeschichte der griechisch-römischen Antike, Denkschriften der österreichischen Akademie der Wissenschaften, philosophisch-historische Klasse* 469: 231–256.

Israelowich, U. (2012) *Society, Medicine and Religion in the Sacred Tales of Aelius Aristides.* Leiden and Boston, MA: Brill.

Jackson, D.F. (2012) Greek Medicine in the Fifteenth Century. *Early Science and Medicine* 17: 378–390.

Jackson, R. (2018) Les instruments de Galien. In Verbank Piérard *et al.* (eds): 128–147.

Jacquart, D. (1998) *La médecine médiévale dans le cadre parisien, xiv–xv siècle.* Paris: Fayard.

Jacques, J.M. (1996) La conservation du vin à Pergame au IIe siècle après J.-C. *Revue des Études anciennes* 98: 173–185.

Jacques, J.M. (1997) La méthode de Galien pharmacologue. In Debru (ed.): 103–132.

Jacques, J.M. (1999) Le manuscrit de Florence Laurentianus Gr. 74.5 et les écrits galéniques sur la thériaque et les antidotes. *Revue des Études anciennes* 101: 523–531.

Joffe, S.N. (2014) *Vesalius, the Making, the Madman and the Myth.* Bloomington, IN: AuthorHouse.

Johnston, I. (2006) *Galen, On Diseases and Symptoms.* Cambridge: Cambridge University Press.

Johnston, I. (2016) *Galen, On the Constitution of the Art of Medicine, The Art of Medicine, A Method of Medicine to Glaucon.* Cambridge, MA and London: Harvard University Press.

Johnston, I. (2018) *Galen, Hygiene, Thrasybulus, On the Small Ball.* Cambridge, MA and London: Harvard University Press.

Johnston, I. and Horsley, G.H.R. (2011) *Galen, Method of Medicine.* Cambridge, MA and London: Harvard University Press.

Jones, A. (2017) *A Portable Cosmos. Revealing the Antikythera Mechanism, Scientific Wonder of the Ancient World.* Oxford: Oxford University Press.

Jones, C.P. (1998) Aelius Aristides and the Asclepieion. In Koester (ed.): 63–76.

Jones, C.P. (2012) Galen's Travels. *Chiron* 42: 399–417.

Jouanna, J. (1997) La lecture de l'éthique hippocratique chez Galien. In Flashar, H. and Jouanna, J. (eds): 211–256.

Jouanna, J. (1999) *Hippocrates.* Baltimore, MD: Johns Hopkins University Press.

Jouanna, J. (2003) La notion de nature chez Galien. In Barnes *et al.* (eds): 229–268.

Jouanna, J. (2007) Un pseudo-Galien inédit: Le Pronostic sur l'homme. Contribution à l'histoire de la théorie quaternaire dans la médecine grecque tardive: l'insertion des quatre vents. In David, S. and Geny, D. (eds) *Troïka. Mélanges offerts à Michel Woronoff.* Besançon: Presses universitaires de Franche-Comté: I,303–322.

Jouanna, J. (2009) Bile noire et mélancholie chez Galien: le traité Sur la bile noire est-il authentique? In Brockmann *et al.* (eds): 235–257.

Jouanna, J. (2011) Médecine rationelle et magie: le statut des amulettes et des incantations chez Galien. *Revue des Etudes grecques* 124: 47–78.

Jouanna, J. (2013) *Hippocrate. Tome III. 1e partie, Pronostic.* Paris: Les Belles Lettres.

Jouanna, J. (2017) L'histoire textuelle du *Corpus Hippocratique. Journal des Savants* no. 2: 195–266.

Jouanna, J. (2018) *Hippocrate. Tome I. 2e partie, Le serment, Les serments chrétiens, La loi.* Paris: Les Belles Lettres.

Jouanna-Bouchet, J. (2016) *Scribonius Largus, Compositions médicales.* Paris: Les Belles Lettres.

Joubert, L. (1579) *Traité du ris.* Paris: N. Chesneau.

Kagan, J. (1994) *Galen's Prophecy. Temperament in Human Nature.* London: Free Association Books.

Kahl, O., with Bos, G. (2018) *'Ubaidallāh Ibn Buhtīšū' on Apparent Death. The Kitāb taḥrīm dafn al-aḥyā, Arabic Edition and English Translation.* Leiden: Brill.

Kaufman, D.H. (2015) Galen on the Therapy of Distress and the Limits of Emotional Therapy'. *Oxford Studies in Ancient Philosophy* 47: 275–296.

Kaufman, D.H. (forthcoming) Galen on Reason and Appetite: A Study of the De Moribus. *Apeiron.*

Kessel, G. (2019) Syriac Medicine. In King, D. (ed.) *The Syriac World.* London and New York, NY: Routledge: 438–459.

Keynes, Sir G. (1978) *The Life of William Harvey.* Oxford: Clarendon Press.

Keyser, P.T. (1997) Science and Magic in Galen's Recipes (Sympathy and Efficacy). In Debru (ed.): 175–198.

Kieffer, J.S. (1964) *Galen's Institutio logica.* Baltimore, MD: Johns Hopkins University Press.

King, D. (2018) *Experiencing Pain in Imperial Greek Culture.* Oxford: Oxford University Press.

King, H. (1998) *Hippocrates' Woman.* London: Routledge.

King, H. (2018) 'First behead your viper': Acquiring Knowledge in Galen's Poison Stories. In Grell, O.P., Cunningham, A., and Arrizabalaga, J. (eds) *"It All Depends on the Dose": Poisons and Medicines in European History.* Abingdon, UK: Routledge: 25–42.

König, J. (2005) *Athletics and Literature in the Roman Empire.* Cambridge: Cambridge University Press.

König, J. (2009) Conventions of Prefatory Self-presentation in Galen's On the Order of My Own Books. In Gill *et al.* (eds): 35–58.

König, J., Oikonomopoulou, K., and Woolf, G. (eds.) (2013) *Ancient Libraries.* Cambridge: Cambridge University Press.

König, J. and Whitmarsh, T. (eds) (2007) *Ordering Knowledge in the Roman Empire.* Cambridge: Cambridge University Press.

König, J. and Woolf, G. (eds) (2017) *Authority and Experience in Ancient Scientific Culture.* Cambridge: Cambridge University Press.

Koester, H. (ed.) (1998) *Pergamon, Citadel of the Gods. Archaeological Record, Literary Description, and Religious Development.* Harrisburg: Trinity Press International.

Koetschet, P. (2019a) From Commentary to Polemic: The Reception of Galen by Abū Bakr al-Rāzī. In Bouras-Vallianatos and Zipser (eds): 196–214.

Koetschet, P. (2019b) Abū Bakr al-Rāzī contre Galien ou comment «s'élever du niveau des médecins à celui des philosophes». In Crignon and Lefebvre (eds): 147–170.

Koetschet, P. (2019c) *Abū Bakr al-Rāzī, Doutes sur Galien (Édition, traduction, commentaire).* Berlin: W. De Gruyter.

Kollesch, J. (2019) *Kleine Schriften zur antiken Medizin. CMG Suppl.* VI. Berlin: W. De Gruyter.

Kollesch, J. and Nickel, D. (eds) (1993) *Galen und das hellenistische Erbe.* Stuttgart: Steiner.

Kotrc, R.F. (1970) *Galen's Phlebotomy against the Erasistrateans in Rome.* Dissertation, Washington State University, Seattle.

Kovačič, F. (2001) *Der Begriff der Physis bei Galen vor dem Hintergrund seiner Vorgänger.* Stuttgart: Steiner.

Kräupl Taylor, F. (1979) *The Concepts of Illness, Disease and Morbus.* Cambridge: Cambridge University Press.

Kraus, P. (1939) Kitāb al-Akhlāq li-Jālīnus. *Bulletin of the Faculty of Arts of the Egyptian University* 5(1): 1–51.

Kraus, P. and Walzer, R. (1951) *Galeni Compendium Timaei Platonis.* London: Oxford University Press.

Kudlien, F. (1965) Zum Thema, Homer und die Medizin. *Rheinisches Museum* 108: 293–299.

Kudlien, F. (1971) Galens Urteil über die Thukydideische Pestbeschreibung. *Episteme* 5: 132–133.

Kudlien, F. (1974) Ein vergessener griechischer Dichter der Kaiserzeit. *Rheinisches Museum* 117: 280–287

Kudlien, F. (1981) Galen's Religious Belief. In Nutton (ed.): 117–130.

Kudlien, F. and Durling, R.J. (eds) (1991) *Galen's Method of Healing.* Leiden: Brill.

Kühn, K.G. (1821–33) *Claudii Galeni Opera Omnia.* Leipzig: C. Knobloch, 20 vols in 22.

Kupreeva, I. (2014) Galen's Theory of Elements. In Adamson *et al.* (eds): 197–212.

Laguna, A. (1548) *Epitome omnium Galeni Pergameni operum.* Venice: H. Scotus.

Laguna, A. (1604) *Epitome omnium Galeni Pergameni operum.* Strasbourg: L. Zetzner.

Laín Entralgo, P. (1970) *The Therapy of the Word in Classical Antiquity.* New Haven, CT: Yale University Press.

Lamoreaux, J.C. (2016) *Hunayn ibn Isḥāq on his Galen Translations: a Parallel English-Arabic text.* Provo, UT: Brigham Young University Press.

Lang, P. (2013) *Medicine and Society in Ptolemaic Egypt.* Leiden and Boston, MA: Brill.

Langermann, T.Z. (2019) Maimonides and Galen. In Bouras-Vallianatos and Zipser (eds): 244–262.

Langslow, D. (2000) *Medical Latin in the Roman Empire.* Oxford: Oxford University Press.

Larrain, C.J. (1992) *Galens Kommentar zu Platons Timaios.* Stuttgart: B.G. Teubner.

Laskaris, J., Rosen, R., and Singer, P.N. (eds) (forthcoming) *The Oxford Handbook to Galen.* Oxford: Oxford University Press.

Lazaris, S. (2019) Medieval Portraits of Galen. In Bouras-Vallianatos and Zipser (eds): 609–637.

Lehoux, D. (2017) The Authority of Galen's Witnesses. In König and Woolf (eds): 261–282.

Leigh, R. (2015) *On Theriac, to Piso, Attributed to Galen*. Leiden: Brill.

Leith, D. (2008) The diatritos and Therapy in Graeco-Roman Medicine. *Classical Quarterly* 58: 581–600.

Leith, D. (2014) Galen's Refutation of Atomism. In Adamson *et al.* (eds): 213–234.

Levey, M. and Souryal, S. (1968) Galen's On the Secrets of Women and The Secrets of Men. *Janus* 55: 208–219.

Leoniceno, N. (1508) *In libros Galeni e greca in linguam latinam a se translatos*. Venice: J. Pentius de Leucho.

Lewis, O. (2015) Marcellinus De pulsibus: A Neglected Treatise on the Ancient "Art of the Pulse." *Scripta Classica Israelitica* 35: 193–214.

Lewis, O. (2016) The Practical Applications of Ancient Pulse-lore and its Influence on the Patient–Doctor Interaction. In Petridou and Thumiger (eds): 345–364.

Lewis, O. (2017) *Praxagoras of Cos on Arteries, Pulse and Pneuma*. Leiden and Boston, MA: Brill.

Liewert, A. (2015) *Die meteorologische Medizin des Corpus Hippocraticum*. Berlin: De Gruyter.

Lind, L.R. (1975) Studies in pre-Vesalian Anatomy, Biography, Translations, Documents. *Memoirs of the American Philosophical Society* 104.

Littmann, R.J. and Littman, M.L. (1973) Galen and the Antonine Plague. *American Journal of Philology* 94: 243–255.

Lloyd, G.E.R. (1979) *Magic, Reason and Experience. Studies in the Origin and Development of Greek Science*. Cambridge: Cambridge University Press.

Lloyd, G.E.R. (1983) *Science, Folklore and Ideology*. Cambridge: Cambridge University Press.

Lloyd, G.E.R. (1991) *Methods and Problems in Greek Science. Selected Papers*. Cambridge: Cambridge University Press.

Lloyd, G.E.R. (1996) Theories and Practices of Demonstration in Galen. In Frede, M. and Striker, G. (eds) *Rationality in Greek Thought*. Oxford: Clarendon Press: 255–277.

Lloyd, G.E.R. (2005) Mathematics as a Model of Method in Galen. In Sharples, R. (ed.) *Philosophy and the Sciences in Antiquity*. Aldershot: Ashgate: 110–130.

Lloyd, G.E.R. (2008) Galen and his Contemporaries. In Hankinson (ed.): 34–48.

Lloyd, G.E.R. (2009) Galen's un-Hippocratic Case Histories. In Gill *et al.* (eds): 115–131.

Long, A.A. (1996) Ptolemy *On the Criterion; an Epistemology for the Practicing Scientist*. In Dillon and Long (eds): 176–207.

Long, B. (2019) Arabic–Latin Translations: Transmission and Transformation. In Bouras-Vallianatos and Zipser (eds): 343–358.

López Férez, J.A. (ed.) (2015) *Galeno, lengua, composición literaria, léxico, estilo*. Madrid: Ediciones Clásicas.

Lorusso, V. (2005) Nuovi frammenti di Galeno (In Hipp. Epid, VI comm. VII; In Plat. Tim. Comm.). *Zeitschrift für Papyrologie und Epigraphik* 152: 43–56.

Ludwig, W. (1999) *Vater und Sohn im 16. Jahrhundert: der Briefwechsel von Wolfgang Reichart, genannt Rychardus, mit seinem Sohn Zenon (1520–1543)*. Hildesheim: Weidmann.

Lytton, D.C. and Resuhr, L.M. (1978) Galen on Abnormal Swellings. *Journal of the History of Medicine and Allied Sciences* 53: 531–549.

Maclean, I. (2002), *Logic, Signs and Nature in the Renaissance: The Case of Learned Medicine*. Cambridge: Cambridge University Press.

MacLeod, R. (2004) *The Library of Alexandria, Centre of Learning in the Ancient World*. London: I. B.Tauris.

Maddison, F., Pelling, M., and Webster, C. (eds) (1977) *Essays on the Life and Work of Thomas Linacre c.1460–1524*. Oxford: Clarendon Press.

Magri, R. (2002) *Il medico delle isole: primo libro della vita di Claudio Galeno: romanzo*. Milan: Ares.

Magri, R. (2004) *Il medico dell'imperatore: secondo libro della vita di Claudio Galeno: romanzo*. Milan: Ares.

Majno, G. (1975) *The Healing Hand. Man and Wound in the Ancient World.* Cambridge, MA: Harvard University Press.

Manetti, D. (2009) Galen and Hippocratic Medicine: Language and Practice. In Gill *et al.* (eds): 157–174.

Manetti, D. (ed.) (2012). *Studi sul "De indolentia" di Galeno. Atti del seminario fiorentino (22 novembre 2010).* Pisa and Rome: F. Serra.

Manetti, D. and Roselli, A. (1994) Galeno commentatore di Ippocrate. *ANRW* II,37,2: 1527–1634.

Mani, N. (1991) Die wissenschaftlichen Grundlage der Chirurgie (mit besonderer Berücksichtigung der MM). In Kudlien and Durling (eds): 26–50.

Manuli, P. and Vegetti, M. (eds) (1988) *Le Opere psicologiche di Galeno.* Naples: Bibliopolis.

Manzoni, T. (2001) *Il Cervello secondo Galeno.* Ancona: Il Lavoro editoriale.

Marechal, P. (2019) Galen's Constitutive Materialism. *Ancient Philosophy* 39: 1–19.

Marganne, M.H. (1994) *L'opthalmologie dans l'Égypte gréco-romaine d'après les papyrus littéraires grecs.* Leiden, New York, NY, and Cologne: Brill.

Marganne, M.H. (1998) *La chirurgie dans l'Égypte gréco-romaine d'après les papyrus littéraires grecs.* Leiden: Brill.

Margócsy, D., Somos, M., and Joffe, S.N. (2018). *The Fabrica of Andreas Vesalius. A Worldwide Descriptive Census, Ownership and Annotations of the 1543 and 1555 Editions.* Leiden: Brill.

Marinone, N. (1973) *Galeno. La dieta dimagrante.* Turin: Paravia.

Martelli, M. (2012) Galeno grammatico sui nomi stranieri e il *digamma*. Un passo inedito dal *ix* libro del trattato *Sui medicamenti semplici. Annali dell'Università degli Studi di Napoli 'L'Orientale' (Sezione Filologico-Letteraria)* 34: 124–136.

Martelli, M. (2019) Galen in the Late Antique, Byzantine and Syro-Arabic Alchemical Traditions. In Bouras-Vallianatos and Zipser (eds): 577–593.

Mártinez, V.M. and Sensenet, M.F. (2013) Special Libraries in the Ancient World. In König *et al.* (eds): 401–417.

Mattern, S.P. (2008) *Galen and the Rhetoric of Healing.* Baltimore, MD: Johns Hopkins University Press.

Mattern, S.P. (2013) *Prince of Medicine: Galen in the Roman World.* Oxford: Oxford University Press.

Mattern, S.P. (2016) Galen's Anxious Patients: lypē as Anxiety Disorder. In Petridou and Thumiger (eds): 303–323.

Mattern, S.P. (2017) Galen. In Richter, D.S. and Johnson, W.A. (eds) *The Oxford Handbook of the Second Sophistic.* Oxford: Oxford University Press.

May, M.T. (1968) *Galen On the Usefulness of Parts of the Body.* Ithaca, NY: Cornell University Press.

Mazzini, I. (1999) *A. Cornelio Celso, La Chirurgia (libri VII e VIII del De medicina).* Pisa and Rome: Istituti editoriali e poligrafici.

McVaugh, M. (2019) Galen in the Medieval Universities, 1200–1400. In Bouras-Vallianatos and Zipser (eds): 381–392.

Meisami, J.S. (1989) Mas'ūdī on love and the fall of the Barmakids. *Journal of the Royal Asiatic Society* 1: 252–277.

Meyerhof, M. (1929) Autobiographische Bruchstücke Galens aus arabischen Quellen. *Sudhoffs Archiv* 22: 72–86.

Meyerhof, M. and Schacht, J. (1930–1) *Galen, Über die medizinischen Namen, Abhandlungen der Preussischen Akademie der Wissenschaften, philologisch-historische Klasse*, 3.

Miller, K.J. (2018) From Critical Days to Critical Hours: Galenic Refinements of Hippocratic Models. *Transactions of the American Philological Association* 148: 111–138.

Minor, A. (1911) *De Galeni libris περὶ δυσπνοίας.* Dissertation, Marburg.

Mittarelli, G.B. and Costadoni, A. (1764) *Annales Camaldulenses ordinis Sancti Benedicti, Tomus VIII.* Venice: G.B. Pasquali.

Mohaghegh, M. (1971) The Shūkūk of al-Rāzī against Galen and the Problem of the Eternity of the World. In *Proceedings of the 27th International Congress of Orientalists.* Wiesbaden: Steiner Verlag: 240–242.

Mondella, L. (1568) *Theatrum Galeni sive unjversae medicinae....promptuarium.* Basle: E. Episcopius and the heirs of N. Episcopius.

Moraux, P. (1984) *Der Aristiotelismus bei den Griechen. Band II. Der Aristotelismus im I. und II. Jh. n. Chr.* Berlin and New York, NY: W. De Gruyter.

Morison, B. (2008) Logic, Language. In Hankinson (ed.): 66–156.

Mugnai Carrara, D. (1991) *La biblioteca di Nicolò Leoniceno: tra Aristotele e Galeno cultura e libri di un medico umanista.* Florence: L.S. Olschki.

Mulhall, J. (2019) Plague before the Pandemics: The Greek Medical Evidence for Plague before the Sixth Century. *Bulletin of the History of Medicine* 93: 151–179.

Müller, I.W. (1993) *Humoralmedizin: physiologische, pathologische und therapeutische Grundlagen der galenistischen Heilkunst.* Heidelberg: Haug.

Nesselrath, H.-G. (2013) Das Mouseion und die Grosse Bibliothek von Alexandria. In Georges, T., Albrecht, A., and Feldmeier, R. (eds) *Alexandria.* Tübingen: Mohr Siebeck: 65–88.

Nicholls, M.C. (2011) Galen and Libraries in the Peri Alupias. *Journal of Roman Studies* 101: 123–142.

Nicholls, M.C. (2014) A Library at Antium? In Rothschild and Thompson (eds): 65–78.

Nicholls, M.C. (2019) Galen and the Last Days of Commodus. In Petit (ed.): 245–262.

Nickel, D. (2002) On the Authenticity of an 'Excerpt' from Galen's Commentary on the Timaeus. In Nutton (ed.): 73–79.

Nova Academia Florentina (1533) *Opuscula adversus Avicennam et medicos neotericos, qui Galeni disciplina neglecta, barbaros colunt.* Venice: Lucantonio Junta.

Nutton, V. (1973) The Chronology of Galen's Earlier Career. *Classical Quarterly* 23: 158–171; repr. as Ch. II in Nutton (1988).

Nutton, V. (ed.) (1981) *Galen: Problems and Prospects.* London: The Wellcome Institute.

Nutton, V. (1983) The Seeds of Disease: An Explanation of Contagion and Infection from the Greeks to the Renaissance. *Medical History* 27: 1–24; repr. as ch. XI in Nutton (1988).

Nutton, V. (1984a) From Galen to Alexander, Aspects of Medical Practice in Late Antiquity. *Dumbarton Oaks Papers* 38: 1–14; repr. as ch. X in Nutton (1988).

Nutton, V. (1984b) Galen in the Eyes of his Contemporaries. *Bulletin of the History of Medicine* 58: 315–324; repr. as ch. III in Nutton (1988).

Nutton, V. (1986) The Perils of Patriotism. Pliny and Roman Medicine. In French, R.K. and Greenaway, F. (eds) *Science in the Roman Empire. Pliny the Elder, his Sources and Influence.* London: Croom Helm: 30–58; repr. as ch. VII in Nutton (1988).

Nutton, V. (1987) *John Caius and the Manuscripts of Galen.* Cambridge: Cambridge Philological Society.

Nutton, V. (1988) *From Democedes to Harvey: Studies in the History of Medicine.* London: Variorum Reprints.

Nutton, V. (1990a) The Patient's Choice: A New Treatise by Galen. *Classical Quarterly* 40: 235–257.

Nutton, V. (1990b) The Anatomy of the Soul in Early Renaissance Medicine. In Dunstan, G.R. (ed.) *The Human Embryo.* Exeter: University of Exeter Press: 136–157.

Nutton, V. (1991) Style and Context in the Method of Healing. In Kudlien and Durling (eds): 1–25.

Nutton, V. (1993a) Wittenberg Anatomy, In Grell, O.P. and Cunningham, A. (eds) *Medicine and the Reformation.* London: Routledge: 11–32.

Nutton, V. (1993b) Galen and Egypt. In Kollesch and Nickel (eds): 11–31.

Nutton, V. (1993c) Galen at the Bedside: The Methods of a Medical Detective. In Bynum, W.F. and Porter, R.S. (eds), *Medicine and the Five Senses.* Cambridge: Cambridge University Press: 7–16, 275–276.

Nutton, V. (1995) Galen ad multos annos. *Dynamis* 15: 25–40.
Nutton, V. (1997) Galen on Theriac: Problems of Authenticity. In Debru (ed.): 133–151.
Nutton, V. (1998) An Early Reader of Vesalius' Fabrica. *Vesalius* 3: 73–74.
Nutton, V. (2000) Medical Thoughts on Urban Pollution. In Hope, V.M. and Marshall, E. (eds) *Death and Disease in the Ancient City*. London: Routledge: 65–73.
Nutton, V. (ed.) (2002a) *The Unknown Galen, Bulletin of the Institute of Classical Studies, Suppl.* 77, London: Institute of Classical Studies.
Nutton, V. (2002b) In Defence of Kühn. In Nutton (ed.): 1–7.
Nutton, V. (2003) André Vésale et l'anatomie parisienne. *Cahiers de l'Association Internationale des Études Françaises* 55: 239–249.
Nutton, V. (2007) Galen in Byzantium. In Grünbart, M., Kislinger, E., Muthesius, A., and Stathakopoulos, D. (eds) *Material Culture and Well-being in Byzantium, Österreichische Akademie der Wissenschaften, phil.-hist. Klasse, Denkschriften*, Bd. 356, *Veröffentlichen zur Byzanzforschung* 11: 171–176.
Nutton, V. (2008) The Fortunes of Galen. In Hankinson (ed.) 2008a: 355–390.
Nutton, V. (2009a) Galen's Library. In Gill *et al.* (eds): 19–34.
Nutton, V. (2009b) Biographical Accounts of Galen, 1340–1660. In Rütten, T. (ed.) *Geschichte der Medizingeschichtsschreibung. Historiographie unter dem Diktat literarischer Gattungen von der Antike bis zur Aufklärung*. Remscheid: Gardez! Verlag: 201–232.
Nutton, V. (2009c) Galen's Authorial Voice. In Taub, L. and Doody, A. (eds) *Authorial Voices in Greco-Roman Technical Writing*. Trier: Wissenschaftliche Verlag: 53–62.
Nutton, V. (2010) Galen in Context. In Cairns, F. and Griffin, M. (eds) *Papers of the Langford Latin Seminar* 14: 1–18.
Nutton, V. (2011) Picturing Medicine: The Dresden Galen. In Krause, K. and Schellewald, B. (eds) *Bild und Text im Mittelalter*. Cologne, Weimar and Vienna: Böhlau Verlag: 347–361
Nutton, V. (2012a) From Noah to Galen. A Medieval Latin History of Medicine. In Csepregi, I. and Burnett, C. (eds) *Ritual Healing. Magic, Ritual and Medical Therapy from Antiquity until the Early Modern Period*. Florence: SISMEL – Edizioni del Galluzzo: 53–69.
Nutton, V. (2012b) The Commentary on the Hippocratic Oath Ascribed to Galen. In Fortuna, S., Garofalo, I., Lami, A., and Roselli, A. (eds) *Sulla tradizione indiretta dei testi medici greci: i commenti. Atti del iv seminario internazionale di Siena (Certosa di Pontignano, 3–4 giugno, 2011)*. Pisa and Rome: Fabrizio Serra Editore: 91–100.
Nutton, V. (2012c) Vesalius Revised: his Annotations to the 1555 Fabrica. *Medical History* 56: 415–443.
Nutton, V. (2012d) Galen's Rhetoric of Certainty. In Coste, J., Jacquart, D., and Pigeaud, J. (eds) *La rhétorique médicale à travers les siècles. Actes du colloque international de Paris, 9 et 10 octobre, 2008*. Geneva: Droz: 39–49.
Nutton, V. (2013a) *Ancient Medicine*, ed. 2. London: Routledge.
Nutton, V. (2013b) Galien dans son contexte; épigraphie, archéologie et codicologie. *Comptes rendus de l'Académie des Inscriptions & Belles-Lettres* 4: 1481–1491.
Nutton, V. (2013c) Galenic Madness. In Harris, W.V. (ed.): 119–128.
Nutton, V. (2013d) Niccolò in Context. *Medicina nei Secoli* 25: 941–956.
Nutton, V. (2013e) *Galen, Avoiding Distress*. In Singer, P.N.: 43–106.
Nutton, V. (2014a) Introduction. In Garrison, D.S. and Hast, M.H. *Vesalius on the Fabric of the Human Body*. Basle: Karger: LXXV–CIX.
Nutton, V. (2014b) Rhodiapolis and Allianoi: Two Missing Links in the History of Hospitals? *Early Christianity* 5: 371–389.
Nutton, V. (2015a) What's in a Nomen: Vlatadon 14 and an Old Theory Resurrected. In Holmes, B. and Fischer, K.D. (eds) *The Frontiers of Ancient Science. Essays in Honor of Heinrich von Staden, Beiträge zur Altertumskunde* 338. Berlin, Munich and Boston: De Gruyter: 453–462.
Nutton, V. (2015b) De virtutibus centaureae: A Pseudo-Galenic Text on Pharmacology. *Galenos* 8: 149–175.

Nutton, V. (2016) Folk Medicine in the Galenic Corpus. In Harris, W.V. (ed.): 272–279.

Nutton, V. (2017) *Johann Guinter and Andreas Vesalius, Principles of Anatomy According to the Opinion of Galen*. London: Routledge.

Nutton, V. (2018) *An Autobibliography by John Caius*. London: Routledge.

Nutton, V. (2019) Renaissance Galenism, 1540–1640: Flexibility or an Irrelevance? In Bouras-Vallianatos and Zipser (eds): 472–486.

Nutton, V. (2020) Galenism and Anti-Galenism in Renaissance Anatomy. In Pietrobelli: 215–227.

Nutton, V. (forthcoming 1) Galenic Anatomy in the Long Renaissance. In Laskaris, J., Rosen, R., and Singer, P.N. (eds) *The Oxford Handbook to Galen*. Oxford: Oxford University Press.

Nutton, V. (forthcoming 2) *Galen and the Latin De voce: A New Edition and English Translation*.

Nutton, V. with Bos, G. (2011) *Galen, On Problematical Movements*. Cambridge: Cambridge University Press.

Oberhelman, S.M. (1983) Galen, On Diagnosis from Dreams. *Journal of the History of Medicine and Allied Sciences* 38: 36–47.

Oberhelman, S.M. (1994) Aretaeus of Cappadocia – the Pneumatic Physician of the First Century A.D. *ANRW*, II, 37, 2: 941–966.

O'Boyle, C. (1998) *The Art of Medicine. Medical Teaching at the University of Paris 1250–1400*. Cambridge: Cambridge University Press.

O'Malley, C.D. (1964). *Andreas Vesalius of Brussels, 1514–1564*. Berkeley and Los Angeles, CA: University of California Press.

O'Rourke Boyle, M. (2018) *Cultural Anatomies of the Heart in Aristotle, Augustine, Aquinas, Calvin and Harvey*. London: Palgrave Macmillan.

Ogden, D. (2017) *The Legend of Seleucus. Kingship, Narrative and Mythmaking in the Ancient World*. Cambridge: Cambridge University Press.

Ohlemutz, W. (1968) *Die Kulte und Heiligtümer der Götter in Pergamon*. Darmstadt: Wissenschaftliche Buchgesellschaft.

Ongaro, G. (1994) L'insegnamento clinico di Giovanni Battista Da Monte (1458–1551): una rivisione critica. *Physis. Rivista internazionale di storia della scienza* n.s. 31: 358–369.

Orengo, A. (2019) The Reception of Galen in the Armenian Tradition. In Bouras-Vallianatos and Zipser (eds): 559–576.

Ormos, I. (1993) Bemerkungen zur editorischen Bearbeitung der Galenschrift "Über die Sektion toter Lebewesen". In Kollesch and Nickel (eds): 165–172.

Otte, C. (2001) *Galen, De plenitudine*. Wiesbaden: Steiner.

Palmieri, N. (2002) La médecine alexandrine et son rayonnement occidental (VIe–VIIe s. ap. J.-Ch.). *Lettre d'informations. Médecine antique et médiévale* n.s. 1: 5–23.

Palmieri, N. (ed.) (2008) L'Ars medica (Tegni) de Galien: lectures antiques et médiévales. *Mémoires du Centre Jean Palerne* XXXII.

Parker, H.N. (2012) Galen and the Girls: Sources for Women Medical Writers Revisited. *Classical Quarterly* 62: 359–386.

Pastore, A. and Peruzzi, E. (eds) (2006) *Girolamo Fracastoro. Fra medicina, filosofia e scienze della natura*. Florence: Leo S. Olschki.

Patterson, J.F. (2017) The Hippocratic Critical Days. *Syllecta Classica* 28: 111–145.

Perilli, L. (2007) Da medico a lessicografo: Galeno e il Glossario Ippocratico. In Müller, C.W., Brockmann, C., and Brunschön, C. (eds) *Ärzte und Ihre Interpreten. Medizinische Fachtexte der Antike als Forschungsgegenstand der klassischen Philologie. Fachkonferenz zu Ehren von Diethard Nickel*. Munich and Leipzig: K G Saur: 165–202.

Perilli, L. (2012) A Risky Enterprise: The Aldine Edition of Galen, the Failures of the Editors, and the Shadow of Erasmus of Rotterdam. *Early Science and Medicine* 17: 446–466.

Perilli, L. (2018) Aldus Manutius' Unfulfilled Dream: Galen's Journey from Campo Sant'Agostin to Western Culture. In Canalis and Ciavolella: 47–81.

Petit, C. (2009) *Galien. Tome III, Le médecin. Introduction*. Paris: Les Belles Lettres.

Petit, C. (2017) Galen, Pharmacology and the Boundaries of Medicine: A Reassessment. In Lehmhaus, L. and Martelli, M. (eds) *Collecting Recipes. Byzantine & Jewish Pharmacology in Dialogue.* Wiebaden: Harrassowitz: 51–79.

Petit, C. (2018) *Galien de Pergame ou la rhétorique de la Providence.* Leiden: Brill.

Petit, C. (ed.) (2019) *Galen's Treatise ΠΕΡΙ ΑΛΥΠΙΑΣ (De Indolentia) in Context.* Leiden: Brill.

Petridou, G. (2018) Contesting Religious and Medical Expertise in the Hieroi Logoi. The therapeutai of Pergamum as Religious and Medical Entrepreneurs. In Gordon, R.L., Petridou, G., and Rūpke, J. (eds) *Beyond Priesthood: Religious Entrepreneurs and Innovators in the Imperial Era.* Berlin: W. De Gruyter: 183–208.

Petridou, G. (ed.) (2017) Embodying Ancient Religion and Medicine. *Religion in the Roman Empire* 3(2).

Petridou, G. and Thumiger, C. (eds) (2016) *Homo Patiens – Approaches to the Patient in the Ancient World.* Leiden and Boston, MA: Brill.

Petsalis-Diomidis, A. (2010) *Truly beyond Wonders. Aelius Aristides and the Cult of Asklepios.* Oxford: Oxford University Press.

Photos-Jones, E., Edwards, C., Häner, F., Lawton, L., Keane, C., Leanord, A., and Perdikatsis, V. (2017) Archaeological medicinal earths as antibacterial agents: the case of the Basel Lemnian sphragides. *Geological Society, London, Special Publications* 452(1): 141–153.

Photos-Jones, E. and Hall, A.J. (2011) *Lemnian Earth and the Earths of the Aegean: An Archaeological Guide to Medicines, Pigments and Washing Powders.* Glasgow: Potingair Press.

Photos-Jones, E., Venieri, D., Knapp, C.W., Jones, A.X., Lawton, L., Gounaki, I., and Christidis, G., (forthcoming) The True Nature of Lemnian Earth: Understanding the Clay–fungus Interface.

Pielmeyer, K. (1981) *Statuten der deutschen medizinischen Fakultäten im Mittelalter.* Dissertation, University of Bonn.

Pietrobelli, A. (2009) Le modèle des démonstrations géométriques dans la médecine de Galien. *Bulletin de l'Association Guillaume Budé* no.2 : 110–130.

Pietrobelli, A. (2013) Galien agnostique: un texte caviardé par la tradition. *Revue des Études grecques* 126: 103–135.

Pietrobelli, A. (2017) Galen's Religious Itineraries. *Religion in the Roman Empire* 3: 221–241

Pietrobelli, A. (2019a) Galen's Early Reception (Second-third Centuries). In Bouras-Vallianatos and Zipser (eds): 11–37.

Pietrobelli, A. (2019b) *Galien, Commentaire au Régime des maladies aiguës d'Hippocrate, Livre I.* Paris: Les Belles Lettres.

Pietrobelli, A. (2020) (ed.) *Contre Galien.* Paris: Honoré Champion.

Pigeaud, J. (1987) *Folies et cures de la folie chez les médecins de l'Antiquité grécoromaine. La manie.* Paris: Les Belles Lettres.

Pigeaud, J. (2006) *La crise.* Nantes: Éditions Céciledefaut.

Pigeaud, J. (2008) *Mélancholie: La malaise de l'individu.* Paris: Payot.

Pinault, J.R. (1992) *Hippocratic Lives and Legends.* Leiden, Boston and Cologne: Brill.

Pirson, F. (2017) Die Siedlungsgeschichte Pergamons; Überblick und kritische Revision. *Istanbuler Mitteilungen* 67: 43–127.

Podolak, P. (2010) *Soranos von Ephesos, Peri psyches: Sammlung der Testimonien, Kommentar und Einleitung.* Berlin and New York, NY: W. De Gruyter.

Polito, R. (1994) I quattri libri sull'anima di Sorano e lo scritto De anima di Tertulliano. *Rivista di Storia della Filosofia* 3: 423–468.

Popović, M. (2007) *Reading the Human Body. Physiognomics and Astrology in the Dead Sea Scrolls and Hellenistic-Early Roman Period.* Leiden: Brill.

Pormann, P. (ed.) (2008) *Rufus of Ephesus. On Melancholy.* Tūbingen: J.C.B. Mohr.

Potter, P. (1993) Apollonius and Galen on "Joints". In Kollesch and Nickel (eds): 117–124.

Potter, P. (1998) The editiones principes of Galen and Hippocrates and their Relationship. In Fischer, K.D., Nickel, D., and Potter, P. (eds) *Text and Tradition.* Leiden, Boston and New York: Brill.

Powell, O. (2003) *Galen On the Properties of Foodstuffs (De Alimentorum Facultatibus)*. Cambridge: Cambridge University Press.

Prantera, A. (1991) *The Side of the Moon*. London: Bloomsbury.

Pressouyre, L. (1966) Le cosmos platonicien de la Cathédrale d'Anagni. *Mélanges d'Archéologie et d'Histoire* 78: 551–593.

Radt, W. (2016) *Pergamon. Geschichte und Bauten einer antiken Meropole*, ed. 3. Mainz: Philipp von Zabern.

Raiola, T. (2011) 'Asini per uccelli': una noterella al testo di de indolentia 61. *Galenos* 5: 21–26.

Raiola, T. (2015) *Nel tempo di una vita. Studi sull'autobiografia in Galeno. AION Quaderni* 19. Pisa and Rome: Fabrrizio Serra Editore.

Raiola, T. (2018) *Sabini medici eiusque discipulorum fragmenta*. Pisa: Fabrizio Serra.

Raiola, T. and Mascolo, A. (2014) Galeno e la Campania (De meth, med. V.12). *Annali dell'Università degli Studi di Napoli `L'Orientale' (Sezione Filologico-Letteraria)* 35: 124–136.

Ramelli, I. (2015) Ethos and *Logos*: A Second-century Debate between "Pagan" and Christian Philosophers. *Vigiliae Christianae* 69: 123–156.

Rat, G. (1899) *Shihāb-ad-dīn Āhmad al-Abshīhī, Kitāb al-Mustaṭraf.* Paris: E. Leroux.

Reardon, B.P. (1971) *Courants littéraires grecs des IIe et IIIe siècles après J.-C.* Paris: Les Belles Lettres.

Reedy, J. (1968) *Galen, De tumoribus praeter naturam*. Dissertation, University of Michigan.

Regenbogen, O. (1961) *Kleine Schriften*. Munich: C.H. Beck.

Renberg, G.H. (2017) *Where Dreams May Come. Incubation Sanctuaries in the Greco-Roman World*. Religions in the Graeco-Roman World 184. Leiden and Boston, MA: Brill.

Rescher, N. (1965) Galen and the Fourth Figure of the Syllogism. *Journal of the History of Philosophy* 3: 27–41.

Rescher, N. (1966) *Galen and the Syllogism*. Pittsburgh, PA: Pittsburgh University Press.

Rescher, N. and Marmura, M.E. (1965) *Alexander against Galen on Motion*. Islamabad: Islamic Research Institute.

Richardson, W.F. and Carman, J.B. (1998–2009) *Vesalius, On the Fabric of the Human Body*. San Francisco, CA and Novato: Norman Publishing.

Riddle, J. (1985) *Dioscorides on Pharmacy and Medicine*. Austin, TX: University of Texas Press.

Riethmüller, J.W. (2005) *Asklepios: Heiligtümer und Kulte*. Heidelberg: Verlag Archäologie und Geschichte.

Robert, L. (1938) *Etudes épigraphiques et philologiques*. Paris: E. Champion.

Robert, L. (1940) *Les gladiateurs dans l'Orient grec*. Paris: E. Champion.

Robert, L. (1980) *À travers l'Asie Mineure*. Paris: École française d'Athènes.

Roby, C. (2016) Galen's Role in Pain Diagnosis: Sensation, Consensus and Metaphor. In Petridou and Thumiger (eds): 304–322.

Rocca, J. (2002) The Brain beyond Kühn; Reflections on Anatomical Procedures, Book IX. In Nutton (ed.): 87–100.

Rocca, J. (2003) *Galen on the Brain. Anatomical Knowledge and Physiological Speculation in the Second Century AD*. Leiden: Brill.

Rocca, J. (2008) Anatomy. In Hankinson (ed.): 242–262.

Rocca, J. (ed.) (2017). *Teleology in the Ancient World. Philosophical and Medical Approaches*. Cambridge: Cambridge University Press.

Rocca, J. (2018) Galen and Middle Platonism: The Case of the Demiurge. In Tarrant, H., Layne, D.A., Baltzly, D., and Renaud, F. (eds) *Brill's Companion to the Reception of Plato in Antiquity*, Leiden and Boston, MA: Brill: 206–222.

Röhr, J. (1923) Die okkullte Kraftbegriff im Altertum. *Philologus, Suppl.* 17(1).

Roselli, A. (1999) Notes on the Doxai of Doctors in Galen's Commentaries *on Hippocrates*. In van der Eijk (ed.): 359–381.

Rosen, R. (2010) Galen and the Compulsion to Instruct. In Horstmanshoff (ed.): 325–342.

Rosen, R. (2017) Anatomy and Aporia on the Construction of Fetuses. In König, J. and Woolf, G. (eds): 283–305.

Rosenthal, F. (1956) An Ancient Commentary on the Hippocratic Oath. *Bulletin of the History of Medicine* 30: 52–87; repr. in Rosenthal, F. (1990) *Science and Medicine in Islam*, Guildford: Variorum.

Rosenthal, F. (1975) *The Classical Heritage in Islam*. London: Routledge.

Rothschild, C.K. (2014) The Apocolocyntosis of Commodus or the Anti-Imperial Tendenz of Galen's De Indolentia. In Rothschild and Thompson (eds): 175–200.

Rothschild, C.K. and Thompson, T.W. (eds) (2014) *Galen's De Indolentia. Essays on a Newly Discovered Letter*. Tübingen: Mohr Siebeck.

Roussel, F. (2002) *Nature et nature de l'homme chez Galien. Physique et physiologie*. PhD Dissertation, Université de Paris IV.

Ruffy, M.V. (2011) Symposium, Physical and Social Health in Plutarch's Table Talk. In Klotz, F. and Oikonomopoulou, F. (eds) *The Philosopher's Banquet. Plutarch's Table Talk in the Intellectual Culture of the Roman Empire*. Oxford: Oxford University Press: 131–160.

Ruffy, M.V. (2012) *Les vertus thérapeutiques du banquet. Médecine et idéologie dans les Propos de Table de Plutarque*. Paris: Les Belles Lettres.

Ryholt, K. (2011) New Light on the Legendary King Nechepsos of Egypt. *Journal of Egyptian Archaeology* 97: 61–72.

Samama, E. (2003) *Les médecins dans le monde grec. Sources épigraphiques sur la naissance d'un corps médical*. Geneva: Droz.

Savage-Smith, E. (2002) Galen's Lost Ophthalmology and the *Summaria Alexandrinorum*. In Nutton (ed.): 121–138.

Savage-Smith, E., Swain, S., and van Gelder, G.J. (eds) (2020) *A Literary History of Medicine*. Leiden: Brill.

Savino, S. (2019) 'Galenic' Forgeries of the Renaissance: An Overview on Commentaries Falsely Attributed to Galen. In Bouras-Vallianatos and Zipser (eds): 453–471.

Schacht, J. and Meyerhof, M. (1937a) *The Medico-philosophical Controversy between Ibn Butlan of Baghdad and Ibn Ridwan of Cairo. A Contribution to the History of Greek Learning among the Arabs*. Cairo: The Egyptian University.

Schacht, J. and Meyerhof, M. (1937b) Maimonides against Galen on Philosophy and Cosmogony. *Bulletin of the Faculty of Arts of the University of Egypt* 5: 52–88.

Schiefsky, M. (2012) Galen and the Tripartite Soul. In Barney, R., Brennan, T., and Brittain, C. (eds) *Plato and the Divided Self*. Cambridge: Cambridge University Press: 331–347.

Schlange-Schöningen, H. (2003) *Die römische Gesellschaft bei Galen. Biographie und Sozialgeschichte*. Berlin: De Gruyter.

Schlange-Schöningen, H. (2013) Herrschaftskritk bei Galen. In Holmes and Fischer (eds): 655–674.

Schiefsky, M. (2013) Herrschaftskritk bei Galen. In Holmes and Fischer (eds): 655–674.

Schöne, H. (1933) Galenos' Schrift über die Siebenmonatskinder. *Quellen und Studien zur Geschichte der Naturwissenschaften und der Medizin* 3(4): 120–138.

Schrenk, L.P. (1989) Byzantine Evidence for Galen's *On Medica. l Experience. Medical Experience Byzantinische Zeitschrift* 82: 251–257.

Schrier, O.J. (1995) Hunayn ibn Ishaq on Tragedy and Comedy, a New Fragment of Galen. *Mnemosyne* 48: 344–348.

Scolnicov, S. (2017) Atemporal Teleology in Plato. In Rocca (ed.): 45–57.

Sconocchia, S. (1993) L'opera di Scribonio Largo e la letteratura medica latina del 1 sec. d. C. *ANRW* 37(1): 845–922.

Sharples, R.W. and van der Eijk, P.J. (trans.) (2008) *Nemesius, On the Nature of Man*. Liverpool: Liverpool University Press.

Sider, D. and McVaugh, M. (1979) Galen On Tremor, Palpitation, Spasm and Rigor. *Transactions and Studies of the College of Physicians of Philadelphia* 1(3): 183–210.

Siegel, R.E. (1968) *Galen's System of Physiology and Medicine: An Analysis of his Doctrines and Observations on Bloodflow, Humors and Internal Diseases*. Basle and New York, NY: Karger.

Sider, D. and McVaugh, M. (1970) *Galen on Sense Perception: His Doctrines, Observations and Experiments on Vision, Hearing, Smell, Taste, Touch and Pain, and their Historical Sources.* Basle and New York, NY: Karger.

Sider, D. and McVaugh, M. (1976) *Galen On the Affected Parts.* Basle: Karger.

Simon, M. (1906) *Galen, Sieben Bücher Anatomie.* Leipzig: Heinrich.

Singer, C. (1952) Galen's Elementary Course on Bones. *Proceedings of the Royal Society of Medicine* 4: 767–776.

Singer, C. (1956) *Galen On Anatomical Procedures: Translation of the Surviving Books.* London, Oxford and New York: Oxford University Press.

Singer, P.N. (1991) Aspects of Galen's Platonism. In López Férez, J.A. (ed.) *Galeno. Obra, pensamento e influencia.* Madrid: UNED: 41–55.

Singer, P.N. (1997) *Galen. Selected Works.* Oxford: Oxford University Press.

Singer, P.N. (ed.) (2013) *Galen. Psychological Writings.* Cambridge: Cambridge University Press.

Singer, P.N. (2014) Galen and the Philosophers: Philosophical Engagement, Shadowy Contemporaries, Aristotelian Transformations. In Adamson *et al.* (eds): 7–32.

Singer, P.N. (2017) The Essence of Rage. Galen on Emotional Disturbances and their Physical Correlates. In Seaford, R., Wilkins, J., and Wright, M. *Selfhood and the Soul. Essays on Ancient Thought and Literature in Honour of Christopher Gill.* Oxford: Oxford University Press: 161–196.

Singer, P.N. (2019a) Note on MS Vlatadon 14: A Summary of the Main Findings and Problems. In Petit (ed.): 10–37.

Singer, P.N. (2019b) New light and Old Texts: Galen on his own Books. In Petit (ed.): 91–131.

Singer, P.N. and van der Eijk, P.J., with the assistance of Tassinari, P. (2018) *Galen. Works on Human Nature. Volume 1. Mixtures (De temperamentis).* Cambridge: Cambridge University Press.

Siraisi, N.G. (1990) *Medieval and Early Renaissance Medicine: An Introduction to Knowledge and Practice.* Chicago, IL: Chicago University Press.

Siraisi, N.G. (2001) *Medicine and the Italian Universities, 1250–1600.* Leiden, Boston and Cologne: Brill.

Skaarup, B.O. (2015) *Anatomy and Anatomists in Early Modern Spain.* Farnham and Burlington, VT: Ashgate.

Skoda, F. (1987) *Métaphore et médecine.* Paris: Peeters-Selaf.

Smith, W.D. (1979) *The Hippocratic Tradition.* Ithaca, NY: Cornell University Press.

Spawforth, A.J. and Walker, S. (1985) The World of the Panhellenion. I. Athens and Eleusis. *The Journal of Roman Studies* 75: 78–104.

Spawforth, A.J. and Walker, S. (1986) The World of the Panhellenion. II. Three Dorian Cities. *The Journal of Roman Studies* 76: 88–105.

Stathakopoulos, D. (2019) Galen in Non-medical Byzantine Texts. In Bouras-Vallaniatos and Zipser (eds): 140–159.

Stauber, R. (1908) *Die Schedelsche Bibliothek. Studien und Darstellungen aus dem Gebiete der Geschichte* 6. Freiburg im Breisgau: Herdersche Verlagshandlung.

Stern, S.M. (1956) Some Fragments of Galen's on Dispositions (Περὶ ἠθῶν) in Arabic. *Classical Quarterly* 6: 91–101.

Stewart, K.A. (2019) *Galen's Theory of Black Bile: Hippocratic Tradition, Manipulation, Innovation.* Leiden: Brill.

Stolberg, M. (2015) *Uroscopy in Early Modern Europe.* Farnham and Burlington, VT: Ashgate.

Strocka, V.M. (2012) Bauphasen des kaiserzeitlichen Asklepieions von Pergamon. Mit einem Beitrag von Michael Wörrle. *Istanbuler Mitteilungen* 62:199–287.

Strohmaier, G. (1970) Asklepios und das Ei. Zur Ikonographie in einem arabisch erhaltenen Kommentar zum hippokratischen Eid. In Altheim, R. and Stier, H.U. (eds) *Beiträge zur Alten Geschichte und deren Nachleben.* Berlin: W. De Gruyter: II, 143–153.

Strohmaier, G. (2007) La longévité de Galien et les deux places de son tombeau. In Boudon-Millot *et al.* (eds): 393–404.

Strohmaier, G. (2019) Avicenna between Galen and Aristotle. In Bouras-Vallianatos and Zipser (eds): 215–226.

Surianus, H. (1502) *Claudii Galeni Opera Omnia.* Venice: B. Benalius.

Swain, S. (1996) *Hellenism and Empire.* Oxford: Clarendon Press.

Swain, S. (2007a) Beyond the Limits of Greek Biography: Galen from Alexandria to the Arabs. In McGing, B. and Mossman, J. (eds), *The Limits of Ancient Biography.* Cardiff: The Classical Press of Wales: 395–420.

Swain, S. (2007b) *Seeing the Face, Seeing the Soul: Polemon's Physiognomy from Classical Antiquity to Medieval Islam.* Oxford: Oxford University Press.

Swain, S. (2008) Social Stress and Political Pressure. On Melancholy in context. In Pormann (ed.): 113–138.

Tacoma, L.E. (2016) *Moving Romans. Migration to Rome in the Principate.* Oxford: Oxford University Press.

Tassinari, P. (2019) Galen in the Modern World: From Kühn to the Corpus Medicorum Graecorum. In Bouras-Vallianatos and Zipser (eds): 508–536.

Tecusan, M.M. (2004) *The Fragments of the Methodists*, vol. 1. Leiden: Brill.

Temkin, O. (1932) Geschichte des Hippokratismus im ausgehenden Altertum. *Kyklos* 4: 1–80.

Temkin, O. (1934) Galen's Advice for an Epileptic Boy. *Bulletin of the History of Medicine* 2: 179–189.

Temkin, O. (1956) *Soranus' Gynaecology*, Baltimore, MD: John Hopkins University Press.

Temkin, O. (1971) *The Falling Sickness*, ed. 2. Baltimore, MD: Johns Hopkins University Press.

Temkin, O. (1973) *Galenism. Rise and Decline of a Medical Philosophy.* Ithaca, NY and London: Cornell University Press.

Temkin, O. (1977) *The Double Face of Janus.* Baltimore, MD: Johns Hopkins University Press.

Temkin, O. (1991) *Hippocrates in a World of Pagans and Christians.* Baltimore, MD: Johns Hopkins University Press.

Temkin, O. (2002) *'On Second Thought' and Other Essays in the History of Medicine and Science.* Baltimore, MD and London: Johns Hopkins University Press.

Theoharides, T.C. (1971) Galen, *On Marasmus. Journal of the History of Medicine* 26: 369–390.

Thillet, P. (1984) A*lexandre d'Aphrodise: Traité du destin.* Paris: Les Belles Lettres.

Thom, J.C. (1995) *The Pythagorean Golden Verses, with Introduction and Commentary.* Leiden, New York and Cologne: Brill.

Thorndike, L (1923) *A History of Magic and Experimental Science*, vol. 1. New York, NY: Columbia University Press.

Thorndike, L. (1946) Translations of the Works of Galen from the Greek by Niccolò da Reggio (c. 1308–1345). *Byzantina Metabyzantina* 1: 213–235.

Thumiger, C. (2017) *A History of the Mind and Mental Health in Classical Greek Medical Thought.* Cambridge: Cambridge University Press.

Tieleman, T. (1996) *Galen and Chrysippus on the Soul: Argument and Refutation in the De placitis.* Leiden: Brill.

Tieleman, T. (1997) The Hunt for Galen's Shadow: Alexander of Aphrodisias, De anima 94.7–100 Bruns Reconsidered. In Algra, K.A. (ed.) *Polyhistor: Studies in the History and Historiography of Ancient Philosophy Presented to J. Mansfeld.* Leiden: Brill: 256–283.

Tieleman, T. (2003) Galen's Psychology. In Barnes *et al.* (eds) 131–161

Tieleman, T. (2008) Methodology. In Hankinson (ed.): 49–65.

Tieleman, T. (2009) Galen and the Stoics, or the Art of not Naming. In Gill *et al.* (eds): 282–299.

Tieleman, T. (2013) Miracle and Natural Cause in Galen. In Alkier, S. and Weissenrieder, A. (eds) *Miracles Revisited. New Testament Miracle Stories and their Concepts of Reality.* Leiden and Boston, MA: Brill: 102–113.

Tieleman, T. (2018) Galen and Doxography. In Mansfeld, J. and Runia, D.R. (eds) *Aetiana IV. Paper of the Melbourne Colloquium on Ancient Doxography.* Leiden and Boston, MA: Brill: 453–472.

Toledo-Pereyra, L. (1973) Galen's Contribution to Surgery. *Journal of the History of Medicine and Allied Sciences* 28: 356–375.

Toomer, G.J. (1985) Galen on the Astronomers and Astrologers. *Archive for the History of Exact Science* 32: 193–206.

Totelin, L.M.V. (2004) Mithridates' Antidote: A Pharmacological Ghost. *Early Science and Medicine* 9: 1–19.

Touwaide, A. (1994) Galien et la toxicologie. *ANRW* II,37,2: 1887–1986.

Touwaide, A. (1997) La thérapeutique médicamenteuse de Dioscoride à Galien. In Debru (ed.): 255–282.

Touwaide, A. (2010) Research Breakthrough: 2000-year-old Medicine Revealed. On-line at https://medicaltraditions.org/institute/news/168-research-breakthrough-2000-year-old-medicine-revealed, accessed 11 July 2019.

Touwaide, A. (2012) Quid pro Quo. Revisiting the Practice of Substitution in Ancient Pharmacy. In Van Arsdall, A. and Graham, T. (eds) *Herbs and Healers from the Ancient Mediterranean through the Medieval West. Essays in Honor of John M. Riddle.* Farnham and Burlington, VT: Ashgate: 19–62.

Touwaide, A. (2014) Collecting Books, Acquiring Medicines: Knowledge Acquisition in Galen's Therapeutics. In Rothschild and Thompson (eds): 79–88.

Trompeter, J. (2018) The Actions of Spirit and Appetite: Voluntary Motion in Galen. *Phronesis* 63: 176–207.

Tucci, P.L. (2013) Galen and the Library at Antium. *Classical Philology* 108: 240–251.

Ullmann, M. (1977) Galens Kommentar zu der Schrift De aere aquis locis. In Joly, R. (ed.) *Actes du Colloque hippocratique de Mons.* Mons: Université de Mons: 353–365.

Ullmann, M. (1978) *Die Medizin im Islam*. Leiden: Brill.

Urso, A.M. (2019) Translating Galen in the Mediaeval West: The Greek–Latin Translations. In Bouras-Vallianatos and Zipser (eds): 359–380.

Van den Bergh S (1954) *Averroes' Tahafut al-tahafut*. London: Luzac.

van der Eijk, P.J. (1997) Galen's Use of the Concept of "Qualified Experience" in his Dietetic and Pharmacological Works. In Debru (ed.): 35–58. repr. in van der Eijk (2005).

van der Eijk, P.J. (ed.) (1999) *Ancient Histories of Medicine. Essays in Medical Doxography and Historiography in Classical Antiquity.* Leiden, Boston and Cologne: Brill.

van der Eijk, P.J. (2005) *Medicine and Philosophy in Classical Antiquity. Doctors and Philosophers on Nature, Soul, Health and Disease.* Cambridge: Cambridge University Press.

van der Eijk, P.J. (2008) Therapeutics. In Hankinson (ed.): 283–303.

van der Eijk, P.J. (2009) "Aristotle! What a Thing for You to Say!". In Gill *et al.* (eds): 261–281.

van der Eijk, P.J. (2013) Cure and (In)curability of Mental Disorders in Ancient Medical and Philosophical Thought. In Harris, W.V. (ed.): 307–338.

van der Eijk, P.J. (2014) Galen on the Nature of Human Beings. In Adamson *et al.* (eds): 89–134.

van der Eijk, P.J. (2017) The Place of Disease in a Teleological World-view. Plato, Aristotle, Galen. In Rocca (ed.): 217–241.

Van der Ploeg, G. (2018) *The Impact of the Roman Empire on the Cult of Asclepius.* Leiden and Boston, MA: Brill.

Van Hee, R. (ed.) (2014) *Art of Vesalius.* Antwerp and Apeldoorn: Garant.

Van Nuffelen, P. (2014) Galen, Divination and the Status of Medicine. *Classical Quarterly* 64: 337–352.

Vegetti, M. (2007) *Dialoghi con gli antichi*. Sankt Augustin: Academia Verlag.

Vegetti, M. (2013) *Galeno. Nuovi scritti autobiografici*. Rome: Carrocci editore.

Verbank Piérard, A., Boudon-Millot, V., and Gourevitch, D. (eds) (2018) *Au temps de Galien. Un médecin grec dans l'Empire romain*. Paris: Somogy, Éditions d'Art.

Vesalius, A. (1543) *De humani corporis fabrica*. Basle: J. Oporinus.

Vesalius, A. (1555) *De humani corporis fabrica*. 2 ed. Basle: J. Oporinus.

Vieillefond, J.R. (1970) *Les `Cestes' de Julius Africanus: Étude sur l'ensemble des fragments avec édition, traduction et commentaires*. Paris: Librairie Marcel Didier.

Vogt, S. (2005) '… er schrieb in Versen, und er tat recht daran.' Lehrdichtung im Urteil Galens. In Fögen, T. (ed.) *Ancient Technical Texts.* Berlin and New York, NY: W. De Gruyter: 51–78.

Vogt, S. (2008) Drugs and Pharmacology. In Hankinson (ed.): 304–322.

Volk, R. (1990) *Der medizinische Inhalt der Schriften des Michael Psellos.* Munich: Institut für Byzantinistik und neugriechische Philologie der Universität.

von Müller, I. (1897) Über Galens Werk vom wissenschaftlichen Beweis. *Abhandlungen der kgl. bayerischen Akademie der Wissenschaften* 20(2).

Von Staden, H. (1989) *Herophilus. The Art of Medicine in Early Alexandria.* Cambridge: Cambridge University Press.

Von Staden, H. (1992) The Discovery of the Human Body: Human Dissection and its Cultural Context in Ancient Greece. *Yale Journal of Biology and Medicine* 65: 223–241.

Von Staden, H. (1997a) Galen and the Second Sophistic. In Sorabji, R. (ed.) *Aristotle and After.* London: Duckworth: 33–54.

Von Staden, H. (1997b) Inefficacy, Error and Failure: Galen on δόκιμα φάρμακα ἄπρακτα. In Debru (ed.): 59–84.

Von Staden, H. (2002) Division, Dissection and Specialization: Galen's On the Parts of the Medical Techne. In Nutton (ed.): 19–48.

Von Staden, H. (2003) Galen's Daimon: Reflections on 'Rational' and 'Irrational'. In Palmieri (ed.): 15–44.

Von Staden, H. (2004) Galen's Alexandria. In Harris, W.V. and Ruffini (eds): 179–216.

Von Staden, H. (2009) Staging the Past, Staging Oneself: Galen on Hellenistic Exegetical Traditions. In Gill *et al.* (eds): 132–156.

Von Staden, H. (2011) The Physiology and Therapy of Anger: Galen on Medicine, the Soul, and Nature. In Opwis, F. and Reisman, D. (eds) *Islamic Philosophy, Science, Culture, and Religion. Studies in Honor of Dimitri Gutas.* Leiden: Brill: 63–87.

Von Staden, H. (2017) "A Woman does not become Ambidextrous". Galen and the Culture of Scientific Commentary. In Gibson, R.K. and Kraus, C.S. (eds) *The Classical Commentary. Histories, Practices, Theory, Mnemosyne, Supplement* 232. Boston, MA and Leiden: Brill: 109–139.

Vons, J. (ed.) (2016) *La Fabrique de Vésale. La mémoire d'un livre.* Paris: Bibliothèque interuniversitaire de Santé.

Walbridge, J. (2014) *The Alexandrian Epitomes of Galen. Volume 1. On Medical Sects for Beginners. The Small Art of Medicine. On the Elements According to the Opinion of Hippocrates.* Provo, UT: Brigham Young University Press.

Walzer, R. (1935) Galens Schrift über die Siebenmonatskinder. *Rivista di Studi orientali* 15: 323–328.

Walzer, R. (1944) *Galen, On Medical Experience.* Oxford: Clarendon Press.

Walzer, R. (1949) *Galen on Jews and Christians.* Oxford: Clarendon Press.

Walzer, R. (1962) *From Greek into Arabic.* London: B. Cassirer.

Walzer, R. and Frede, M. (1985) *Galen, Three Treatises on the Nature of Science.* Indianapolis: Hackett.

Wasserstein, A. (1982) Galen's Commentary on the Hippocratic Treatise Airs, Waters and Places in the Hebrew Translation of Solomon ha-Me'ati. *Proceedings of the Israel Academy of Sciences and Humanities* 6(3).

Watson, G. (1966) *Theriac and Mithridatium: A Study in Therapeutics.* London: The Wellcome Historical Medical Library.

Wee, J.Z. (ed.) (2017) *The Comparable Body: Analogy and Metaphor in Ancient Mesopotamian, Egyptian and Greco-Roman Medicine.* Leiden: Brill.

Weisser, U. (1989) Das Corpus Hippocraticum in der arabischen Medizin. In Baader, G. and Winau, R. (eds) *Die hippocratischen Epidemien: Theorie-Praxis-Tradition: Verhandlungen des Ve Colloque international hippocratique.* Stuttgart: Fritz Steiner: 387–408.

Wenkebach, E. (1938) Galenos von Pergamon: Allgemeine Ertüchtigung durch Ballspiel. Eine sporthygienishe Schrift aus dem zweiten Jahrhundert n. Chr. *Archiv für die Geschichte der Medizin* 31: 254–297.

Wilkins, J. (2007) Galen and Athenaeus in the Hellenistic Library. In König and Whitmarsh (eds): 69–87.

Wilkins, J. (2011) Galen the Scholar. In Millett, P., Oakley, S.P., and Thompson, R.J.E. (eds) *Ratio et res ipsa: Classical Essays presented by Former Pupils to James Diggle on his Retirement*. Cambridge: Cambridge Philological Society: 45–60.

Wilkins, J. (2013) *Galien*, Tome V, *Sur les facultés des aliments.* Paris: Les Belles Lettres.

Wilkins, J. (2016) Treatment of the Man: Galen's Preventive Medicine in the De sanitate tuenda. In Petridou and Thumiger (eds): 413–421.

Wille, I. (1960) *Die Schrift Galens Περ τῶν ἐν τα ς νόσοις καιρῶν und ihre Überlieferung*. Dissertation, University of Kiel.

Woolf, G. (1994) Becoming Roman, Staying Greek: Culture, Identity and the Civilizing Process in the Greek East. *Proceedings of the Cambridge Philological Society* 40: 116–143.

Wootton, D. (2007) *Bad Medicine. Doctors doing Harm since Hippocrates.* Oxford: Oxford University Press.

Wörrle, M. (2019) Neue Freunde von Antoninus Pius. Ein Kaiserpriester und ein proconsul Asiae in Hierapolis. *Chiron* 49: 475–488.

Xenofontos, S. (2016) Casting Light on the Connection between Pseudo-Plutarch's On the Education of Children and Galen's Exhortation to the Study of Medicine. *Latomus* 75: 71–77.

Xenofontos, S. (2018) Galen's Exhortation to the Study of Medicine: An Educational work for Prospective Medical Students. In Bouras-Vallianatos, P. and Xenofontos, S. (eds) *Greek Medical Literature and its Readers: From Hippocrates to Islam and Byzantium.* Abingdon and New York, NY: Routledge: 67–93.

Yegül, F.K. (2010) *Bathing in the Roman World.* Cambridge: Cambridge University Press.

Yoeli-Tlalim, R. (2019) Galen in Asia? In Bouras-Vallianatos and Zipser (eds): 594–608.

Zadorojnyi, A.V. (2013) Libraries and Paideia in the Second Sophistic. Plutarch and Galen. In König *et al.* (eds): 377–400.

Ziegenaus, O. and De Luca, G. (1968–84) *Das Asklepieion von Pergamum, Altertümer von Pergamon* XI. Berlin: W. de Gruyter.

Zipser, B. (2019) Galen in Byzantine iatrosophia. In Bouras-Vallaniatos and Zipser (eds): 111–123.

Zonta, M. (1995) *Un interprete ebreo della filosofia di Galeno.* Turin: S. Zamorani.

Index

For Product Safety Concerns and Information please contact our EU representative GPSR@taylorandfrancis.com
Taylor & Francis Verlag GmbH, Kaufingerstraße 24, 80331 München, Germany

www.ingramcontent.com/pod-product-compliance
Lightning Source LLC
LaVergne TN
LVHW080751300926
849162LV00008BA/1793

* 9 7 8 0 3 6 7 3 5 7 2 2 1 *